W9-DFE-174

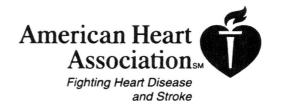

American Heart
Association℠
*Fighting Heart Disease
and Stroke*

Monograph Series

HORMONAL, METABOLIC, AND CELLULAR INFLUENCES ON CARDIOVASCULAR DISEASE IN WOMEN

Previously published:

Cardiovascular Applications of Magnetic Resonance
Edited by Gerald M. Pohost, MD

Cardiovascular Response to Exercise
Edited by Gerald F. Fletcher, MD

Congestive Heart Failure: Current Clinical Issues
Edited by Gemma T. Kennedy, RN, PhD, and Michael H. Crawford, MD

Atrial Arrhythmias: State of the Art
Edited by John P. DiMarco, MD, PhD and Eric N. Prystowsky, MD

Invasive Cardiology: Current Diagnostic and Therapeutic Issues
Edited by George W. Vetrovec, MD and Blase Carabello, MD

Syndromes of Atherosclerosis: Correlations of Clinical Imaging and Pathology
Edited by Valentin Fuster, MD, PhD

Exercise and Heart Failure
Edited by Gary J. Balady, MD and Ileana L. Piña, MD

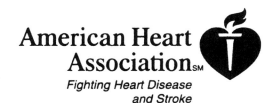

American Heart
Association™
*Fighting Heart Disease
and Stroke*

Monograph Series

HORMONAL, METABOLIC, AND CELLULAR INFLUENCES ON CARDIOVASCULAR DISEASE IN WOMEN

Edited by

Trudy M. Forte, PhD

*Donner Laboratory
Lawrence Berkeley Laboratory
Berkeley, California*

Futura Publishing
Company, Inc.
Armonk, NY

Library of Congress Cataloging-in-Publication Data

Hormonal, metabolic, and cellular influences on cardiovascular
  disease in women/edited by Trudy M. Forte.
        p.   cm. — (American Heart Association monograph series)
    Includes bibliographical references and index.
    ISBN 0-87993-668-1
    1. Cardiovascular system—Diseases—Etiology.   2. Women—
Diseases—Etiology.   3. Cardiovascular system—Diseases—Sex
factors.   4. Estrogen—Physiological effect.   5. Hormones,
Sex—Physiological effect.   I. Series.
    [DNLM: 1. Heart Diseases—etiology—congresses.   2. Heart
Diseases—metabolism—congresses.   3. Atherosclerosis—
physiopathology—congresses.   4. Estrogens—metabolism—
congresses.   5. Risk Factors—congresses.   6. Women—
congresses.   WG 210 H812 1997]
    RC669.H67   1997
    616.1'071'082—dc21
    DNLM/DLC
    for Library of Congress   97-12112
                                                                                           CIP

Copyright © 1997
Futura Publishing Company, Inc.

Published by
Futura Publishing Company, Inc.
135 Bedford Road
Armonk, New York 10504

LC #: 97-12112
ISBN #: 0-87993-668-1

Every effort has been made to ensure that the information in this
book is as up to date and accurate as possible at the time of publication. However, due to the constant developments in medicine, neither the author, nor the editor, nor the publisher can accept any legal
or any other responsibility for any errors or omissions that may
occur.

Printed in the United States of America on acid-free paper.

Preface

Heart disease is the major cause of death in women; however, until ~10 years ago most basic and clinical research on heart disease focused on the male population. The root cause of heart disease in women generally has been overlooked. This is partly due to the fact that the onset of heart disease in women is 10–15 years later in life than in men. Women generally are considered protected from premature heart attacks because of the protective role afforded by the hormone, estrogen. After menopause, however, heart disease in women rises sharply. The present text provides insights into the status of our knowledge on important parameters influencing the etiology of heart disease in women.

Not surprisingly, estrogen, and its putative beneficial effects in decreasing heart disease in women. It is long recognized that estrogen has a significant role in regulating lipid levels in women; however, the important new emerging area of vascular biology suggests that estrogen also has a key role in maintaining normal vascular reactivity. Estrogen has ability to modulate metabolic events in the artery wall including regulation of blood flow, stimulation of endothelial cell nitric oxide production, regulation of cell proliferation, and calcification of the artery. It appears that progesterone may compromise some of the beneficial effects of estrogen, but our present knowledge suggests that the mechanism of antagonism by progestins is not completely understood.

In considering the more clinical aspects of prevention of heart disease in women, this text reviews the information available on the use of estrogen replacement therapy. Evidence is strong that estrogen replacement therapy postmenopausally reduces cardiovascular disease mortality. It is apparent, however, that there is still a paucity of information on very basic issues such as the most beneficial form of estrogen to use. Furthermore, the question of the nature and degree of impact of progestins on the beneficial effect of estrogen is not completely resolved. Along with the latter, this text indicates that the effect of progestin type, dose, route of administration, and continuous versus sequential intake are little understood.

The present text has highlighted research areas in basic and clinical aspects of cardiovascular disease in women where there is a paucity of information; it is hoped that this summary will stimulate research in those areas.

Contributors

Michael R. Adams, DVM   Professor, Department of Comparative Medicine, Bowman Gray School of Medicine of Wake Forest University, Winston-Salem, NC

Mary S. Anthony, MS   Research Assistant, Department of Comparative Medicine, Bowman Gray School of Medicine of Wake Forest University, Winston-Salem, NC

Melissa A. Austin, PhD   Department of Epidemiology, School of Public Health and Community Medicine, Division of Metabolism, Endocrinology and Nutrition, University of Washington, Seattle, WA

Mihaela Balica, MD   Resident in Internal Medicine, Departments of Medicine and Physiology, UCLA School of Medicine, Los Angeles, CA

Carole L. Banka, PhD   Assistant Member, Department of Immunology, The Scripps Research Institute, La Jolla, CA

Dustan A. Barber, RPh, PhD   Senior Resident Fellow, Department of Surgery, Mayo Clinic and Foundation, Rochester, MN

Kristina Boström, MD, PhD   Clinical Instructor, Departments of Medicine and Physiology, UCLA School of Medicine, California, Los Angeles, CA.

Hannia Campos, PhD   Assistant Professor, Department of Nutrition, Harvard School of Public Health, Boston, MA

Richard O. Cannon III, MD   Cardiology Branch, National Heart, Lung, and Blood Institute, National Institutes of Health, Bethesda, MD

Gautam Chaudhuri, MD, PhD   Professor, Departments of Obstetrics and Gynecology and Molecular and Medical Pharmacology, UCLA School of Medicine, Los Angeles, CA

Thomas B. Clarkson, DVM   Professor and Chairman, Department of Comparative Medicine, Bowman Gray School of Medicine of Wake Forest University, Winston-Salem, NC

Orla M. Conneely, PhD   Associate Professor, Department of Cell Biology, Baylor College of Medicine, Houston, TX

Linda D. Cowan, PhD   Professor, University of Oklahoma Health Sciences Center, Oklahoma City, OK

Linda L. Demer, MD, PhD   Chief, Division of Cardiology, Departments of Medicine and Physiology, UCLA School of Medicine, Los Angeles, CA

Marie L. Foegh, MD, DSc   Adjunct Professor, Department of Surgery, Georgetown University Medical Center, Washington, DC

Trudy M. Forte, PhD   Donner Laboratory, Lawrence Berkeley National Laboratory, Berkeley, CA

Oscar Go, PhD   Assistant Professor, College of Public Health, University of Oklahoma Health Sciences Center, Oklahoma City, OK

Steven M. Haffner, MD   Professor, University of Texas Health Sciences Center, San Antonio, TX

David M. Herrington, MD, MHS   Associate Professor, Section of Cardiology, Department of Internal Medicine, Bowman Gray School of Medicine of Wake Forest University, Winston-Salem, NC

John E. Hokanson, MPH, PhD   Research Scientist, Departments of Medicine and Epidemiology, School of Medicine, University of Washington, Seattle, WA

Barbara V. Howard, PhD   President, Medlantic Research Institute, Washington, DC

Helena Judge, BA   Project Manager, Department of Nutrition, Harvard School of Public Health, Boston, MA

Lewis H. Kuller, MD, DrPH   Professor and Chairperson, Department of Epidemiology, Graduate School of Public Health, University.of Pittsburgh, Pittsburgh, PA

John C. LaRosa, MD   Chancellor, Tulane University Medical Center, New Orleans, LA

Holly Lassila, DrPH   Postdoctoral Fellow, University of Pittsburgh, Pittsburgh, PA

Douglas W. Losordo, MD   Departments of Medicine and Biomedical Research, Division of Cardiology, St. Elizabeth's Medical Center, Tufts University School of Medicine, Boston, MA

Karen Matthews, PhD   Professor, Department of Epidemiology, University of Pittsburgh, Pittsburgh, PA

Elaine N. Meilahn, DrPH   Senior Lecturer, London School of Hygiene and Tropical Medicine, London, UK

Virginia M. Miller, PhD   Associate Professor, Departments of Physiology and Surgery, Mayo Clinic and Foundation, Rochester, MN

Joel D. Morrisett, PhD   Professor of Medicine, Baylor College of Medicine, Houston, TX

Lauren Nathan, MD   Assistant Professor, Department of Obstetrics and Gynecology, UCLA School of Medicine, Los Angeles, CA

Mauro L. Nava, PhD   Research Associate, Department of Medicine, Baylor College of Medicine, Houston, TX

Shehla Pervin, PhD   Postdoctoral Fellow, Departments of Obstetrics and Gynecology and Molecular and Medical Pharmacology, UCLA School of Medicine, Los Angeles, CA

Peter W. Ramwell, PhD   Professor, Department of Physiology and Biophysics, Georgetown University School of Medicine, Washington, DC

Thomas C. Register, PhD   Assistant Professor, Department of Comparative Medicine, Bowman Gray School of Medicine of Wake Forest University, Winston-Salem, NC

Maryanne Reilly, RN   Research Nurse II, Department of Obstetrics/Gynecology, Baylor College of Medicine, Houston, TX

David C. Robbins, MD   Director, Medlantic Research Institute, Penn Medical Laboratory, Washinton, DC

Michael E. Rosenfeld, PhD   Associate Professor, Department of Pathobiology and Program in Nutritional Sciences, University of Washington, Seattle, WA

Frank M. Sacks, MD   Associate Professor, Department of Nutrition, Harvard School of Public Health; Department of Medicine, Brigham and Women's Hospital; and Department of Medicine, Harvard Medical School, Boston, MA

Philip M. Sarrel, MD   Professor, Department of Obstetrics, Gynecology and Psychiatry, Yale School of Medicine, New Haven, CT

Gary C. Sieck, PhD   Professor, Departments of Anesthesiology and Physiology, Mayo Clinic and Foundation, Rochester, MN

Rajan Singh, PhD   Postdoctoral Fellow, Departments of Obstetrics and Gynecology and Molecular and Medical Pharmacology, UCLA School of Medicine, Los Angeles, CA

Carolyn L. Smith, PhD   Assistant Professor, Department of Cell Biology, Baylor College of Medicine, Houston, TX

Michael C. Snabes, MD   Medical Resident, Department of Obstetrics/Gynecology, Baylor College of Medicine, Houston, TX

Leon Speroff, MD   Professor, Department of Obstetrics and Gynecology, Oregon Health Sciences University, Portland, OR

Ioakim Spyridopoulos, MD   Assistant Professor, Departments of Medicine and Biomedical Research, Division of Cardiology, St Elizabeth's Medical Center, Tufts University School of Medicine, Boston, MA

Janice D. Wagner, DVM, PhD   Assistant Professor, Department of Comparative Medicine, Bowman Gray School of Medicine of Wake Forest University,Winston-Salem, NC

Brian W. Walsh, MD   Director, Department of Obstetrics and Gynecology, Menopause Center, Brigham and Women's Hospital, Boston, MA

Karol E. Watson, MD   Clinical Instructor, Departments of Medicine and Physiology, UCLA School of Medicine, Los Angeles, CA

J. Koudy Williams, DVM   Associate Professor, Department of Comparative Medicine, Bowman Gray School of Medicine of Wake Forest University, Winston-Salem, NC

Rena Wing, PhD   Professor, Department of Epidemiology, University of Pittsburgh, Pittsburgh, PA

Jeunliang L. Yeh, PhD   Associate Professor, University of Oklahoma Health Sciences Center, Oklahoma City, OK

Ronald L. Young, MD   Associate Professor, Department of Obstetrics/Gynecology, Baylor College of Medicine, Houston, TX

Li Zhang, MD   Research Associate, Department of Comparative Medicine, Bowman Gray School of Medicine of Wake Forest University, Winston-Salem, NC

Contents

Chapter 1

Estrogen and the Pathophysiology of Atherosclerosis
Potential Effects of Estrogen on the Cell Biology of the Artery Wall

Michael E. Rosenfeld, PhD

To date, there is still no clear understanding of the mechanisms by which estrogen is protective of cardiovascular diseases. This is especially true with respect to how estrogen may impact directly on the cells of the artery wall and alter the development of atherosclerotic lesions. This brief review is designed to set the stage for many of the chapters to follow by providing some insights into which aspects of the atherogenic process may be responsive to estrogen. I have first included a brief discussion of why it is likely that estrogen has direct effects on cells within the artery wall. In this regard, this chapter discusses some of the conflicting results from animal studies that have made a clear interpretation of the mechanism(s) by which estrogen works at the level of the artery wall difficult. In some cases, the data suggest that estrogen acts primarily by lowering plasma lipoproteins, in other cases, the data are more indicative of there being direct effects on the artery wall. I have further included a brief discussion of known estrogen effects on cell proliferation and associated gene expression from nonvascular systems that may provide additional hints as to the potential estrogenic effects on vessel wall biology. Finally, I have provided an overview of our current understanding of the cellular events that occur during the initiation and progression of atherosclerosis and have speculated as to how estrogen might alter these processes, thus contributing to its overall protection against cardiovascular diseases.

From: Forte TM, (ed). *Hormonal, Metabolic, and Cellular Influences on Cardiovascular Disease in Women.* Armonk, NY: Futura Publishing Company, Inc.; © 1997.

Conflicting Evidence for Protective Effects of Estrogen at the Level of the Artery Wall

There have been a considerable number of studies of the effects of estrogen on the development of atherosclerosis in hypercholesterolemic animal models conducted over the past 20 years. Early studies of coronary atherosclerosis in chicks[1] and rats[2] and spontaneous aortic atherosclerosis in pigeons[3] clearly demonstrated that exogenous estrogen administration is inhibitory of lesion formation. More recent studies in hypercholesterolemic rabbits,[4–8] baboons,[9] and cynomologus monkeys[10] have provided additional evidence for the protective effects of estrogen on coronary and aortic atherosclerosis.

As noted, there is still no consistent interpretation concerning the mechanism(s) by which estrogen is protective of atherosclerosis. This, in large part, is due to significant differences in experimental designs and conflicting results from previous experimental studies. In studies by Kushwaha and Hazzard,[4] where intact female rabbits fed cholesterol containing diets were administered estradiol-17β via weekly intramuscular (IM) injections, the authors reported a significant effect of the estradiol in lowering plasma cholesterol levels, (especially in the very low-density lipoprotein (VLDL) and intermediate density lipoprotein (IDL) fractions) as well as a profound inhibition of cholesteryl-ester accumulation in the aorta. In a more recent study by Henriksson et al.,[6] in which all male rabbits fed a high-cholesterol diet (1%) were administered estradiol via diet as well as weekly IM injections, the authors also observed a significant reduction in plasma cholesterol, VLDL cholesterol (VLDL-C), and an increase in high-density lipoprotein cholesterol (HDL-C) that accompanied the profound reduction in the area of aortic atherosclerosis. Furthermore, in two recent studies of ovariectomized female rabbits that received estrogen replacement via diet[7] or daily IM injections,[11] both groups report significant reductions in plasma cholesterol levels as well as inhibition of aortic atherosclerosis[7] or intimal hyperplasia and foam cell formation after arterial grafting.[11] Studies using ovariectomized baboons[9] also have demonstrated a significant reduction in plasma lipids after estrogen administration.

There is considerable evidence that estrogen regulates lipoprotein binding and clearance by the liver that could account for the observed reductions in plasma lipoproteins. Studies of estradiol treated rats and rabbits have demonstrated increased clearance of low-density lipoprotein (LDL),[12] and increased binding of LDL and VLDL to liver membranes or perfused liver.[6,13,14] Recent data indicate that this increased binding is due to a specific upregulation of the expression of the apolipoprotein (apo) B/E receptor in the liver.[14-17] In humans, the evidence also strongly suggests that estrogen administration lowers plasma LDL and VLDL levels[18] and stimulates the expression of the apo B/E receptor in the liver.[19] Thus, taken together, these data suggest that estrogen inhibits the formation of atherosclerosis primarily via its capacity to reduce plasma cholesterol levels.

In contrast, Hough and Zilversmit,[5] observed no effect of estradiol on plasma lipids in intact female rabbits, but observed a significant reduction in aortic cholesteryl-ester content. Similarly, in a recent study of the effects of 17α-dihydroequilin (DHES), conjugated estrogen, and ethynyl estradiol on hypercholesterolemic, ovariectomized rabbits,[8] the authors report either no effects or an elevation of LDL-C with the estrogens despite a profound inhibitory effect on aortic atherosclerosis. These observations are further supported by the study of the protective effects of estrogen on atherosclerosis in cynomologus monkeys cited above[10] where there were also no alterations of plasma lipids reported. The fact that there are examples of protective effects of estrogen that are independent of effects on plasma lipids strongly suggests that estrogen also exerts some direct effect on cells within the artery wall or those interacting with the artery wall. This possibility is supported by additional recent data. For example, in a series of studies on estrogen and progesterone replacement therapy in ovariectomized cynomologus monkeys, Wagner et al.[20,21] have demonstrated that hormone replacement significantly reduces the accumulation and subsequent cellular degradation of LDL in the coronary arteries without altering plasma lipoprotein levels (See Chapter 10). Combined contraceptive steroid therapy in hypercholesterolemic rabbits has further been reported to inhibit collagen and elastin synthesis.[22,23] However, in both cases, it is still unclear to what extent the effect is due to the progesterone component of the combined therapy. Nevertheless, a study by Subbiah[24] on the effects of estradiol on pigeon artery, as well as data obtained in the study by Hough and Zilversmit in rabbits,[5] suggests that there is a specific estrogen-mediated stimulation of cholesteryl-ester hydrolysis (cholesteryl-ester hydrolase activity) and efflux of cholesterol from the artery wall. Unfortunately, it is still unknown which cell types may be stimulated and whether this is due to a direct effect of estrogen on the expression or activity of the hydrolytic enzymes in these cells.

As noted above, recent studies have further demonstrated an inhibitory effect of estrogen on the formation of a neointima in aortic allografts and after balloon injury in hypercholesterolemic rabbits,[11,25,26] (See Chapter 7). Although there were reductions in plasma lipoproteins that accompanied the inhibitory effects on neointima formation, it is unlikely that a reduction in plasma lipids could entirely explain these effects. Thus, these data provide preliminary evidence that estrogen may affect cellular migration and proliferation in the artery. This is further supported by in vitro observations by Fischer-Dzoga et al.[27] that estradiol specifically inhibits the proliferative response of rabbit aortic smooth muscle cells to hyperlipidemic serum and the formation of stainable collagen and elastin. Finally, as also will be discussed later in this text (See Chapter 6), there is a considerable volume of data showing effects of estrogen on arterial reactivity, primarily with regard to endothelial dependent vasodilatory mechanisms.[28]

Probably the strongest evidence for a direct estrogen effect on artery wall cells is the demonstration of the presence of estrogen receptors in artery wall cells both in vitro and in vivo. Initial autoradiographic studies of the distribution of labeled estradiol demonstrated the presence of specific estrogen binding sites in the aorta from normal and cholesterol-fed rabbits[29] and nuclear localization in smooth muscle cells of all of the major muscular arteries of baboons.[30] Scatchard analyses of the binding of labeled estradiol by cultured rat aortic smooth muscle cells[31] and by cytoplasmic preparations of homogenized dog coronary arteries[32] have demonstrated specific high-affinity binding sites. Radioligand binding assays as well as gel retardation assays have further confirmed the presence of functional estrogen receptors in cultured human vascular smooth muscle cells[33] (See also Chapter 5). Immunocytochemical analyses with monoclonal antibodies against human estrogen receptors[33] have demonstrated specific staining within most normal human coronary arteries of both pre- and postmenopausal women and reduced positivity in corresponding atherosclerotic coronary arteries. Immunocytochemistry has also been used to demonstrate estrogen receptors in smooth muscle cells of the uterine arteries of humans and rabbits.[34] Finally, there is recent evidence that macrophages also contain estrogen receptors.[35] Scatchard analyses of the binding of labeled estradiol by J111 monocytic leukemic cells and mouse peritoneal macrophages demonstrate high-affinity binding sites in both types of cells. It has also been demonstrated recently that T cells (suppressor/cytotoxic T cells) express estrogen receptors.[36]

Estrogen Effects on Cell Proliferation and Gene Expression in Nonarterial Cells

There is a huge volume of reports in the literature of effects of estrogen on gene expression and cell proliferation primarily in cells of the reproductive tract and bones. Table 1 is a partial compilation of some of the data in the literature from the past several years showing which cells and tissues have been reported to exhibit increased or decreased proliferation in response to estrogen and, further, what genes or gene products have been reported to be estrogen responsive in these cell types. In general, most of the data indicate that there is an increase in cell proliferation in response to estrogen. This may be due to the fact that several of the estrogen responsive genes are growth factors and their receptors such as insulin-like growth factor I,[37,38] epidermal growth factor and receptor,[38-41] and transforming-growth factor α.[41-44] Furthermore, it appears that estrogen inhibits the expression of transforming growth factor-β which in some cell systems exerts an antimitotic effect.[43-45]

Estrogen has also been reported to affect cellular differentiation in a variety of different cell types and in this capacity may play a role in the regulation of inflammatory cell differentiation during atherogenesis. These known effects on differentiation include myeloid cells,[46] mast cells,[47] T cells,[48] vaginal epithelial cells,[49] and osteoblast differentiation to osteoclasts.[50,51]

What are the Potential Mechanisms by Which Estrogen May Directly Affect the Artery Wall at Different Stages in the Development of Atherosclerosis?

Our current understanding of the biochemical and cellular events that occur during the initiation and progression of atherosclerotic lesions suggests that there are many stages of the atherogenic process that may be responsive to estrogen. Table 2 lists in semichronological order many of these key cellular events.

Based on the elegant studies of Schwenke and Carew,[52,53] it appears that the first stage in the atherogenic process probably involves the trapping and retention of lipoproteins at lesion prone sites. The data suggest that even a small elevation of the atherogenic lipoproteins in the plasma coupled with a connective tissue composition at specific lesion prone sites that facilitates trapping and retention of the particles may be sufficient to change the mass action toward a net influx into the artery wall. This trapping and increased retention in turn could allow for spontaneous and/or cell mediated oxidation of the particles.[54] The formation of oxidized lipoproteins at very early stages of the process may trigger

TABLE 1

Known Effects of Estrogen on Cell Proliferation and Gene Expression In Nonvascular Tissues

| Increased cell proliferation | Gene expression | | References |
	Increased	Decreased	
Cells of Reproductive Tract			
Breast cancer cell lines	PS-2	Estrogen rec	37,41,42,45,
MCF-7	EGF	c-erb B2	98–106
ZR-75-1	EGF-Rec	Retinoic acid rec	
T-47D	TGF-α	TGF-β	
CAMA-1	TGF-α rec		
	IGF-I rec		
	HMFGM		
	Ras p21		
	Neu		
	c-Jun		
	c-Fos		
	c-Myc		
	cathepsin D		
	PNR-1		
	PNR-2		
	PNR-25		
Uterus			
Rat, mouse,	IGF-1	TGF-β	39,40,43,44,
pig uterus			107–112
Ishikawa cells	EGF-rec	IL-6	
ZIF 268	TGF-α		
	IL-1 α		
	IL-1 β		
	c-Fos		
	c-Jun		
	c-Myc		
Ovarian cancer cell lines			
BG-1			113–116
PEO4			
Leydig cell line		Leukotrienes	
B-IF cells			
Other Tissues or Cells			
Liver			
Rat, frog	Vit D rec		117,118
	Vitellogenin		
			continues

Increased cell proliferation	Gene expression		References
	Increased	Decreased	

Other Tissues or Cells continued

Increased cell proliferation	Increased	Decreased	References
Kidney			
Rat	Retinal BP	Vit D rec	119–121
Hamster prox. tubule			
Hamster H301 cells			
Pituitary			
Rat	Prolactin		122,123
GH3 cells			
MtT/F4 cells			
Hypothalamus			
Rat			125
RCF-8 cells			
(SV-40 transformed)			
Bone			
ROS 17/2.8 cells	Vit D rec		51,97,126,
MC3T3-E1 cells	Osteocalcin		
RCT-3 cells	IGF-1		
Primary cultures—rat	Collagen		
Diaphyseal cells			
Calvarial cells			
Trabecular cells			

Decreased cell proliferation			
Mouse vaginal epithelial cells			49,124,
HELA cells (transfected with HuER)			127–129
3T3-A31 (transfected with HuER)			
KSE-1 esophogeal carcinoma cells			
RCA-6 cells (rat hypothalamus)			

an inflammatory activation of the endothelium and/or attract inflammatory cells into the intima, thus setting in motion the subsequent fibroproliferative responses characteristic of the atherogenic process in general.[55] Estrogen could alter this process in several ways. First, as will be discussed later (See Chapter 12), because estrogen has antioxidant and lipophilic properties, the presence of estrogen molecules within the lipid core of the atherogenic lipoproteins could inhibit oxidation.[56,57] Inhibition of oxidation could in turn reduce the trapping and retention of the particles within the matrix, the activation of the endothelium, and the subsequent chemotactic attraction of leukocytes into the intima.[58] In addition, estrogen may also directly alter the composition of connective tissue molecules synthesized and secreted by resident intimal smooth muscle cells, further reducing lipoprotein

---

TABLE 2

Chronology of the Major Cellular Events in the Development and Progression of Atherosclerotic Lesions

Stages in the Atherogenic Process

1. Trapping, retention, and oxidation of lipoproteins at lesion prone sites
   Result: Initiation of the atherogenic process.
2. Activation of the endothelium
   Result: Expression of adhesion molecules and chemokines.
3. Monocyte and lymphocyte adherence and diapedesis
   Result: Formation of the initial fatty streak.
4. Monocyte differentiation and activation
   Result: Macrophage foam cell formation and proliferation, secretion of cytokines, growth factors, and chemokines.
5. Smooth muscle cell migration, proliferation, and connective tissue synthesis
   Result: Formation of the fibrous cap.
6. Modulation of the production of vasoactive factors
   Result: Alterations in vascular tone.
7. Cellular necrosis and apoptosis, coalescence of extracellular lipid, calcification
   Result: Development of the necrotic core and formation of an unstable plaque.
8. Neovascularization
   Result: Further infiltration of inflammatory cells and plasma components, continued destabilization of the plaque.
9. Plaque fissure and remodeling
   Result: Mural thrombus formation and reorganization, compensatory enlargement, formation of complex/complicated lesions.
10. Plaque rupture
    Result: Unstable angina and terminal thrombotic events.

---

trapping and retention.[22,23] As has been noted above[20,21] (See Chapter 10), after trapping in the matrix, estrogen may also directly reduce the cellular uptake and degradation of the atherogenic lipoproteins.

The second major stage of lesion development involves the adherence of leukocytes to the endothelium followed by diapedesis into the intimal space.[55,59] There is as yet only preliminary evidence suggesting that estrogen may reduce monocyte adherence to endothelial cells (See Chapter 8). However, if there is an inhibitory effect, it is possible that it is directly due to inhibition of the expression of monocyte and endothelial cell adhesion molecules such as VLA-4 and VCAM-1, respectively. Although there have not yet been reports of a consensus sequence for the estrogen response element within the promoters for these adhesion molecule genes, there is recent in vitro data suggesting that estradiol-17β inhibits expression of VCAM-1 in human umbilical vein endothelial cells treated with IL-1/β.[60] An alternative possibility is that estrogen alters endothelial and/or macrophage production of nitric oxide (NO); this in turn may affect monocyte adhesion as suggested by several recent studies.[61,62] Estrogen may also alter the expression by endothelial cells of monocyte chemokines, such as MCP-1, either by directly reducing its expression or by inhibiting expression induced by oxidative mechanisms.[63]

A third stage in the atherogenic process involves the expansion of the fatty streak with the continuous influx of lymphocytes and monocytes and the differentiation, activation, and conversion of the monocytes into macrophage-derived foam cells.[55,59] As noted, estrogen may alter this stage by inhibiting monocyte differentiation into tissue macrophages[46,50,51] and thus conversion into foam cells. To date, evidence is still lacking for a direct effect of estrogen on scavenger receptor expression in macrophages. However, as previously noted, estrogen does increase cholesteryl-ester hydrolysis in the aorta of cholesterol-fed rabbits,[5,24] suggesting a potential effect on the expression of macrophage hydrolytic enzymes and an impairment of foam cell formation. It is also feasible that estrogen may inhibit the inflammatory activation of macrophages within the fatty streak. Activation, in this case, refers to the induction of expression of cytokines and growth regulatory molecules as well as proliferation. This potential effect of estrogen is supported by many of the studies included in Table 1 and by two recent publications showing modulation of PDGF-A and MCP-1 expression by estrogen in vitro in several monocytic cell lines.[64,65] Ovariectomy in mice has also been reported to lead to an increased expression and production of IL-1 and TNF by mononuclear cells in the bone marrow.[66]

Although T lymphocytes populate experimental and human fatty streaks and advanced lesions,[67,68] it is still unclear how immune mechanisms contribute to the atherogenic process. There are several possibilities that now are supported by experimental data. Evidence suggests that oxidized lipids and lipoproteins are immunogenic and can induce both autoantibody production in vivo[54] and some T cell clonal proliferation in vitro.[69] Again, estrogen could have an impact here by virtue of its antioxidant properties. It is also clear that many atherosclerotic lesions contain infectious organisms (eg, chlamydia pneumoniae[70]) and that the presence of T lymphocytes may be an additional protection against these infectious agents. Although most of the T cells within human lesions appear to be CD4 positive and thus of the T helper variety, there are also CD8-positive T killer cells.[68] Interestingly, there is recent evidence that estrogen may modulate killer cell mediated cytotoxicity.[71]

A hallmark of the conversion of fatty streaks to more advanced atherosclerotic lesions is the formation of a fibrous cap.[59,67] This process clearly involves an increase in the number of smooth muscle cells within the intima and likely requires both increased migration and proliferation as well as stimulation of connective tissue synthesis. Based on the disparate effects of estrogen on cell proliferation and related gene expression shown in Table 1, it is possible that estrogen may have an impact on the formation of the fibrous cap by altering both smooth muscle proliferation and collagen and elastin synthesis.[22,23] There have been a number of reports of the expression of some of the estrogen responsive growth factors in the artery wall in vivo or by artery wall cells in vitro that support a role for estrogen in regulating vascular cell proliferation. Insulin-like growth factor-I (IGF-I) expression primarily by smooth muscle cells in the rat aorta has been reported by several groups[72-74] and has also been reported recently for macrophages[75] and for platelets.[76] Bornfeldt et al.[77,78] have demonstrated that IGF-I is mitogenic and chemotactic for arterial smooth muscle cells in vitro. TGF-α and β expression in arterial tissue or by arterial cells in vitro has also been demonstrated previously.[72,79-81] Because there have been no systematic evaluations of the effects of estrogen on changes in the cellular and connective tissue composition of atherosclerotic lesions, it is unclear whether estrogen is likely to stimulate or inhibit fibrous cap formation. It is also not known whether the formation of a fibrous cap is a normal protective mechanism or whether its presence contributes to the progression of lesions. Nevertheless, as cited above,[11,25,26] estrogen appears to reduce neointima formation after balloon injury and in aortic allografts in rabbits, suggesting that it may inhibit smooth muscle migration and/or proliferation and thus the formation of the fibrous cap.

There is a large volume of data demonstrating that hypercholesterolemia and the resulting atherosclerosis in several animal models and in humans alters the production and/or responsiveness of arteries to vasoactive factors.[28] There are also rapidly accumulating data (See Chapter 6) showing that estrogen improves the impaired arterial responsiveness, especially with regard to endothelium-dependent vasodilation.[82-84] It is still unclear, however, how alterations in vascular tone impact on the atherogenic process and whether the effects of estrogen are direct effects on cells producing vasoactive factors or on smooth muscle cell responses to these mediators. The failure of an artery to dilate or contract properly could contribute to alterations in blood pressure, to vasospasm, to compensatory remodeling, and to the extent of plaque stenosis. On a cellular level, one possibility is that estrogen directly alters expression and activity of the enzymes involved in prostacyclin and NO synthesis and/or the production and secretion of these vasodilators.[28,85] As yet, it is unclear whether this might include all of the enzymes in the cyclooxygenase pathway and both the constitutive NO synthase found in endothelial cells as well as the inducible form found in macrophages.[86] In both cases, however, positive estrogenic effects would potentially increase the availability of prostacyclin and/or NO and the vasodilatory response. Another untested possibility is that by acting as an antioxidant, estrogen may reduce the amount of reactive oxygen capable of scavenging NO,[87] thus further increasing its availability for stimulating vasodilation.

The primary hallmark of an advanced atherosclerotic lesion is the formation of a necrotic core.[67] The necrotic core generally refers to an acellular region consisting of lipid, necrotic cell debris and, in many cases, calcium-phosphate deposits, centrally located at the base of the plaque. Although it is still unclear as to whether the necrotic core forms as a result of the necrotic and/or apoptotic death of foam cells and/or from the coalescence of extracellular lipid, it is clear that the presence of a necrotic core has profound clinical implications. This is because the formation of a necrotic core frequently destablizes a plaque leading to rupture and the subsequent formation of large, occlusive thrombi that cause unstable angina and myocardial infarctions.[67,88] Again, there is not yet direct evidence that estrogen retards the formation of the necrotic core. However, if estrogen inhibits foam cell formation by stimulating cholesteryl-ester hydrolysis, this in turn would impact on necrotic core formation by limiting a possible source of lipid and necrotic cell debris. A reduction in cholesteryl-ester deposition in foam cells also would inhibit oxidative stress-induced necrotic and/or apoptotic cell death by reducing the availability of oxidizable lipids within the cell. Increased formation of lipid hydroperoxides would contribute to a depletion of the cell's pool of endogenous antioxidants and hasten the cell's demise.

It is also unclear as to how estrogen might affect the deposition of calcium-phosphate within the plaques, in large part because we still do not have many leads as to what induces calcification within the vessel wall. Calcification-related proteins, such as osteopontin and bone morphogenic protein, are expressed by arterial wall cells,[89–92] but it is still unknown whether estrogen plays a role in the regulation of their expression. Recent studies have also suggested that there may be specialized smooth muscle-like cells that form nodules of cells that may facilitate calcification within the artery wall.[89,92] Formation of these nodules and their subsequent calcification is stimulated by TGF-β in vitro and as cited previously[(93)] estrogen may alter this process by inhibiting TGF-β expression (See Chapter 9).

Another hallmark of an advanced lesion is the formation of neovessels.[67] These small arterioles and capillary-like vessels are frequently located adjacent to a necrotic core and often are surrounded by loci of monocytic cells. It is still unknown exactly what induces the formation of these neovessels, but many studies have demonstrated that inflammatory cells, especially macrophages, are rich sources of angiogenic factors.[94] The formation of these neovessels may also contribute to plaque destablization and, by being the conduit for entry of monocytic cells into the depths of the plaque, could contribute to the severity of inflammatory and immune responses occurring within the plaques. Again, experimental support for an effect of estrogen on angiogenesis is limited, but a recent report indicates that estradiol-17β promotes angiogenic activity in human umbilical vein endothelial cells in vitro and that vascularization of matrigel plugs is inhibited in ovariectomized mice in vivo.[95] Despite a lack of current experimental support, an additional possibility for a role for estrogen in protecting against plaque rupture may be in inhibiting the expression, secretion, and/or activity of cellular metalloproteinases. This family of proteolytic enzymes has been suggested to play a role in the breakdown of the connective tissue matrix of advanced plaques thus contributing to a reduction in tensile strength and destablization leading to the eventual rupture of the plaques.[88]

One of the last stages of the disease process involves the formation of complicated/complex lesions. These very advanced lesions show clear evidence of the integration of organized thrombi into the body of the plaques, suggesting that episodic plaque fissure or rupture has occurred previously.[67] I have already dealt with the possible ways that estrogen may reduce plaque rupture. However, the protective effects of estrogen may also involve alterations in the expression of prothombotic factors such as tissue factor by cells within the lesions. To date, there is still no evidence that estrogen alters expression of tissue factor, but given that it may be expressed by macrophages within the lesions,[96] estrogenic effects on macrophage activation again would contribute to a protective effect on this process.

In summary, it is now clear that estrogen may impart its protective effects on cardiovascular disease by altering one or more of the cellular and biochemical events associated with the initiation and progression of atherosclerosis. Our mandate for the future is to determine which stages are estrogen responsive and investigate from a mechanistic perspective how estrogen might alter these atherogenic processes.

References

1. Pick R, Stamler J, Rodband, S. Inhibition of coronary atherosclerosis by estrogen in cholesterol-fed chickens. *Circulation* 1952;6:276–281.
2. Moskowitz MS, Moskowitz AA, Bradford W. Changes in serum lipids and coronary arteries of the rat in response to estrogen. *Arch Pathol* 1956;61:245–263.
3. Hanash KA, Kottke BA, Greene LF, et al. Effects of conjugated estrogens on spontaneous atherosclerosis in pigeons. *Arch Pathol* 1972; 93:184–189.
4. Kushwaha RS, Hazzard WR. Exogenous estrogens attenuate dietary hypercholesterolemia and atherosclerosis in the rabbit. *Metabolism* 1981;30:359–366.
5. Hough JL, Zilversmit DB. Effect of 17-beta estradiol on aortic cholesterol content and metabolism in cholesterol-fed rabbits. *Arteriosclerosis* 1986;6:57–63.
6. Henriksson P, Stamberger M, Eriksson M, et al. Oestrogen-induced changes in lipoprotein metabolism: Role in prevention of atherosclerosis in the cholesterol-fed rabbit. *Eur J Clin Invest* 1989;19:395–403.
7. Haarbo J, Leth-Espensen P, Stender S, et al. Estrogen monotherapy and combined estrogen-progestogen replacement therapy attenuate aortic accumulation of cholesterol in ovariectomized cholesterol-fed rabbits. *J Clin Invest* 1991;87:1274–1279.
8. Sulistiyani, Adelman SJ, Chandrasekaren A, et al. Effect of 17α-dihydroequilin sulfate, a conjugated equine estrogen, and ethynylestradiol on atherosclerosis in cholesterol-fed rabbits. *Arterio Thromb Vasc Biol* 1995;15:837–846.
9. Kushwaha RS, Lewis DS, Carey KD, et al. Effects of estrogen and progesterone on plasma lipoproteins and experimental atherosclerosis in the baboon (Papio sp.). *Arterioscler Thromb* 1991;11:23–31.
10. Adams MR, Kaplan JR, Manuck SB, et al. Inhibition of coronary artery atherosclerosis by 17-beta estradiol in ovariectomized monkeys. Lack of an effect of added progesterone. *Arteriosclerosis* 1990;10:1051–1057.
11. Cheng LP, Kuwahara M, Jacobsson J, et al. Inhibition of myointimal hyperplasia and macrophage infiltration by estradiol in aorta allografts. *Transplantation* 1991;52:967–972.
12. Chao Y, Windler EE, Chen GC, et al. Hepatic catabolism of rat and human lipoproteins in rats treated with 17 alpha-ethinyl estradiol. *J Biol Chem* 1979;254:11360–11366.
13. Kovanen PT, Brown MS, Goldstein JL. Increased binding of low density lipoprotein to liver membranes from rats treated with 17 alpha-ethinyl estradiol. *J Biol Chem* 1979;254:11367–11373.
14. Floren CH, Kushwaha RS, Hazzard WR, et al. Estrogen-induced increase in uptake of cholesterol-rich very low density lipoproteins in perfused rabbit liver. *Metabolism* 1981;30:367–375.

15. Ma PTS, Yamamoto P, Goldstein JL, et al. Increased mRNA for low density lipoprotein receptor in livers of rabbits treated with 17 alpha-ethinyl estradiol. *Proc Natl Acad Sci USA* 1986;83:792–796.
16. Demacker PNM, Mol MJ, Stalenhoef AFH. Increased hepatic lipase activity and increased direct removal of very-low density lipoprotein remnants in Watanabe heritable hyperlipemic (WHHL) rabbits treated with ethinyl estradiol. *Biochem J* 1990;274:647–651.
17. Demacker PNM, Staels B, Stalenhoef AFH, et al. Increased removal of β-very low density lipoproteins after ethinyl estradiol is associated with increased mRNA levels for hepatic lipase, lipoprotein lipase, and the low density lipoprotein receptor in Watanabe Heritable Hyperlipidemic rabbits. *Arterioscler Thromb* 1991;11:1652–1659.
18. Wallace RB, Hoover J, Barrett-Connor E, et al. Altered plasma lipid and lipoprotein levels associated with oral contraceptive and oestrogen use. *Lancet* 1979;21:111–114.
19. Nanjee MN, Koritnik DR, Thomas J, et al. Hormonal determinants of apolipoprotein B,E, receptor expression in human liver. Positive association of receptor expression with plasma estrone concentration in middle-aged/elderly women. *Biochim Biophys Acta* 1990;N046:151–158.
20. Wagner JD, Clarkson TB, St. Clair RW, et al. Estrogen and progesterone replacement therapy reduces low density lipoprotein accumulation in the coronary arteries of surgically postmenopausal cynomolgus monkeys. *J Clin Invest* 1991;N8:1995–2002.
21. Wagner JD, St. Clair RW, Schwenke DC, et al. Regional differences in arterial low density lipoprotein metabolism inn surgically postmenopausal cynomolgus monkeys. Effects of estrogen andd progesterone replacement therapy. *Arterioscler Thromb* 1992;N2:717–726.
22. Fischer GM, Cherian K, Swain ML. Increased synthesis of aortic collagen and elastin in experimental atherosclerosis: Inhibition by contraceptive steroids. *Atherosclerosis* 1981;N9:463–467.
23. Fischer GM, Swain ML. Effects of estradiol and progesterone on the increased synthesis of collagen in atherosclerotic rabbit aortas. *Atherosclerosis* 1985;N4:177–185.
24. Subbiah MTR. Effect of estrogens on the activities of cholesteryl ester synthetase and cholesteryl ester hydrolases in pigeon aorta. *Steroids* 1977;N0:259–265.
25. Jacobsson J, Cheng L, Lyke K, et al. Effect of estradiol on accelerated atherosclerosis in rabbit heterotopic aortic allografts. *J Heart Lung Transplant* 1992;N1:1188–1193.
26. Foegh ML, Asotra S, Howell MH, et al. Estradiol inhibition of arterial neointima hyperplasia after balloon injury. *J Vasc Surg* 1994;N9:722–726.
27. Fischer-Dzoga K, Wissler RW, Vesselinovitch D. The effect of estradiol on the proliferation of rabbit aortic medial tissue culture cells induced by hyperlipemic serum. *Exp Mol Pathol* 1983;N9:355–363.
28. Mendelsohn ME, Karas RH. Estrogen and the blood vessel wall. *Curr Opin Cardiol* 1994;N:619–626.
29. Malinow MR, Pellegrino AA, Lange G. Distribution of oestradiol-6,7-H3 in the arteries of normal and cholesterol-fed rabbits. *Acta Endocrinol* 1959;N1:500–504.
30. McGill HC, Sheridan PJ. Nuclear uptake of sex steroid hormones in the cardiovascular system of the baboon. *Circ Res* 1981;N8:238–244.

31. Nakao J, Chang WC, Murota SI, et al. Estradiol-binding sites in rat aortic smooth muscle cells in culture. *Atherosclerosis* 1981;N8:75–80.
32. Harder DR, Coulson PB. Estrogen receptors and effects of estrogen on membrane electrical properties of coronary vascular smooth muscle. *J Cell Physiol* 1979;N00:375–382.
33. Losordo DW, Kearney M, Kim EA, et al. Variable expression of the estrogen receptor in normal and atherosclerotic coronary arteries of premenopausal women. *Circulation* 1994;N9:1501–1510.
34. Perrot-Applanat M, Groyer-Picard MT, Garcia E, et al. Immunocyto-chemical demonstration of estrogen and progesterone receptors in muscle cells of uterine arteries in rabbits and humans. *Endocrinology* 1988;N23:1511–1519.
35. Gulshan S, McCruden AB, Stimson WH. Oestrogen receptors in macrophages. *Scand J Immunol* 1990;N1:691–697.
36. Stimson WH. Oestrogen and human T lymphocytes: Presence of specific receptors in the T-suppressor/cytotoxic subset. *Scand J Immunol* 1988;N8:345–350.
37. van der Burg B. Sex steroids and growth factors in mammary cancer. *Acta Endocrinol* 1991;N25(suppl 1):38–41.
38. Sahlin L, Rodriguez-Martinez H, Stanchev P, et al. Regulation of the uterine expression of messenger ribonucleic acids encoding the oestrogen receptor and IGF-I peptides in the pig uterus. Abstract. *Zentralbl Veterinarmed* 1990;N7:795–800.
39. Ignar-Trowbridge DM, Nelson KG, Bidwell MC, et al. Coupling of dual signaling pathways: Epidermal growth factor action involves the estrogen receptor. *Proc Natl Acad Sci USA* 1992;N9:4658–4662.
40. Gardner RM, Verner G, Kirkland JL, et al. Regulation of uterine epidermal growth factor (EGF) receptors by estrogen in the mature rat and during the estrous cycle. *J Steroid Biochem* 1989;N2:339–343.
41. Gabelman BM, Emerman JT. Effects of estrogen, epidermal growth factor, and transforming growth factor-alpha on the growth of human breast epithelial cells in primary culture. *Exp Cell Res* 1992;N01:113–118.
42. Fontana JA, Nervi C, Shao ZM, et al. Retinoid antagonism of estrogen-responsive transforming growth factor alpha and pS2 gene expression in breast carcinoma cells. *Cancer Res* 1992;N2:3938–3945.
43. Anzai Y, Gong Y, Holinka CF, et al. Effects of transforming growth factors and regulation of their mRNA levels in two human endometrial adenocarcinoma cell lines. *J Steroid Biochem Mol Biol.* 1992; 42:449-455.
44. Murphy LJ, Gong Y, Murphy LC. Regulation of transforming growth factor gene expression in human endometrial adenocarcinoma cells. *J Steroid Biochem Mol Biol* 1992;N1:309–314.
45. Arrick BA, Korc M, Derynck R. Differential regulation of expression of three transforming growth factor beta species in human breast cancer cell lines by estradiol. *Cancer Res* 1990;N0:299–303.
46. Burk O, Klempnauer KH. Estrogen-dependent alterations in differentiation state of myeloid cells caused by a v-myb/estrogen receptor fusion protein. *EMBO J* 1991;N0:3713–3719.
47. Gaytan F, Bellido C, Carrera G, et al. Differentiation of mast cells during postnatal development of neonatally estrogen-treated rats. *Cell Tissue Res* 1990;N59:25–31.

48. Okuyama R, Abo T, Seki S, et al. Estrogen administration activates extrathymic T cell differentiation in the liver. *J Exp Med* 1992; N75:661–669.
49. Tsai PS, Uchima FD, Hamamoto ST, et al. Proliferation and differentiation of prepubertal mouse vaginal epithelial cells in vitro and the specificity of estrogen-induced growth retardation. *In Vitro. Cell Dev Biol* 1991;N7A:461–468.
50. Kaye AM, Weisman Y, Harell A, et al. Hormonal stimulation of bone cell proliferation. *J Steroid Biochem Mol Biol* 1990;N7:431–435.
51. Liel Y, Kraus S, Levy J, et al. Evidence that estrogens modulate activity and increase the number of 1,25-dihydroxyvitamin D receptors in osteoblast-like cells (ROS 17/2.8). *Endocrinology* 1992;N30:2597–2601.
52. Schwenke DC, Carew TE. Initiation of atherosclerotic lesions in cholesterol-fed rabbits. I. Focal increases in arterial LDL concentration precede development of fatty streak lesions. *Arteriosclerosis* 1989;N: 895–907.
53. Schwenke DC, Carew TE. Initiation of atherosclerotic lesion in cholesterol-fed rabbits. II. Selective retention of LDL vs. selective increases in LDL permeability in susceptible sites of arteries. *Arteriosclerosis* 1989;N:908–918.
54. Steinberg D, Parthasarathy S, Carew TE, et al. Beyond cholesterol. Modifications of low-density lipoprotein that increase its atherogenicity. *N Engl J Med* 1989;N20:916–924.
55. Ross R. The pathogenesis of atherosclerosis: A perspective for the 1990s. *Nature* 1993;N62:801–809.
56. Lacort M, Leal AM, Liza M, et al. Protective effect of estrogens and catecholestrogens against peroxidative membrane damage in vitro. *Lipids* 1995;N0:141–146.
57. Wiseman H. Tamoxifen and estrogens as membrane antioxidants. *Methods Enzymol* 1994;N34:590–602.
58. Quinn MT, Parthasarathy S, Fong L, et al. Oxidatively modified low density lipoproteins: A potential role in the recruitment and retention of monocyte/macrophages during atherogenesis. *Proc Natl Acad Sci USA* 1987;N4:2995–2998.
59. Stary HC, Chandler AB, Glagov S, et al. A definition of initial, fatty streak, and intermediate lesions of atherosclerosis. *Circulation* 1994; N9:2462–2478.
60. Nakai K, Itoh C, Hotta K, et al. Estradiol-17 beta regulates the induction of VCAM-1 mRNA expression by interleukin-1 beta in human umbilical vein endothelial cells. *Life Sci* 1994;N4:221–227.
61. Tsoa PS, McEvoy LM, Drexler H, et al. Enhanced endothelial adhesiveness in hypercholesterolemia is attenuated by L-arginine. *Circulation* 1994;N9:2176–2182.
62. Gauthier, TW, Scalia, R, Murohara, T, et al. Nitric oxide protects against leukocyte-endothelium interactions in early stages of hypercholesterolemia. *Arterioscler Thromb Vasc Biol* 1995;N5:1652-1659.
63. Satriano JA, Shuldiner M, Hora K, et al. Oxygen radicals as second messengers for expression of the monocyte chemoattractant protein, JE/MCP-1, and the monocyte colony-stimulating factor, CSF-1, in response to tumor necrosis factor-α and immunoglobulin G: Evidence for involvement of reduced nicotinamide adenine dinucleotide phosphate (NADPH)-dependent oxidase. *J Clin Invest* 1993;N2:1564–1571.

64. Shanker G, Sorci-Thomas M, Adams MR. Estrogen modulates the inducible expression of platelet-derived growth factor mRNA by monocyte/macrophages. *Life Sci* 1995;N6:499–507.
65. Frazier-Jessen MR, Kovacs EJ. Estrogen modulation of JE/monocyte chemoattractant protein-1 mRNA expression in murine macrophages. *J Immunol* 1995;N54:1838–1845.
66. Kitazawa R, Kimble RB, Vannice JL, et al. Interleukin-1 receptor antagonist and tumor necrosis factor binding protein decrease osteoclast formation and bone resorption in ovariectomized mice. *J Clin Invest* 1994;N4:2397–2406.
67. Stary HC, Chandler AB, Glagov S, et al. A definition of advanced types of atherosclerotic lesions and a histological classification of atherosclerosis. *Arterioscler Thromb Vasc Biol* 1995;N5:1512–1531.
68. Hansson GK, Jonasson L, Seifert PS, et al. Immune mechanisms in atherosclerosis. *Arteriosclerosis* 1989;N:567–578.
69. Stemme S, Faber B, Holm J, et al. T lymphocytes from human atherosclerotic plaques recognize oxidized low density lipoprotein. *Proc Natl Acad Sci USA* 1995;N2:3893–3897.
70. Kuo CC, Grayston JT, Campbell LA, et al. Chlamydia pneumoniae (TWAR) in cornary arteries of young adults (15-34 years old). *Proc Natl Acad Sci USA* 1995;N2:6911–6914.
71. Baral E, Nagy E, Berczi I. Modulation of natural killer cell-mediated cytotoxicity by tamoxifen and estradiol. *Cancer* 1995;N5:591–599.
72. Sarzari R, Brecher P, Chobanian AV. Growth factor gene expression in aorta from normotensive and hypertensive rats. *J Clin Invest* 1989;N3:1404–1408.
73. Delafontaine P, Lou H, Alexander RW. Regulation of insulin-like growth factor I messenger RNA levels in vascular smooth muscle cells. *Hypertension* 1991;N8:742–747.
74. Cercek B, Fishbein MC, Forrester JS, et al. Induction of insulin-like growth factor I messenger RNA in rat aorta after balloon denudation. *Circ Res* 1990;N6:1755–1760.
75. Rom WN, Basset P, Fells GA, et al. Alveolar macrophages release an insulin-like growth factor I-type molecule. *J Clin Invest* 1988;N2:1685–1693.
76. Karey KP, Sirbasku DA. Human platelet-derived mitogens II. Subcellular localization of insulin-like growth factor I to the alpha granule and release in response to thrombin. *Blood* 1989;N4:1093–1100.
77. Bornfeldt KE, Gidlof RA, Wasteson A, et al. Binding and biological effects of insulin, insulin analogues and insulin-like growth factors in rat aortic smooth muscle cells. Comparison of maximal growth promoting activities. *Diabetologia* 1991;N4:307–313.
78. Bornfeldt KE, Arnqvist HJ, Capron L. In vivo proliferation of vascular smooth muscle in relation to diabetes mellitus, insulin-like growth factor I and insulin. *Diabetologia* 1992;N5:104–108.
79. Ross R, Masuda J, Raines EW, et al. Localization of PDGF-B protein in macrophages in all phases of atherogenesis. *Science* 1990;N48:1009–1012.
80. Majesky MW, Giachelli CM, Reidy MA, et al. Rat carotid neointimal smooth muscle cells reexpress a developmentally regulated mRNA phenotype during repair of arterial injury. *Circ Res* 1992;N1:759–768.
81. Strandjord T, Clark J, Madtes D. Expression of TGF-alpha, EGF, and EGF receptor in fetal rat lung. *Am J Physiol* 1994;N67:L384–389.

82. Bell DR, Rensberger HJ, Koritnik DR, et al. Estrogen pretreatment directly potentitates endothelium-dependent vasorelaxation of porcine coronary arteries. *Am J Physiol* 1995;N68:H377–383.
83. Lieberman EH, Gerhard MD, Uehata A, et al. Estrogen improves endothelium-dependent, flow-mediated vasodilation in postmenopausal women. *Ann Intern Med* 1994;N21:936–941.
84. Williams JK, Honore EK, Washburn SA, et al. Effects of hormone replacement therapy on reactivity of atherosclerotic coronary arteries in cynamalogous monkeys. *J Am Coll Cardiol* 1994;N4:1757–1761.
85. Redmond EM, Cherian MN, Wetzel RC. 17 beta-Estradiol inhibits flow- and acute hypoxia-induced prostacyclin release from perfused endocardial endothelial cells. *Circulation* 1994;N0:2519–2524.
86. Nathan C, Xie Q. Regulation of biosynthesis of nitric oxide. *J Biol Chem* 1994;N69:13725–13728.
87. Rubbo H, Radi R, Trujillo M, et al. Nitric oxide regulation of superoxide and peroxynitrite-dependent lipid peroxidation. *J Biol Chem* 1994;N6066–26075.
88. Falk E. Why do plaques rupture? *Circulation* 1992;N6(suppl 6):30–42.
89. Bostrom K, Watson KE, Horn S, et al. Bone morphogenetic protein expression in human atherosclerotic lesions. *J Clin Invest* 1993;N1:1800–1809.
90. Fitzpatrick LA, Severson A, Edwards WD, et al. Diffuse calcification in human coronary arteries. Association of osteopontin with atherosclerosis. *J Clin Invest* 1994;N4:1597–1604.
91. Shanahan CM, Cary NR, Metcalfe JC, et al. High expression of genes for calcification-regulating proteins in human atherosclerotic plaques. *J Clin Invest* 1994;N3:2393–2402.
92. Bostrom K, Watson KE, Stanford WP, et al. Atherosclerotic calcification: Relation to developmental osteogenesis. *Am J Cardiol* 1995;N5:88B–91B.
93. Watson KE, Bostrom K, Ravindranath R, et al. TGF-beta 1 and 25-hydroxycholesterol stimulate osteoblast-like vascular cells to calcify. *J Clin Invest* 1994;N3:2106–2113.
94. Nathan C. Secretory products of macrophages. *J Clin Invest* 1987;N9:319–326.
95. Morales DE, McGowan KA, Grant DS, et al. Estrogen promotes angiogenic activity in human umbilical vein endothelial cells in vitro and in a murine model. *Circulation* 1995;N1:755–763.
96. Wilcox JN, Smith KM, Schwartz SM, et al. Localization of tissue factor in the normal vessel wall and in the atherosclerotic plaque. *Proc Natl Acad Sci USA* 1989;N6:2839–2843.
97. Keeting PE, Scott RE, Colvard DS, et al. Lack of a direct effect of estrogen on proliferation and differentiation of normal human osteoblast-like cells. *J Bone Miner Res* 1991;N:297–304.
98. Santos GF, Scott GK, Lee WM, et al. Estrogen-induced post-transcriptional modulation of c-myc proto-oncogene expression in human breast cancer cells. *J Biol Chem* 1988;ℱ3:9565–9568.
99. Warri AM, Laine AM, Majasuo KE, et al. Estrogen suppression of erbB2 expression is associated with increased growth rate of ZR-75-1 human breast cancer cells in vitro and in nude mice. *Int J Cancer* 1991;N9:616–623.
100. Koga M, Sutherland RL. Retinoic acid acts synergistically with 1,25-dihydroxyvitamin D3 or antioestrogen to inhibit T-47D human breast cancer cell proliferation. *J Steroid Biochem Mol Biol* 1991;N9:455–460.

101. Mizukami Y, Tajiri K, Nonomura A, et al. Effects of tamoxifen, medroxyprogesterone acetate and estradiol on tumor growth and oncogene expression in MCF-7 breast cancer cell line transplanted into nude mice. *Anticancer Res* 1991;N1:1333–1338.
102. Bezwoda WR, Meyer K. Effect of alpha-interferon, 17 beta-estradiol, and tamoxifen on estrogen receptor concentration and cell cycle kinetics of MCF 7 cells. *Cancer Res* 1990;N0:5387–5391.
103. Weisz A, Cicatiello L, Persico E, et al. Estrogen stimulates transcription of c-jun protooncogene. *Mol Endocrinol* 1990;N:1041–1050.
104. Dati C, Antoniotti S, Taverna D, et al. Inhibition of c-erbB-2 oncogene expression by estrogens in human breast cancer cells. *Oncogene* 1990;N:1001–1006.
105. Johnson MD, Westley BR, May FE. Oestrogenic activity of tamoxifen and its metabolites on gene regulation and cell proliferation in MCF-7 breast cancer cells. *Br J Cancer* 1989;N9:727–738.
106. van der Burg B, Rutteman GR, Blankenstein MA, et al. Mitogenic stimulation of human breast cancer cells in a growth factor-defined medium: Synergistic action of insulin and estrogen. *J Cell Physiol* 1988; N34:101–108.
107. Kirkland JL, Murthy L, Stancel GM. Progesterone inhibits the estrogen-induced expression of c-fos messenger ribonucleic acid in the uterus. *Endocrinology* 1992;N30:3223–3230.
108. Weisz A, Bresciani F. Estrogen induces expression of c-fos and c-myc protooncogenes in rat uterus. *Mol Endocrinol* 1988;N:816–824.
109. De Sanford M, Wood GW. Interleukin-1, interleukin-6, and tumor necrosis factor alpha are produced in the mouse uterus during the estrous cycle and are induced by estrogen and progesterone. *Dev Biol* 1992;N51:297–305.
110. Suva LJ, Harm SC, Gardner RM, et al. In vivo regulation of Zif268 messenger RNA expression by 177 beta-estradiol in the rat uterus. *Mol Endocrinol* 1991;N:829–835.
111. Papa M, Mezzogiorno V, Bresciani F, et al. Estrogen induces c-fos expression specifically in the luminal and glandular epithelia of adult rat uterus. *Biochem Biophys Res Commun* 1991;N75:480–485.
112. Tabibzadeh SS, Santhanam U, Sehgal PB, et al. Cytokine-induced production of IFN-beta 2/IL-6 by freshly explanted human endometrial stromal cells. Modulation by estradiol-17 beta. *J Immunol* 1989;N42: 3134–3139.
113. Pavlik EJ, Nelson K, van Nagell JR Jr, et al. The growth response of BG-1 ovarian carcinoma cells to estradiol, 4OH-tamoxifen, and tamoxifen: Evidence for intrinsic antiestrogen activation. *Gynecol Oncol* 1991;N2:245-249.
114. Nash JD, Ozols RF, Smyth JF, et al. Estrogen and anti-estrogen effects on the growth of human epithelial ovarian cancer in vitro. *Obstet Gynecol* 1989;N3:1009–1016.
115. Nishizawa Y, Nishii K, Koga M, et al. Effects of estrogen on cell proliferation and leukotriene formation in transformed mouse Leydig cells cultured under serum-free conditions. *Cancer Res* 1990;N0: 3866–3871.
116. Nishizawa Y, Sato B, Miyashita Y, et al. Autocrine regulation of cell proliferation by estradiol and hydroxytamoxifen of transformed mouse Leydig cells in serum-free culture. *Endocrinology* 1988;N22:227–235.

117. Duncan WE, Glass AR, Wray HL. Estrogen regulation of the nuclear 1,25-dihydroxyvitamin D3 receptor in rat liver and kidney. *Endocrinology* 1991;N29:2318–2324.
118. Wahli W, Martinez E, Corthesy B, et al. Cis- and trans-acting elements of the estrogen-regulated vitellogenin gene B1 of Xenopus laevis. *J Steroid Biochem* 1989;N4:17–32.
119. Whitman MM, Harnish DC, Soprano KJ, et al. Retinol-binding protein mRNA is induced by estrogen in the kidney but not in the liver. *J Lipid Res* 1990;N1:1483–1490.
120. Oberley TD, Lauchner LJ, Pugh TD, et al. Specific estrogen-induced cell proliferation of cultured Syrian hamster renal proximal tubular cells in serum-free chemically defined media. *Proc Natl Acad Sci USA* 1989;N6:2107–2110.
121. Soto AM, Bass JC, Sonnenschein C. Estrogen-sensitive proliferation pattern of cloned Syrian hamster kidney tumor cells. *Cancer Res* 1988;N8:3676–3680.
122. Rhode PR, Gorski J. Growth and cell cycle regulation of mRNA levels in GH3 cells. *Mol Cell Endocrinol* 1991;N2:11–22.
123. Jin L, Song JY, Lloyd RV. Estrogen stimulates both prolactin and growth hormone mRNAs expression inn the MtT/F4 transplantable pituitary tumor. *Proc Soc Exp Biol Med* 1989;N92:225–229.
124. Rasmussen JE, Torres-Aleman I, MacLusky NJ, et al. The effects of estradiol on the growth patterns of estrogen receptor-positive hypothalamic cell lines. *Endocrinology* 1990;N26:235-240.
125. Tremollieres, FA, Strong, DD, Baylink, DJ, et al. Insulin-like growth factor II and transforming growth factor beta 11 regulate insulin-like growth factor I secretion in mouse bone cells. *Acta Endocrinol* 1991; N25:538–546.
126. Ernst M, Heath JK, Rodan GA. Estradiol effects on proliferation, messenger ribonucleic acid for collagen and insulin-like growth factor-I, and parathyroid hormone-stimulated adenylate cyclase activity in osteoblastic cells from calvariae and long bones. *Endocrinology* 1989; N25:825–833.
127. Maminta ML, Molteni A, Rosen ST. Stable expression of the human estrogen receptor in HeLa cells by infection: Effect of estrogen on cell proliferation and c-myc expression. *Mol Cell Endocrinol* 1991; N8:61–69.
128. Gaben AM, Mester J. BALB/C mouse 3T3 fibroblasts expressing human estrogen receptor: Effect of estradiol on cell growth. *Biochem Biophys Res Commun* 1991;N76:1473–1481.
129. Ueo H, Matsuoka H, Sugimachi K, et al. Inhibitory effects of estrogen on the growth of a human esophageal carcinoma cell line. *Cancer Res* 1990;N0:7212–7215.

Chapter 2

Estrogen and Heart Disease
Lessons to be Learned from Nonhuman Primates

*Thomas B. Clarkson, DVM
and Mary S. Anthony, MS*

Until relatively recently, animal models had not been used widely to understand gender differences in coronary artery atherosclerosis or pathophysiological influences on progression of the process among females. This lack of comparative research resulted primarily from the lack of a suitable animal model. The complexities of coronary artery atherogenesis in females requires a model with many risk-factor and physiological similarities to women.

Cynomolgus macaque females have been shown to be excellent animal models for research on coronary heart disease for both pre- and postmenopausal women. Some of the characteristics of the model as they relate to human beings are summarized in Figure 1[1]. Like women, premenopausal monkeys have higher plasma concentrations of high-density lipoprotein cholesterol (HDL-C) than do surgically postmenopausal females. The monkey models, again like women, have relative protection from coronary artery atherogenesis premenopausally and experience loss of that protection and more rapidly progressing coronary artery atherogenesis postmenopausally.[2] However, hormone replacement therapy after ovariectomy reduces coronary artery atherosclerosis progression relative to untreated controls in our monkey model[1] and in women.[3]

The cynomolgus female model also shares with women important postmenopausal clinical disorders such as osteopenia[4,5] and retrogressive changes in the genitourinary system[6]. Although the stud-

This work was supported in part by Grant P01 HL-45666 from the National Heart, Lung, and Blood Institute.

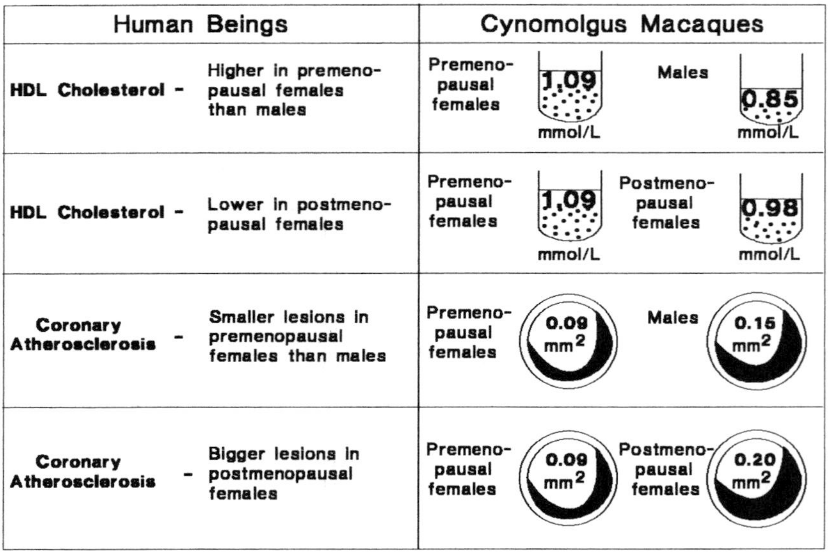

Human Beings		Cynomolgus Macaques	
HDL Cholesterol -	Higher in premeno-pausal females than males	Premeno-pausal females **1.09** mmol/L	Males **0.85** mmol/L
HDL Cholesterol -	Lower in postmeno-pausal females	Premeno-pausal females **1.09** mmol/L	Postmeno-pausal females **0.98** mmol/L
Coronary Atherosclerosis -	Smaller lesions in premenopausal females than males	Premeno-pausal females 0.09 mm²	Males 0.15 mm²
Coronary Atherosclerosis -	Bigger lesions in postmenopausal females	Premeno-pausal females 0.09 mm²	Postmeno-pausal females 0.20 mm²

FIGURE 1. *Cardiovascular parameters in human beings versus the macaque model. Reproduced with permission from Reference 1.*

ies are underway, it is unclear at this time whether cognitive function of estrogen-deficient monkeys may be improved with hormone replacement therapy, an area of intense interest for women's health.

Most of the data presented herein are derived from experiments using this model during the past two decades. We have summarized what we believe to be the clinical implications of this research by questions and answers that highlight the observations and potential mechanisms elucidated by this monkey model.

Premenopausal Considerations

Does Progression of Coronary Artery Plaque Premenopausally Determine the Likelihood of Coronary Heart Disease Events Postmenopausally?

Considerable variability exists in the rates and degree of progression of premenopausal coronary artery atherosclerosis. We have focused our efforts on understanding processes that influence premenopausal atherosclerosis, based on the premise that the extent of coronary artery atherosclerosis at the onset of menopause will be a major determinant of the progression associated with estrogen deficiency and finally with the occurrence or lack of occurrence of clinical events. In Figure 2, we have illustrated this premise[7].

It seems useful to think of the extent of coronary artery atherosclerosis at the time of the onset of menopause and its subsequent influence on coronary heart disease in much the same way as peak bone mass is viewed as a prognostic indicator of subsequent postmenopausal osteoporosis and risk of fractures. We currently have no data from monkey studies that bear directly on this point, but such studies are underway, and their results should be available in a few years.

What are Some of the Principal Determinants of Premenopausal Coronary Artery Atherosclerosis Progression?

Premenopausal Dyslipoproteinemia: Effect on Risk Factors and Progression of Coronary Artery Atherosclerosis

There is remarkable agreement between the human and nonhuman primate studies relative to the role of low-plasma HDLC concentrations on the extent of coronary artery atherosclerosis and coronary heart disease. In Figure 3, we have depicted the association between plasma HDL-C concentrations and coronary heart disease mortality for women in the Framingham study (Figure 3A)[8] and between HDL-C concentrations and atherosclerotic plaque extent in our monkey model (Figure 3B).

This association of low-plasma HDL-C concentrations and coronary artery atherosclerosis relates to innate concentrations, and we lack definitive data among either women or monkeys that pharmacologically induced increases or decreases have the same relationships. We will discuss later in this chapter the interesting phenomenon whereby HDL-C concentrations can be lowered by an oral contraceptive, but atherosclerosis not worsened, presumably by protective effects of the estradiol component at the level of the artery wall. Interestingly, oral contraceptive treatment also showed an association between HDL-C concentrations and coronary artery atherogenesis, except that lower plasma HDL-C concentrations (relative

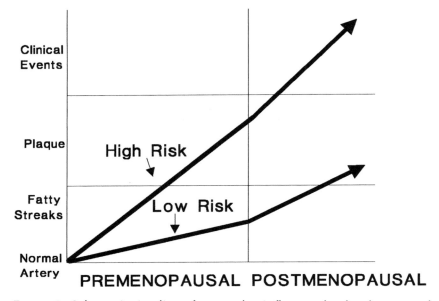

FIGURE 2. *Schematic timeline of events that influence the development of coronary artery atherosclerosis in the premenopausal and postmenopausal periods. Reduced risk factor burden in the premenopausal period may slow the progression of clinically relevant disease, whereas estrogen replacement therapy (ERT) prevents the sharp increase in coronary heart disease risk that occurs postmenopausally. Reproduced with permission from Reference 7.*

to the control group) was associated with a similar or somewhat lower extent of coronary artery atherosclerosis.

Psychosocial Factors and Incidence of Premenopausal CHD Events

Psychosocial Stress

We have used our monkey model to explore premenopausal situations that might result in pathophysiologically significant estrogen deficiency. The most pronounced finding has been that chronic stress (described below) in some of these monkeys results in ovarian dysfunction, estrogen deficiency, exacerbated coronary artery atherosclerosis, and abnormalities in coronary artery vasomotion.

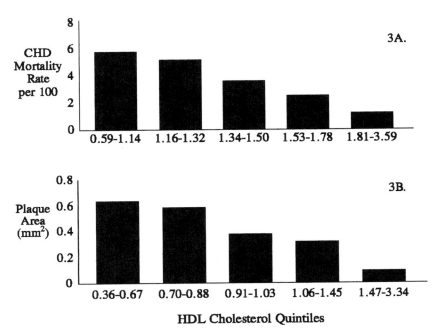

FIGURE 3. A: *Association between coronary heart disease (CHD) mortality rate and quintiles of high-density lipoprotein (HDL) cholesterol concentrations (mmol/L) in women from Framingham. Adapted with permission from Reference 8.* **B:** *Association between coronary artery intimal area and HDL-C quintiles (mmol/L) in a study of premenopausal female cynomolgus monkeys.*

Cynomolgus monkeys arrange themselves in stable social hierarchies; for example, when the monkeys are arranged in four-monkey subsets, animals rank one, two, three, or four, respectively. Low-ranked monkeys (three or four in the dominance hierarchy of a four-monkey group) are stressed chronically because they are frequent subjects of aggression, they spend considerable amounts of time alone, and a large proportion of their time is spent in vigilant behavior. This chronic stress results in larger adrenal glands, higher plasma cortisol concentrations, ovarian dysfunction with markedly reduced estradiol production, reduced plasma HDL-C concentrations, and exacerbated coronary artery atherosclerosis (Figure 4).[1,9]

More recently, Williams et al.[10] evaluated coronary artery reactivity in premenopausal monkeys and compared results for those that ranked three or four (stressed) with those that ranked one or two (not stressed). In the stressed monkeys, coronary arteries con-

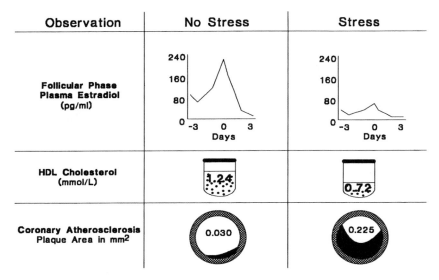

FIGURE 4. *Risk factors for coronary heart disease are more deleterious in premenopausal cynomolgus monkeys subjected to chronic stress (see text for definition) compared with unstressed animals. Stressed animals have lower follicular-phase plasma estradiol concentrations (and hence more anovulatory menstrual cycles), lower plasma concentrations of HDL-C, and more coronary artery atherosclerotic plaque. Reproduced with permission from Reference 7.*

stricted when infused with acetylcholine ($-11\% \pm 3\%$, mean $\pm$ SE), whereas the nonstressed monkeys (one and two) had normal vasomotion and demonstrated coronary artery dilation in response to acetylcholine ($+3\% \pm 2\%$). There were enough monkeys in that study to relate plasma estradiol concentrations to either normal or abnormal coronary artery vasomotion. There appears to be a threshold effect; eg, animals with plasma concentrations of estradiol >80 pg/mL (>293 pmol/L) show normal vasomotion, whereas impaired vasomotion is seen in animals with plasma concentrations less than that amount.

Social Isolation

There is a consistent pattern of increased coronary heart disease mortality associated with decreases in social support (ie, contacts with friends and relatives).[11-13] In previous experiments, we have investigated whether the social isolation induced by single-cage housing might be associated with increased coronary artery athero-sclerosis extent in our monkey model. The premenopausal monkeys were either maintained in social groups with other premenopausal females or were caged individually (social isolation).

There were no differences in plasma lipid or lipoprotein con-centrations between the two groups; however, the female monkeys housed in single cages had significantly more coronary artery ath-erosclerosis than the socially housed animals (mean plaque area: social isolation, 0.13 mm^2; social housing, 0.02 mm^2).[14] The mech-anisms of coronary artery atherosclerosis exacerbation among single-caged females remain uncertain. Apparently it is unrelated to impaired ovarian function, because these females had normal ovar-ian cycles. However, in another study, premenopausal female mon-keys had higher heart rates when they were housed in single cages than when they were housed in stable social groupings (C. Shively, personal communication). Such elevated heart rates are known to potentiate atherogenesis.[15]

Central Obesity and Associated Metabolic Abnormalities in Premenopausal CHD Events

There is considerable interest currently in the association be-tween an android or male-pattern distribution of adipose tissue in women and symptomatic cardiovascular disease. In a study at our institution,[16] central adiposity, as assessed by waist:hip ratios, was significantly related to coronary artery atherosclerosis of women as determined by quantitative angiography. That observation seemed to provide a better understanding of the excess cardiovascular mor-tality among women with central obesity, as observed in several pro-spective studies.[17–19] To better understand this phenomenon, it seemed important to us to characterize a monkey model of the dis-order. We found that female monkeys with a relatively high ratio of central to peripheral fat deposition had about three times more ex-tensive coronary artery atherosclerosis (mean plaque area: high-central adiposity, 0.65 mm^2; low-central adiposity, 0.22 mm^2).[20]

Our monkey model seems to share with women certain associ-ated metabolic differences between centrally obese and lean mon-keys, ie, hyperglycemia, insulin resistance, and low-plasma HDL-C concentrations. The cynomolgus monkey model offers an excellent opportunity for a better understanding of both the associated dis-orders themselves and the evaluation of potential interventions.

What are the Benefits of Premenopausal Exogenous Estrogen Administration to Subsets at High Risk for Coronary Artery Atherosclerosis Premenopausally?

Our research has suggested that estrogen-containing contraceptive steroids have clear cardiovascular benefits for at least two subsets of female monkeys at high risk for development of extensive coronary artery atherosclerosis. The two high-risk subsets we have studied involve monkeys with dyslipoproteinemia [elevated total plasma cholesterol (TPC) concentrations and lower HDLC concentrations] and low-ranking monkeys with chronic stress. The results of both those studies will be summarized below.

Dyslipoproteinemia

We have reported a study in which surgically postmenopausal monkeys fed a moderately atherogenic diet were randomly assigned into a control group and into two groups to be treated with either of two oral contraceptives.[21] Both of the oral contraceptives contained ethinyl estradiol; one (Ovral, Wyeth-Ayerst, Princeton, NJ) contained norgestrel as the progestin, whereas the other (Demulen, Searle and Co., San Juan, PR) contained ethynodiol diacetate as the progestin. The dose of the contraceptive steroids was determined on a caloric basis to approximate that usually prescribed for human females. Monkeys with a TPC/HDL-C ratio >4.5 before treatment were considered the high-risk group. Both contraceptive steroids resulted in a dyslipoproteinemia, characterized by marked lowering of plasma HDL-C concentrations and moderate increases in plasma low-density lipoprotein (LDL) concentrations. Despite lowering of the HDL-C concentrations and of the subfractions HDL 2a and HDL 2b, there was no exacerbation of coronary artery atherosclerosis in the groups as a whole. But, of more importance, among the group at high risk based on their pretreatment atherogenic lipoprotein profile, there was a significant reduction in coronary artery atherosclerosis extent with oral contraceptive treatment. The results of the study are summarized in Figure 5.[21]

We have interpreted this protective effect of the ethinyl estradiol as occurring directly at the coronary artery wall independent of the adverse changes that occurred in the plasma lipoprotein profile. Subsequent to that study, we have reported two different studies that may provide mechanistic explanations for direct effects of estrogen at the level of the artery wall. In one, our group showed that the

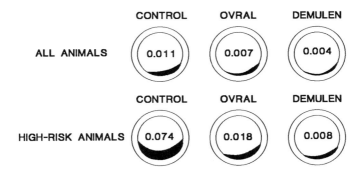

FIGURE 5. *Coronary artery plaque area (mm²) in the three experimental groups described in text. High-risk animals were defined as those with a pretreatment total plasma: HDL-C ratio >4.5. Reproduced with permission from Reference 21.*

ethinyl estradiol/norgestrel compound diminished the coronary artery accumulation of LDL particles among premenopausal monkeys fed a moderately atherogenic diet.[22] In the other, we demonstrated that intravenously administered ethinyl estradiol corrected the paradoxical vasoconstriction after perfusion with acetylcholine that occurs in the coronary arteries of estrogen-deficient monkeys.[23]

Chronic Stress

Our recent research has been based on the premise that premenopausal estrogen deficiency will exacerbate the progression of coronary artery atherosclerosis so that clinically evident coronary heart disease is more likely to occur in the postmenopausal period. This is in contrast to what is observed in postmenopausal subjects with normal premenopausal estrogen production. It also was our hypothesis that if stressed female monkeys (or, by inference, stressed women) were given exogenous estrogen in the form of an oral contraceptive during the premenopausal period, coronary atherogenesis would proceed at a reduced rate, and the subjects would be less likely to have subsequent coronary events whether or not they were treated with estrogen replacement therapy postmenopausally. In contrast, among those with no exogenous estrogen treatment premenopausally, coronary atherogenesis would proceed to plaque formation by the perimenopausal/postmenopausal period and some number of clinical events, regardless of whether postmenopausal estrogen replacement therapy was administered (see Figure 2).

We began to test this hypothesis ~5 years ago using cyno-molgus macaque females as models.[24] In that randomized trial, we used 213 premenopausal monkeys fed a moderately athero-genic diet and randomized into two groups, one that received no hormonal treatment and one that received Triphasil (Wyeth-Ayerst, Philadelphia, PA). The treatment period was for 26 months.

The pills were ground finely and administered in the diet on a 28-day cycle. On days 1–6, the pills contained 0.03 mg/day ethinyl estradiol and 0.05 mg/day levonorgestrel; on days 7–11, they con-tained 0.04 mg/day ethinyl estradiol and 0.075 mg/day levonorges-trel; on days 12–21, they contained 0.03 mg/day ethinyl estradiol and 0.125 mg/day levonorgestrel; and on days 22–28, an inert placebo was mixed into the diet. The oral contraceptive was included in the diet on a caloric basis (per 1,800 calories/day) to be equivalent to a woman's dosage. Note that female cynomolgus monkeys have a ca-loric intake nearly 1/5 that of women despite weighing only 1/20 as much as women.

The female monkeys were kept in social groups of four to five monkeys, and the social hierarchy for all groups was determined weekly. Social status was stable during the study, with a correlation between ranks measured in consecutive months being >0.90. The aggregated rankings were used in all analyses, with animals above the median considered not stressed and animals below the median considered to be stressed.

Plasma lipid concentrations were measured nine times during the experiment. As we have reported previously,[25] oral contraceptive treatment resulted in large decreases in plasma HDL-C concentra-tions, and the effect was more striking among stressed than non-stressed monkeys.

Because we are continuing to evaluate the effects of premeno-pausal atherosclerosis extent of postmenopausal coronary artery atherosclerosis progression, we did not necropsy the animals to eval-uate their coronary arteries. Instead, we did a biopsy of the common iliac artery and evaluated its atherosclerosis extent as a surrogate for the coronary arteries. The average correlation between iliac ar-tery atherosclerosis and coronary artery atherosclerosis in previous studies was 0.71. Also, we found similar treatment effects on coro-nary and iliac arteries in previous studies of oral contraceptive treat-ment of cynomolgus macaque females fed a moderately atherogenic diet.[21] From these studies, we calculated the extent of expected cor-onary artery atherosclerosis reductions in premenopausal monkeys with no treatment versus those treated with ethinyl estradiol plus norgestrel, based on examination of either the left or the right iliac artery. We predicted reductions of ~35% based on the iliac artery atherosclerosis extent; indeed, we observed a reduction of 37% in the coronary arteries.

We have summarized some of the most important observations from this study in Figure 6.[24] Treatment with the oral contraceptive had no effect on plaque size when all of the animals were considered. Of more importance, however, is a consideration of the control and oral contraceptive-treated animals in a high-risk category due to chronic stress. We have defined here the high-risk category as subordinate animals (divided at the median for group size). Among monkeys at high risk for exacerbated atherosclerosis due to chronic stress, those treated with the oral contraceptive had less iliac artery atherosclerosis than untreated animals.

The relevance of our studies on premenopausal estrogen deficiency in monkeys to the pathogenesis of coronary artery atherosclerosis of women is becoming more clear. Given the convincing evidence that normal ovarian function and the ovarian production of follicular-phase estradiol inhibit coronary artery atherogenesis, one must assume that sustained or extreme interruptions of normal ovarian function increases a woman's risk for entering the perimenopause and menopause with more advanced atherosclerosis. As a result, such a woman would be more prone to the clinical sequelae of atherosclerosis in the early postmenopausal years. The magnitude of the clinical problem is considerable, as interruptions of normal ovarian function may occur in up to 29% of women <40 years old.[26-31] In fact, up to 20% of women reporting normal menses actually exhibit abnormal hormone profiles[32].

Postmenopausal Considerations

Does the Decreased Morbidity and Mortality From Coronary Heart Disease Among Postmenopausal Women Taking Hormone Replacement Therapy Result From the Decreased Extensiveness of Coronary Artery Atherosclerosis?

Many observational studies have found an association between hormone replacement therapy and reduced occurrence of coronary heart disease morbidity and mortality among postmenopausal women (see Stampfer and Colditz[33] for a meta-analysis of those observations). Despite these seemingly convincing findings, whether postmenopausal replacement of ovarian hormones is responsible or

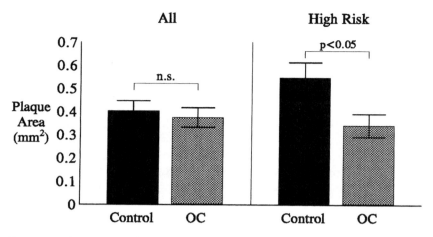

FIGURE 6. *Iliac artery plaque size in untreated premenopausal cynomolgus monkeys versus animals given a triphasic oral contraceptive, depicted as a function of level of chronic stress due to social subordination (see text for description). Adapted with permission from Reference 24.*

whether the results stem in part from patient selection bias remains a controversy. A number of authors have pointed out that post-menopausal women taking hormone replacement therapy are leaner, exercise more, are better educated, have higher incomes, and have better access to medical care,[34–39], all of which might be factors in reduced risk of coronary heart disease.

Cause and effect cannot be established on the basis of observational epidemiological studies alone. The strength of the clinical interpretation of epidemiological associations, however, can be increased by demonstrating effects in controlled trials with suitable animal models and elucidating the biological mechanisms by which the treatments have their effect. These insights can lead to properly designed prospective randomized trials with human participants. We shall discuss each of these points separately as they relate to the association between postmenopausal ovarian hormone treatment and reductions of coronary heart disease mortality.

We have reported the results of a study in which surgically post-menopausal cynomolgus monkeys fed an atherogenic diet received treatment via Silastic implants of estradiol (continuous) or with estradiol (continuous) plus progesterone (cyclically).[40] The hormonal treatments had minimal effects on plasma lipid and lipoprotein concentrations. However, coronary artery atherosclerosis extent was halved by treatment (mean plaque area: controls, 0.227 mm²; estradiol only, 0.101 mm²; estradiol plus progesterone, 0.099 mm²). Interestingly, most investigators believe that postmenopausal women taking estrogen replacement therapy have a 50% decrease in coronary heart disease mortality.

What are the Probable Mechanisms of the Beneficial Effects of Hormone Replacement Therapy on Coronary Heart Disease?

In our studies with ovarian hormone replacement, we sought to determine the proportion of the beneficial effect on atherogenesis that could be ascribed to plasma lipoprotein concentrations and the proportion that was unknown and presumably associated, at least in part, with changes at the coronary artery wall. Our estimate of the allocation of beneficial effect on atherogenesis is schematically illustrated in Figure 7.

To better define the mechanisms by which ovarian hormone replacement reduces atherogenesis beyond altering lipoprotein concentrations, we have measured rates of LDL accumulation within coronary arteries during the early stages of atherogenesis in our monkey model.[41] Use of LDL particles labeled with either

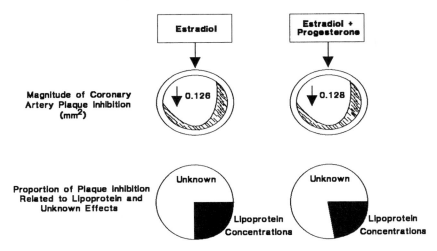

FIGURE 7. *Mechanisms affecting coronary artery atherosclerosis plaque inhibition in surgically postmenopausal cynomolgus monkeys treated with estradiol-17β alone or estradiol-17β plus progesterone. Adapted with permission from Reference 40.*

of two isotopes has enabled us to measure coronary artery LDL metabolism (accumulation and degradation of LDL particles within the walls of coronary arteries). Coronary artery LDL uptake in surgically postmenopausal monkeys was increased five- to sixfold over that in premenopausal females with normal menstrual cycles.[22,41,42] We also noted that the replacement of estradiol plus progesterone restored the postmenopausal animals to premenopausal levels of LDL accumulation. We believe the effect of estradiol on coronary artery LDL metabolism is one of the major mechanisms by which coronary artery atherosclerosis is affected beneficially by estrogen treatment.

Endothelium-dependent vasoconstriction of coronary arteries may promote atherogenesis, especially in association with the adverse effects of nitric oxide depletion on coronary artery cell metabolism. Coronary arteries of estrogen-deficient atherosclerotic monkeys show a paradoxical constriction when infused with acetylcholine; this reaction is changed to vasodilation when estrogen concentrations are adequate in premenopausal[10] or estrogen replacement is given to surgically postmenopausal animals.[43,44] This beneficial effect is prompt, occurring within 20 minutes after the intravenous treatment of monkeys with estrogen[23] and equally prompt after the sublingual treatment of women with estrogen.[45] The potential atherogenic effects of repeated artery constriction may be considerable and nitric oxide depletion may magnify the effect.

Do the Effects of Hormone Replacement Therapy on Atherosclerosis Differ at Different Stages in the Natural History of Plaque Progression and Complication?

We recently have reported results of a large trial with surgically postmenopausal monkeys in which we addressed the question of whether estrogen alone or estrogen plus medroxyprogesterone acetate added to the benefits of diet-induced plasma lipid lowering in affecting coronary artery plaque sizes and arterial remodeling. Estrogen treatment did not induce any regression in the size of the plaques, indicating to us that effects of estrogen on atherogenesis is primarily during periods of plaque progression, with minimal effects on regression of established lesions.[46] When hormone replacement began simultaneous with surgical menopause, plaque size was reduced by half. On the other hand, when hormone replacement (in combination with a low-fat, low-cholesterol diet) began after 2 or more years of diet-induced atherosclerosis induction, no significant regression of atherosclerotic plaques occurred.[46]

Because of the clear benefit of hormone replacement therapy to women with established coronary heart disease, it seems likely that estrogen's beneficial effects on established plaques concern plaque stability and not plaque size.

What is the Likely Future of Postmenopausal Estrogen Replacement Therapy?

The ideal postmenopausal estrogen replacement would be a hormone that is an estrogen agonist for bone, brain, coronary arteries, and the genitourinary system, while at the same time being an estrogen antagonist for breast and the endometrium. It is difficult to predict the likelihood that such a treatment will be available in the near term, although ongoing research with tamoxifen-like drugs[47-49] and with the phytoestrogens from soybeans appears promising.[50]

References

1. Clarkson TB. Estrogens, progestins, and coronary heart disease in cynomolgus monkeys. *Fertil Steril* 1994;62(suppl 2):147S–151S.
2. Adams MR, Kaplan JR, Clarkson TB, et al. Ovariectomy, social status, and atherosclerosis in cynomolgus monkeys. *Arteriosclerosis* 1985;5: 192–200.
3. Sullivan JM, Vander Zwaag R, Lemp GF, et al. Postmenopausal estrogen use and coronary atherosclerosis. *Ann Intern Med* 1988;108:358–363.
4. Jerome CP, Carlson CS, Register TC, et al. Bone functional changes in intact, ovariectomized, and ovariectomized, hormone-supplemented adult cynomolgus monkeys (*Macaca fascicularis*) evaluated by serum markers and dynamic histomorphometry. *J Bone Miner Res* 1994;9: 527–540.
5. Jayo MJ, Jerome CP, Lees CJ, et al. Bone mass in cynomolgus macaques: A cross-sectional and longitudinal study by age. *Calcif Tissue Int* 1994; 54:231–236.
6. Robinson D, Washburn SA, Shively CA. Effect of hypothalamic amenorrhea on urethral epithelium thickness of the cynomolgus macaque monkey: A pilot study. Abstract. *Int Urogynecol J* 1993;4:390.
7. Clarkson TB, Kaplan JR, Shively CA, et al. Benefits of exogenous estrogen in inhibiting stress-related coronary artery atherosclerosis. *Br J Obstet Gynaecol* 1996;103(suppl 13):73–79.
8. Wilson PWF, Abbott RD, Castelli WP. High density lipoprotein cholesterol and mortality: The Framingham Heart Study. *Arteriosclerosis* 1988; 8:737–741.

9. Clarkson TB, Adams MR, Williams JK, et al. Clinical implications of animal models of gender difference in heart disease. In: Douglas PS, ed: *Cardiovascular Health and Disease in Women* Philadelphia: W.B. Saunders; 1993:283–302.

10. Williams JK, Shively CA, Clarkson TB. Determinants of coronary artery reactivity in premenopausal female cynomolgus monkeys with diet-induced atherosclerosis. *Circulation* 1994;90:983–987.

11. Berkman L, Breslow L. *Health and Ways of Living: Findings from the Alameda County Study* New York: Oxford University Press; 1983.

12. Berkman L, Syme SL. Social networks, host resistance, and mortality: A 9-year follow-up study of Alameda County residents. *Am J Epidemiol* 1979;109:186–204.

13. Manuck SB, Kaplan JR, Matthews KA. Behavioral antecedents of coronary heart disease and atherosclerosis. *Arteriosclerosis* 1986;6:2–14.

14. Shively CA, Clarkson TB, Kaplan JR. Social deprivation and coronary artery atherosclerosis in female cynomolgus monkeys. *Atherosclerosis* 1989;77:69–76.

15. Kaplan JR, Manuck SB, Clarkson TB. The influence of heart rate on coronary artery atherosclerosis. *J Cardiovasc Pharmacol* 1987;10(suppl 2):S100–S103.

16. Thompson CJ, Ryu JE, Craven TE, et al. Central adipose distribution is related to coronary atherosclerosis. *Arterioscler Thromb* 1991;11: 327–333.

17. Lapidus L, Bengtsson C, Larsson B, et al. Distribution of adipose tissue and risk of cardiovascular disease and death: A 12-year follow-up of participants in the population study of women in Gothenburg, Sweden. *Br Med J* 1984;288:1401–1404.

18. Stokes J III, Garrison RJ, Kannel WB. The independent contributions of various indices of obesity to the 22-year incidence of coronary heart disease. The Framingham Study. In: Vague J, Björntorp P, Guy-Grand B, et al., eds: *Metabolic Complications of Human Obesities* Amsterdam: Elsevier Science; 1985:49–57.

19. Despres J-P, Moorjani S, Lupien PJ, et al. Regional distribution of body fat, plasma lipoproteins, and cardiovascular disease. *Arteriosclerosis* 1990;10:497–511.

20. Shively CA, Clarkson TB. Regional obesity and coronary artery atherosclerosis in females: A nonhuman primate model. *Acta Med Scand* 1988;723(suppl):71–78.

21. Clarkson TB, Shively CA, Morgan TM, et al. Oral contraceptives and coronary artery atherosclerosis of cynomolgus macaques. *Obstet Gynecol* 1990;75:217–222.

22. Wagner JD, Adams MR, Schwenke DC, et al. Oral contraceptive treatment decreases arterial low density lipoprotein degradation in female cynomolgus monkeys. *Circ Res* 1993;72:1300–1307.

23. Williams JK, Adams MR, Herrington DM, et al. Effects of short-term estrogen treatment on vascular responses of coronary arteries. *J Am Coll Cardiol* 1992;20:452–457.

24. Kaplan JR, Adams MR, Anthony MS, et al. Dominant social status and contraceptive hormone treatment inhibit atherogenesis in premenopausal monkeys. *Arterioscler Thromb Vasc Biol* 1995;15:2094–2100.

25. Parks JS, Pelkey SJ, Babiak J, et al. Contraceptive steroid effects on lipids and lipoproteins in cynomolgus monkeys. *Arteriosclerosis* 1989; 9:261–268.

26. Kinch RAH, Plunkett ER, Smout MS, et al. Primary ovarian failure. A clinicopathological and cytogenetic study. *Am J Obstet Gynecol* 1965; 91:630–644.
27. Russell P, Bannatyne P, Shearman RP, et al. Premature hypergonadotropic ovarian failure. Clinicopathological study of 19 cases. *Int J Gynecol Pathol* 1982;1:185–201.
28. Starup J, Sele V. Premature ovarian failure. *Acta Obstet Gynecol Scand* 1973;52:259–268.
29. Aiman J, Smentek C. Premature ovarian failure. *Obstet Gynecol* 1965; 66:9–14.
30. Prior JC, Vigna YM, Schechter MT, et al. Spinal bone loss and ovulatory disturbances. *N Engl J Med* 1990;323:1221–1227.
31. Wu CH. Ovulatory disorders and infertility in women with regular menstrual cycles. *Curr Opin Obstet Gynecol* 1990;2:398–404.
32. Berga SL, Loucks AB, Rossmanith WG, et al. Acceleration of luteinizing hormone pulse frequency in functional hypothalamic amenorrhea by dopaminergic blockade. *J Clin Endocrinol Metab* 1991;72:151–156.
33. Stampfer MJ, Colditz GA. Estrogen replacement therapy and coronary heart disease: A quantitative assessment of the epidemiologic evidence. *Prevent Med* 1991;20:47–63.
34. Derby CA, Hume AL, Barbour MM, et al. Correlates of postmenopausal estrogen use and trends through the 1980s in two southeastern New England communities. *Am J Epidemiol* 1993;137:1125–1135.
35. Stampfer MJ, Colditz GA, Willett WC, et al. Postmenopausal estrogen therapy and cardiovascular disease. Ten-year follow-up from the Nurses' Health Study. *N Engl J Med* 1991;325:756–762.
36. Criqui MH, Suarez L, Barrett-Connor E, et al. Postmenopausal estrogen use and mortality. Results from a prospective study in a defined, homogeneous community. *Am J Epidemiol* 1988;128:606–614.
37. Barrett-Connor E, Wingard DL, Criqui MH. Postmenopausal estrogen use and heart disease risk factors in the 1980s: Rancho Bernardo, Calif, revisited. *JAMA* 1989;261:2095–2100.
38. Rosenberg L, Shapiro S, Kaufman DW, et al. Patterns and determinants of conjugated estrogen use. *Am J Epidemiol* 1979;109:676–686.
39. Ravnikar VA, Compliance with hormone therapy. *Am J Obstet Gynecol* 1987;156:1332–1334.
40. Adams MR, Kaplan JR, Manuck SB, et al. Inhibition of coronary artery atherosclerosis by 17-beta estradiol in ovariectomized monkeys: Lack of effect of added progesterone. *Arteriosclerosis* 1990;10:1051–1057.
41. Wagner JD, Clarkson TB, St. Clair RW, et al. Estrogen and progesterone replacement therapy reduces low density lipoprotein accumulation in the coronary arteries of surgically postmenopausal cynomolgus monkeys. *J Clin Invest* 1991;88:1995–2002.
42. Wagner JD, St. Clair RW, Schwenke DC, et al. Regional differences in arterial low density lipoprotein metabolism in surgically postmenopausal cynomolgus monkeys: Effects of estrogen and progesterone replacement therapy. *Arterioscler Thromb* 1992;12:717–726.
43. Williams JK, Adams MR, Klopfenstein HS. Estrogen modulates responses of atherosclerotic coronary arteries. *Circulation* 1990;81: 1680–1687.
44. Williams JK, Honoré EK, Washburn SA, et al. Effects of hormonal replacement therapy on reactivity of atherosclerotic coronary arteries in cynomolgus monkeys *J. Am Coll Cardiol* 1994;27:1757–1761.

45. Rosano GMC, Sarrel PM, Poole-Wilson PA, et al. Oestrogen improves exercise-induced myocardial ischaemia in female patients with coronary artery disease. *Lancet* 1993;342:133–136.
46. Williams JK, Anthony MS, Honoré EK, et al. Regression of atherosclerosis in female monkeys. *Arterioscler Thromb Vasc Biol* 1995;15:827–836.
47. Tanaka Y, Sekiguchi M, Sawamoto T, et al. Pharmacokinetics of droloxifene in mice, rats, monkeys, premenopausal and postmenopausal patients. *Eur J Drug Metab Pharmacokin* 1994;19:47–58.
48. Black LJ, Sato M, Rowley ER, et al. Raloxifene (LY139481 HCl) prevents bone loss and reduces serum cholesterol without causing uterine hypertrophy in ovariectomized rats. *J Clin Invest* 1994;93:63–69.
49. Love RR, Mazess RB, Barden HS, et al. Effects of tamoxifen on bone mineral density in postmenopausal women with breast cancer. *N Engl J Med* 1992;326:852–856.
50. Anthony MS, Clarkson TB, Hughes CL Jr., et al. Soybean isoflavones improve cardiovascular risk factors without affecting the reproductive system of peripubertal rhesus monkeys. *J Nutr* 1996;126:43–50.

Chapter 3

Effects of Estrogens and Progestins on the Pathogenesis of Atherosclerosis in Nonhuman Primates

Michael R. Adams, DVM,
Thomas C. Register, PhD,
Janice D. Wagner, DVM, PhD,
and J. Koudy Williams, DVM

In human populations where coronary heart disease is a major public health problem, its incidence is much lower in premenopausal women than in men of similar age. This sex difference in coronary heart disease risk is paralleled by a difference in extent and severity of coronary artery atherosclerosis.[1] It is widely believed that ovarian estrogen is responsible for this relative sparing of the coronary arteries in women. This belief is supported by compelling evidence that estrogen replacement therapy is associated with a marked reduction in angiographically defined extent of coronary artery atherosclerosis[2] and risk of coronary heart disease in postmenopausal women.[3] The mechanisms by which this effect is mediated are poorly understood. Among multiple possibilities are inhibitory effects on atherosclerosis progression, inhibitory effects on coronary thrombosis, and beneficial effects on vasomotor function of coronary arteries. Also unclear are effects of combination hormone replacement therapies, ie, estrogen plus progestin, on atherosclerosis and coronary risk.

We summarize here the experimental evidence regarding effects of sex hormone deficiency and hormone replacement therapy on the

Supported in part by Grants P01 HL-45666 and R01 HL-38964 from the National Heart, Lung, and Blood Institute.

From: Forte TM, (ed). *Hormonal, Metabolic, and Cellular Influences on Cardiovascular Disease in Women.* Armonk, NY: Futura Publishing Company, Inc.; © 1997.

initiation and progression of atherosclerosis in monkeys and mechanisms by which sex hormones influence the pathogenesis of atherosclerosis.

Animal Model Studies

Effects of Estrogen on Coronary Artery Atherosclerosis

Overview

This discussion emphasizes coronary arteries because the gender difference in atherosclerosis extent is confined to coronary arteries,[1] experimental evidence indicates that effects of sex hormones are confined to coronary arteries and, perhaps, femoral arteries,[1,4,5] and effects on coronary arteries are of greatest relevance to coronary heart disease, the major clinical sequela of atherosclerosis in human beings. Effects on aortic atherosclerosis, for example, may be of limited relevance and, in fact, may lead to misleading conclusions regarding coronary heart disease.

Some of the initial evidence that estrogen inhibits the progression of coronary artery atherosclerosis came from a series of studies done in the 1950s at the Michael Reese Research Institute. Among the important findings from these studies was the resistance of hens to development of coronary artery atherosclerosis relative to roosters.[6] Furthermore, ligation of the hen oviduct, which results in a marked elevation in plasma cholesterol concentrations, had no effect on the relative resistance of hens to atherosclerosis, whereas ovariectomy resulted in a marked exacerbation of atherosclerosis.[6] In addition, exogenous estradiol in physiological doses inhibited progression of atherosclerosis[7] and promoted its regression[8] in this species. Subsequent studies using White Carneau pigeons resulted in similar conclusions regarding inhibitory effects of physiological doses of estrogen on coronary atherosclerosis.[9]

The subject of sex hormones and atherosclerosis received relatively little attention until 1977, when McGill and colleagues studied the effects of exogenous estrogens on atherosclerosis extent in ovariectomized baboons.[10] These investigators determined that ovariectomy was not associated with increased extent or severity of diet-induced atherosclerosis. Nor were there any significant effects of treatment with either physiological or pharmacological estrogen replacement therapy. It is important to note that, unlike many other primate species, the baboon is relatively resistant to diet-induced hyperlipidemia and atherosclerosis. Furthermore, there is no sex difference in the extent of diet-induced coronary artery atherosclerosis in baboons.

The Cynomolgus Macaque Model

In our laboratory, we have used the cynomolgus macaque to study effects of reproductive steroids on coronary artery atherosclerosis. This nonhuman primate species has been used in atherosclerosis research for ~30 years principally because of its susceptibility to diet-induced atherosclerotic involvement of main branch coronary arteries. We chose it for our research because, in addition to its susceptibility to atherosclerosis, its reproductive physiology is very similar to that of human beings; the female has a 28-day menstrual cycle and circulating sex hormone patterns that are similar to those of women.[3] Also, a natural menopause occurs in aged monkeys.

In an initial study of the relation between endogenous sex steroids and atherosclerosis, we studied cynomolgus macaques fed a moderately atherogenic diet for 30 months containing 40% of calories as fat and 0.4 mg of cholesterol per calorie. There were four experimental groups: males (n=15); intact, nonpregnant females (n=23); surgically postmenopausal (ie, ovariectomized) females (n=21); and pregnant females (n=27). Total plasma cholesterol (TPC) and plasma high-density lipoprotein (HDL) cholesterol concentrations as well as blood pressure were determined periodically. After 30 months, all animals were necropsied and extent of atherosclerosis (lesion cross-sectional area) was determined morphometrically.

As in a previous study,[11] males had more extensive coronary artery atherosclerosis relative to intact nonpregnant females.[12] Males also had significantly lower plasma HDL cholesterol concentrations and higher systolic blood pressure. Ovariectomy (ie, estrogen deficiency) resulted in a more atherogenic plasma lipoprotein pattern (decreased plasma HDL cholesterol and increased TPC concentrations), and a twofold increase in coronary artery atherosclerosis extent.[13] The hyperestrogenic state of pregnancy was associated with a marked reduction in extent of coronary artery atherosclerosis.[14] In this group of animals, both TPC and HDL cholesterol concentrations were decreased markedly during pregnancy. These findings are summarized in Figure 1.[15]

The results of this study provide indirect evidence regarding effects of endogenous sex hormones on atherosclerosis extent. Males

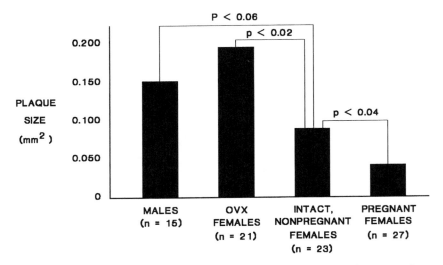

FIGURE 1. *Coronary artery plaque extent in four groups of cynomolgus macaques with diet-induced atherosclerosis. Although ovariectomized (OVX) had a far more atherogenic profile (ie, lower plasma concentrations of high-density lipoprotein and higher plasma concentrations of low-density lipoproteins), their plaque extent did not differ from that of males. Reproduced with permission from Reference 15.*

and ovariectomized females did not differ in regard to coronary artery atherosclerosis extent and also had consistently low-plasma estradiol concentrations in the range of 20 pg/mL. Atherosclerosis extent was reduced by approximately one-half in intact, nonpregnant females, which had much higher plasma estradiol concentrations, fluctuating in the normal range of 60–300 pg/mL depending on time of the menstrual cycle. Relative to these intact females, atherosclerosis extent was reduced by ~50% in pregnant females, a group that also showed sustained dramatic elevations in plasma estradiol concentrations in the range of 300–1,000 pg/mL.

Experimental Effects of Hormone Therapy

Study 1

Direct evidence for an inhibitory effect of endogenous estrogen on progression of coronary artery atherosclerosis is provided by the results of a subsequent study.[16] In this study, ovariectomized monkeys fed an atherogenic diet were assigned randomly to one of three treatment groups: no hormone replacement (n=17), continually administered estradiol-17β estradiol plus cyclically administered progesterone (n=20), and continuously administered 17-β estradiol (n=18). Physiological patterns of plasma estradiol and progesterone concentrations were maintained by administering the hormones in sustained-release subcutaneous Silastic implants. The experiment lasted 30 months. At necropsy, coronary artery atherosclerosis was inhibited similarly (reduced by approximately one-half) in animals in both hormone replacement groups (Figure 2). Antiatherogenic effects of hormone replacement were independent of variations in TPC, lipoprotein cholesterol, apoprotein A-I and B concentrations; average low-density lipoprotein (LDL) particle size; and HDL subfractional heterogeneity. Similarly, effects of hormone replacement on atherosclerosis could not be accounted for by other risk variables, ie, blood pressure or carbohydrate tolerance.

Whereas effects of hormone replacement observed in this study are consistent with results of epidemiological studies that associate estrogen use with reduced risk of coronary heart disease, the hormones administered and their mode of administration are quite different. For this reason, we conducted a second study of the effects

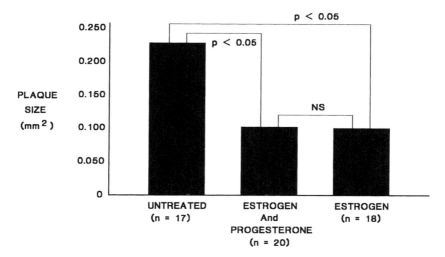

FIGURE 2. *Effect of hormone replacement therapy on coronary artery plaque extent in surgically postmenopausal cynomolgus macaques fed a moderately atherogenic diet. Hormone treatment reduced plaque extent by half. NS, not significant. Reproduced with permission from Reference 15.*

of the compounds most commonly prescribed for prevention or treatment of postmenopausal symptoms.

Study 2

In this study, ovariectomized monkeys were fed an atherogenic diet and assigned randomly to one of four treatment groups: no treatment (n=21), conjugated equine estrogens (human equivalent of 0.625 mg/day) (n=25), medroxyprogesterone acetate (MPA; human equivalent of 2.5 mg/day) (n=19), and conjugated equine estrogens and MPA (n=26). Treatment continued for 30 months. Preliminary analysis of these data[17] indicate that treatment with estrogen alone resulted in a 70% decrease ($P < 0.01$) in atherosclerosis extent, whereas treatment with estrogen and MPA or MPA alone resulted in an atherosclerosis extent that did not differ from that of untreated controls and was increased 170% and 290%, respectively, relative to animals treated with estrogen alone ($P < 0.01$; Figure 3). Preliminary analysis also indicates that these effects are largely independent of variation in plasma lipoproteins.

The results of these two studies (Figure 3) agree incompletely with the epidemiological data. Although the results of Study 1 are consistent with the protective effect of estrogen monotherapy or combination estrogen/sequential MPA therapy against coronary heart disease, the effects seen in Study 2 (combined hormone replacement with estrogen and continuous MPA) are inconsistent. How might this be explained? Unlike the epidemiological data for estrogen monotherapy and coronary heart disease risk, the data for combined hormone therapy with MPA are somewhat limited. Some[18] (and Stampfer M, personal communication), although not all,[19,20] indicate a decrease in risk similar to that seen with estrogen alone. However, these data are limited by the fact that the predominant prescribing pattern represented in the data for combined hormone replacement was continuous estrogen plus sequential MPA administration (ie, 7–14 days per month). In recent years, there has been an increase in the prescription of combined continuous replacement therapy, similar to that used in our second monkey study. Observational data for the effects of this form of therapy on coronary risk are not yet available. The monkey data suggest that this form of therapy may result in increased risk relative to users of estrogen alone of estrogen and sequentially administered progestin.

Our findings also suggest that inhibitory influences of hormone replacement on atherogenesis and coronary heart disease

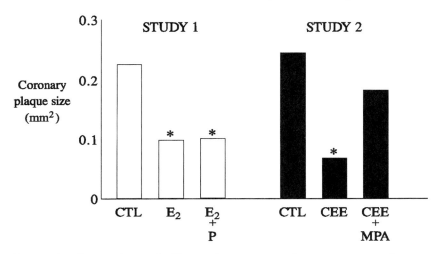

FIGURE 3. *Comparison of effects of two types of estrogen monotherapy and combined hormone replacement therapy on atherosclerosis in ova-riectomized cynomolgus monkeys. Study 1: CTL, untreated controls; E$_2$, estradiol-17β administered continuously by subcutaneous implant; P, progesterone administered sequentially by subcutaneous implant. Study 2: CTL, untreated controls; CEE, conjugated equine estrogens (human equivalent of 0.625 mg/day); MPA, oral medroxyprogesterone acetate (human equivalent of 2.5 mg/day). *P < 0.05 compared with untreated controls in each study. Adapted with permission from Reference 16.*

must be mediated either through nonlipoprotein risk factors not measured in these studies (or not yet described) or through a direct influence on cellular or biochemical events occurring in the arterial intima. Subsequent studies in our laboratory have addressed further the effects of sex hormones on pathophysiological processes of the arterial wall.

Effect of Sex Hormones on Arterial Pathophysiology

Sex Hormones and Arterial Lipoprotein Metabolism

Although effects of estrogen replacement on atherosclerosis are incompletely accounted for by plasma lipoprotein patterns, evidence exists that estrogens may influence directly arterial lipoprotein metabolism. Studies in rabbits[21-23] have suggested that estrogen treatment may decrease arterial lesion formation by directly inhibiting the accumulation and/or hydrolysis of cholesterol in the arterial wall. Hough and Zilversmit[23] investigated the effects of 17-β estradiol cypionate treatment in cholesterol-fed rabbits on net arterial cholesterol influx and hydrolysis of plasma cholesteryl ester. Although there were no significant effects on plasma cholesterol concentrations or lipoprotein patterns, estrogen treatment decreased lesion development significantly. Net cholesteryl ester influx, which was positively correlated with the extent of atherosclerosis, also was decreased in estrogen-treated animals. In addition, the percentage of newly entering cholesteryl ester hydrolyzed by the artery was reduced significantly by estrogen treatment independent of the extent of atherosclerosis. These results indicate that estrogen treatment may decrease arterial lesion formation by directly inhibiting the accumulation of cholesterol and/or hydrolysis of cholesteryl ester in the arterial wall.

To determine the effects of hormone treatment on lipoprotein metabolism in the cynomolgus macaque, we studied LDL coupled to radiolabeled tyramine cellobiose (TC).[24] The labeled TC-LDL, originally described by Pittman et al.,[25] allows quantification of the accumulation of products of LDL degradation and undegraded LDL in tissue or arterial samples. When lipoproteins coupled to iodinated TC are degraded by the cell, the labeled TC remains trapped in the lysosomes, representing the accumulation of products of LDL degradation and undegraded LDL over time.[26,27]

In our laboratory, we studied ovariectomized monkeys fed a moderately atherogenic diet for 18 weeks to study the effects of hormone treatment on early events in atherogenesis. Estrogen and cyclic progesterone were administered via Silastic implants to one group ($n = 9$), resulting in physiological hormone concentrations, whereas controls ($n = 8$) had low to undetectable hormone levels. Radiolabeled LDL was injected 24 hours before necropsy, and whole-body and arterial metabolism was measured. Hormone replacement therapy resulted in significantly reduced accumulation of LDL and products of LDL accumulation in coronary arteries[24] as well as other arterial sites.[27] This occurred despite no significant difference in plasma lipid and lipoprotein concentrations. Furthermore, the reduction in LDL metabolism occurred before any changes in intimal thickening or other indices of endothelial injury, such as increased endothelial cell turnover or numbers of leukocytes adherent to the endothelium.

Thus, studies using both rabbit and monkey models suggest that estrogen treatment inhibits atherosclerosis independently of changes in plasma lipids and lipoproteins. This effect may be occurring through a number of mechanisms. The study of Hough and

Zilversmit[23] and our studies in monkeys[24,27] suggest that estrogen may be acting intracellularly by inhibiting the hydrolysis of cholesterol and degradation of LDL, respectively.

Effects of Estrogen Deficiency on Vasomotor Function in Atherosclerotic Primates

Although the vasodilatory effects of estrogens on normal (non-atherosclerotic) arteries are well known,[28–30] our group was the first to demonstrate that estrogen administered either acutely (20 minutes)[31] or chronically (3 years)[32] can reverse the atherosclerosis-associated impairment of coronary vasodilator function. These findings subsequently were confirmed in studies of human subjects undergoing coronary angiography for the diagnosis of chest pain.[33,34] Although mechanisms involved in this protective effect on coronary reactivity have not been determined with certainty, the available evidence indicates that estrogen acts by augmenting the production of nitric oxide or protecting it from oxidative degradation or modification.[29,30] Estrogen has been found to stimulate expression of nitric oxide synthase by cultured endothelial cells,[35] an effect that may be estrogen receptor dependent.[36]

Progestins antagonize estrogen-induced increases in blood flow and vasodilation in normal (nonatherosclerotic) experimental animals.[37–41] Effects of progestins on atherosclerotic arteries have received attention only recently. We have studied the separate and combined effects of conjugated equine estrogens and MPA on coronary reactivity of atherosclerotic monkeys. As seen previously, estrogen augmented coronary dilator responses[42] and, additionally, augmented coronary blood flow reserve. However, co-administration of MPA resulted in a 50% diminution in the dilator response[42] and complete antagonism of the estrogen-induced improvement in coronary flow reserve (J. K. Williams, unpublished data).

Atherosclerosis results in impaired vasodilator and augmented vasoconstrictor responses to neurohumoral stimuli, which in turn can lead to accelerated progression of atherosclerosis, plaque instability or rupture, thrombosis, myocardial ischemia or myocardial infarction.[43–45] Estrogen treatment preserves vasodilator function and by this means, may retard atherosclerosis progression and reduce the risk of clinical events, ie, myocardial ischemia and infarction. Because MPA antagonizes, in whole or part, the protective effect of estrogen on coronary vasomotor function and blood flow, it also may result in a negation of the estrogen-associated reduction in risk of coronary heart disease.

Sex Hormones and Arterial Pathophysiology

Although sex hormones may influence atherosclerosis indirectly through effects on metabolic risk factors such as lipoproteins, they may have direct effects on cellular or molecular processes occurring in arterial intima that are implicated in the initiation and progression of atherosclerosis. There is plentiful evidence that sex hormones are modulators of immune and inflammatory reactions,[46-49] both of which have been implicated in atherosclerosis initiation and progression. Extracellular matrix elaboration and composition is altered in atherosclerosis, and sex hormones may modulate this process as well. Evidence supporting direct effects on these processes is somewhat limited and largely confined to results from studies of cells in culture. Nonetheless, several studies, including four from our laboratory, have implicated estrogens as modulators of the expression of inflammatory mediators and growth factors. Estrogen seems to, depending on conditions: 1) inhibit or stimulate interleukin-1 (IL-1) expression[50-53] 2) stimulate expression of platelet-derived growth factor-A;[54] 3) inhibit expression of tumor necrosis factor-alpha (TNF-α);[51,55] 4) inhibit expression of monocyte chemotactic protein-1 (MCP-1);[56] and 5) inhibit expression of interleukin-6 (IL-6).[57-59] Transcription factors, such as nuclear factor kappa B (NF-kB) regulate expression of many genes, including IL-1, IL-6, and MCP-1, involved in acute phase and inflammatory responses. Recently, we have found that treatment with conjugated equine estrogens inhibits the activation of NF-kB in the aortic arch of monkeys with very early stages of diet-induced atherosclerosis.[60]

For these studies, ovariectomized monkeys were fed an atherogenic diet for 12 weeks, during which five monkeys were treated with estrogen (the monkey equivalent of 0.625 mg/day of conjugated equine estrogens) and five monkeys were untreated controls. Nuclear extracts isolated from the aortic arches were utilized with a radiolabeled DNA segment containing a tandem repeat of the NF-kB DNA binding site [GGGGACTTTCC] in an electrophoretic mobility shift assay. Nuclear extracts from all control animals and four of five estrogen-treated animals had detectable NF-kB DNA binding activity. Competition studies with cold competitor DNA demonstrated lower activity in samples from the estrogen-treated animals, where 200 ng of competitor completely inhibited binding activity in all samples. In samples from control animals, activity was much greater ($P < 0.05$), with detectable binding present in three of five samples in the presence of 200 ng competitor, and in two of five samples in the presence of 400 and 800 ng competitor. Thus, estrogen may inhibit atherosclerosis progression by modulating activity of this transcription factor, which is known to regulate expression of adhesion molecules and inflammatory mediators implicated in atherosclerosis initiation and progression.

Summary and Conclusions

Although it has long been known that women have a lower incidence of coronary heart disease, clinical and epidemiological studies have not, until recently, investigated the possible role of sex hormones in cardiovascular disease, particularly coronary artery atherosclerosis. We have reviewed the current experimental evidence concerning the roles of sex hormone deficiency and hormone replacement therapy in the initiation and progression of coronary artery atherosclerosis.

Early experimental models of estrogen-deficient animals with coronary artery atherosclerosis used chickens and pigeons. However, nonhuman primate models replaced these earlier models because of greater similarities to human beings. Our studies have focused on the female cynomolgus macaque, especially surgically postmenopausal (ie, estrogen-deficient) animals fed an atherogenic diet. We found that male and ovariectomized female cynomolgus macaques did not differ with respect to coronary artery atherosclerosis, whereas premenopausal females had half the coronary artery atherosclerosis of their ovariectomized counterparts. In two studies of hormone replacement therapy of ovariectomized cynomolgus macaques, we discovered that estrogen replacement therapy, in the form of parenteral estradiol or oral conjugated equine estrogens, resulted in 50% to 70% reductions in the extent of coronary artery atherosclerosis compared with control animals. However, although combined, continuous estradiol/sequential progesterone replacement, administered parenterally, caused a 50% reduction in atherosclerosis extent, treatment with combined continuous, orally administered conjugated equine estrogens and MPA resulted in atherosclerosis, the extent of which was not different from untreated controls. These results indicate that effects of progestin, when given with estrogen, on coronary arteries may depend on type, dose, route of administration, or pattern (continuous versus sequential) of administration and that some forms of progestin cotherapy may antagonize favorable effects of estrogen.

Further investigation has indicated that direct arterial effects of sex hormones may explain their effects on atherosclerosis. Estrogen of either type inhibits the arterial uptake and degradation of plasma LDL, preserves endothelium-dependent vasomotor responses and inhibits the expression of pro-inflammatory and mitogenic cytokines implicated in atherogenesis. Thus, estrogen may directly inhibit the arterial accumulation of cholesterol, inhibit inflammatory and pro-liferative processes of the arterial intima, and promote vasodilation, thereby retarding atherosclerosis progression and reducing the risk of clinically evident coronary heart disease. Effects of progestins on pathophysiological processes of the artery wall are unclear; however, effects on these processes may represent means by which contrasting effects of progestins are mediated.

Acknowledgment

The authors gratefully acknowledge the editorial assistance of Karen Klein.

References

1. McGill HC Jr, Stern MP. Sex and atherosclerosis. *Atheroscler Rev* 1979;4:157–242.
2. Adams MR, Kaplan JR, Clarkson TB, et al. Effects of psychosocial stress, menopause and pregnancy on coronary artery atherosclerosis. In Eaker ED, Packard B, Wenger NK, et al., eds. *Coronary Heart Disease in Women*. New York: Haymarket Doyma; 1987:151–157.
3. Bush TL. The epidemiology of cardiovascular disease in postmeno-pausal women. *Ann NY Acad Sci* 1990;592:263–271.
4. Adams MR, Clarkson TB, Koritnik DR, et al. Contraceptive steroids and coronary artery atherosclerosis in cynomolgus macaques. *Fertil Steril* 1987;47:1010–1018.
5. Clarkson TB, Shively CA, Morgan TM, et al. Oral contraceptives and coronary artery atherosclerosis of cynomolgus monkeys. *Obstet Gynecol* 1990;75:217–222.
6. Stamler J, Pick R, Katz LN. Inhibition of cholesterol-induced coronary atherogenesis in the egg-producing hen. *Circulation* 1954;10:251–254.
7. Pick R, Stamler J, Rodbard S, et al. The inhibition of coronary athero-sclerosis by estrogens in cholesterol-fed chicks. *Circulation* 1952;6: 276–280.
8. Pick R, Stamler J, Rodbard S, et al. Estrogen-induced regression of cor-onary atherosclerosis in cholesterol-fed chicks. *Circulation* 1952;6: 858–861.
9. Prichard RW, Clarkson TB, Lofland HB. Estrogen in pigeon atheroscle-rosis. Estradiol valerate effects at several dose levels on cholesterol-fed male white Carneau pigeons. *Arch Pathol* 1966;82:15–17.

10. McGill HC Jr, Axelrod LR, McMahan CA, et al. Estrogens and experimental atherosclerosis in the baboon (*Papio cynocephalus*). *Circulation* 1977;56:657–662.
11. Hamm TE Jr, Kaplan JR, Clarkson TB, et al. Effects of gender and social behavior on the development of coronary artery atherosclerosis in cynomolgus monkeys. *Atherosclerosis* 1983;48:221–233.
12. Kaplan JR, Adams MR, Clarkson TB, et al. Psychosocial influences on female protection among cynomolgus macaques. *Atherosclerosis* 1984; 53:283–295.
13. Adams MR, Clarkson TB, Kaplan JR, et al. Ovariectomy, social status, and coronary artery atherosclerosis in cynomolgus monkeys. *Arteriosclerosis* 1985;5:192–200.
14. Adams MR, Kaplan JR, Clarkson TB, et al. Pregnancy-associated inhibition of coronary artery atherosclerosis in monkeys: Evidence of a relationship with endogenous estrogen. *Arteriosclerosis* 1987;7:378–384.
15. Adams MR, Washburn SA, Wagner JD, et al. Arterial changes: Estrogen deficiency and effects of hormone replacement. In: Lobo RA, ed. *Treatment of the Postmenopausal Woman: Basic and Clinical Aspects.* New York: Raven Press; 1994:243–250.
16. Adams MR, Kaplan JR, Manuck SB, et al. Inhibition of coronary artery atherosclerosis by 17-beta estradiol in ovariectomized monkeys. Lack of effect of an added progesterone. *Arteriosclerosis* 1990;10: 1051–1057.
17. Adams MR, Golden DL. Atheroprotective effects of estrogen replacement therapy are antagonized by medroxyprogesterone acetate in monkeys. Abstract. *Arterioscler Thromb Vasc Biol* 1997;17:217–221.
18. Psaty B, Heckbert S, Atkins D, et al. The risk of myocardial infarction associated with the combined sue of estrogens and progestins in postmenopausal women. *Arch Intern Med* 1994;154:1333–1339.
19. Nachtigall LE, Nachtigall RH, Nachtigall RD, et al. Estrogen replacement therapy II: A prospective study in the relationship to carcinoma and cardiovascular and metabolic problems. *Obstet Gynecol* 1979; 54:74–79.
20. Rosenberg L, Shapiro S, Kaufman DW, et al. Patterns and determinants of conjugated estrogen use. *Am J Epidemiol* 1979;109:676–686.
21. Kushwaha RS, Hazzard WR. Exogenous estrogens attenuate dietary hypercholesterolemia and atherosclerosis in the rabbit. *Metabolism* 1981; 30:359–366.
22. Haarbo J, Leth-Espensen P, Stender S, et al. Estrogen monotherapy and combined estrogen-progestogen replacement therapy attenuate aortic accumulation of cholesterol in ovariectomized cholesterol-fed rabbits. *J Clin Invest* 1991;87:1274–1279.
23. Hough JL, Zilversmit DB. Effect of 17-beta estradiol on aortic cholesterol content and metabolism in cholesterol-fed rabbits. *Arteriosclerosis* 1986;6:57–63.
24. Wagner JD, Clarkson TB, St. Clair RW, et al. Estrogen and progesterone replacement therapy educes LDL accumulation in the coronary arteries of surgically postmenopausal cynomolgus monkeys. *J Clin Invest* 1991;88:1995–2002.
25. Pittman RC, Carew TE, Glass CK, et al. A radioiodinated, intracellularly trapped ligand for determining the sites of plasma protein degradation in vivo. *Biochem J* 1983;212:791–800.

26. Carew TC, Pittman RC, Marchand ER, et al. Measurement in vivo of irreversible degradation of low density lipoprotein in the rabbit aorta. Predominance of intimal degradation. *Arteriosclerosis* 1984;4:214–224.
27. Wagner JD, St. Clair RW, Schwenke DC, et al. Regional differences in arterial low density lipoprotein metabolism in surgically postmenopausal cynomolgus monkeys: Effects of estrogen and progesterone replacement therapy. *Arterioscler Thromb* 1992;12:716–723.
28. Jiang C, Sarrel PM, Lindsay DC, et al. Endothelium-independent relaxation of rabbit coronary artery by 17-beta estradiol. *Br J Pharmacol* 1991;104:1033–1037.
29. Gisclard V, Miller VM, Vanhoutte PM. Effect of 17-beta estradiol on endothelium-dependent responses in the rabbit. *J Pharmacol Exp Therap* 1988;244:19–22.
30. Miller VM, Gisclard V, Vanhoutte PM. Modulation of endothelium-dependent and vascular smooth muscle responses by oestrogens. *Phlebology* 1988;3(suppl 1):63–69.
31. Williams JK, Adams MR, Klopfenstein HS. Estrogen modulates responses of atherosclerotic coronary arteries. *Circulation* 1990;75:217–222.
32. Williams JK, Adams MR, Herrington DM, et al. Short-term administration of estrogen and vascular responses of atherosclerotic coronary arteries. *J Am Coll Cardiol* 1992;20:452–457.
33. Herrington DM, Braden DA, Downes TR, et al. Estrogen modulates coronary vasomotor responses in postmenopausal women with early atherosclerosis. *Am J Cardiol* 1994;73:951–952.
34. Reis SE, Gloth ST, Blumenthal RS, et al. Ethinyl estradiol acutely attenuates abnormal coronary vasomotor responses to acetylcholine in postmenopausal women. *Circulation* 1994;89:52–60.
35. Schray-Utz B, Zeiher AM, Busse R. Expression of constitutive NO synthase in cultured endothelial cells is enhanced by 17-beta estradiol. Abstract. *Circulation* 1993;88(suppl I):I-80.
36. Sayegh HS, Ohara Y, Navas JP, et al. Endothelial nitric oxide synthase regulation by estrogens. Abstract. *Circulation* 1993;88(suppl I):I-80.
37. Caton D, Abrams RM, Clapp JF, et al. Effect of exogenous progesterone on the rate of blood flow of the uterus of oophorectomized sheep. *Q J Exp Physiol* 1974;59:225–231.
38. Greiss FC, Anderson SG. Effect of ovarian hormones on the uterine vascular bed. *Am J Obstet Gynecol* 1970;107:829–836.
39. Resnik R. The effect of progesterone on estrogen-induced uterine blood flow. *Gynecol Invest* 1976;128:251–254.
40. Sarrel PM. Sexuality and menopause. *Obstet Gynecol* 1990;75:26S–32S.
41. Sarrel PM. Blood flow and ovarian secretions. In: Naftolin F, DeCherney AH, Gutmann JN, et al.. eds. *Ovarian Secretions and Cardiovascular and Neurovascular Function.* New York: Raven Press; 1990:81–89.
42. Williams JK, Honoré EK, Washburn SA, et al. Effects of hormone replacement therapy on reactivity of atherosclerotic coronary arteries in cynomolgus monkeys. *J Am Coll Cardiol* 1994;24:1757–1761.
43. Maseri A, Severi S, DeNes M, et al. "Variant" angina: One aspect of a continuous spectrum of vasospastic myocardial ischemia. Pathogenetic mechanisms, estimated incidence and clinical and coronary arteriographic findings in 138 patients. *Am J Cardiol* 1978;42:1019–1035.
44. Maseri A, L'Abbate A, Bardoli G, et al. Coronary vasospasm as a possible cause of myocardial infarction: A conclusion derived from the study of "preinfarction" angina. *N Engl J Med* 1978;299:1271–1277.

45. Roberts WC, Durry RC, Isner JM. Sudden death in Prinzmetal's angina with coronary spasm documented by angiography: Analysis of three necropsy patients. *Am J Cardiol* 1982;50:203–210.
46. Ahmed SA, Penhale WJ, Talal N Sex hormones, immune responses, and autoimmune diseases: Mechanisms of sex hormone action. *Am J Pathol* 1985;121:531–551.
47. Loy RA, Loukides JA, Polan ML. Ovarian steroids modulate human monocyte tumor necrosis factor alpha messenger ribonucleic acid levels in cultured human peripheral monocytes. *Fertil Steril* 1992;58:733–739.
48. Polan ML, Loukides J, Nelson P, et al. Progesterone and estradiol modulate interleukin-1 beta messenger ribonucleic acid levels in cultured human peripheral monocytes. *J Clin Endocrinol Metab* 1989;69:1200–1206.
49. Schuurs AHWM, Verheul HAM. Effects of gender and sex steroids on the immune response. *J Steroid Biochem* 1990;35:157–172.
50. Hu S-K, Mitcho YL, Rath NC. Effect of estradiol on interleukin-1 synthesis by macrophages. *Int J Immunopharmacol* 1988;10:247–252.
51. Polan ML, Daniele A, Kuo A. Gonadal steroids modulate human monocyte interleukin (IL-1) activity. *Fertil Steril* 1988;49:964–968.
52. Shanker G, Sorci-Thomas M, Register TC, et al. The inducible expression of THP-1 cell interleukin-1 mRNA: Effects of estrogen on differential response to phorbol ester and lipopolysaccharide. *Lymphokine Cytokine Res* 1994;13:1–7.
53. Stock JL, Coderre JA, McDonald B, et al. Effect of estrogen in vitro and in vivo on spontaneous interleukin-1 release by monocytes from postmenopausal women. *J Clin Endocrinol Metab* 1989;68:364–368.
54. Shanker G, Sorci-Thomas M, Adams MR. Estrogen modulates the inducible expression of platelet-derived growth factor mRNA by monocyte/macrophages. *Life Sci* 1995;56:499–507.
55. Shanker G, Sorci-Thomas M, Adams MR. Estrogen modulates the expression of tumor necrosis factor-alpha mRNA in phorbol ester- and lipopolysaccharide-stimulated human monocytic THP-1 cells. *Lymphokine Cytokine Res* 1994;13:377–382.
56. Frazier-Jessen MR, Kovacs EJ. Estrogen modulation of JE/monocyte chemoattractant protein-1 expression in murine macrophages. *J Immunol* 1995;154:1838–1845.
57. Stein B, Yang MX. Repression of the interleukin-6 promoter by estrogen receptor is mediated by NF-kB and C/EBPβ. *Mol Cell Biol* 1995; 15:4971–4979.
58. Girasole G, Jilka RL, Passeri G, et al. 17β-estradiol inhibits interleukin-6 production by bone marrow-derived stromal cells and osteoblasts in vitro: A potential mechanism for the antiosteoporotic effect of estrogens. *J Clin Invest* 1992;89:883–891.
59. Jilka RL, Hangoc G, Girasole G, et al. Increased osteoclast development after estrogen loss: Mediation by interleukin-6. *Science* 1992;257:88–91.
60. Register TC, Bora TA, Adams MR. Estrogen inhibits activation of arterial NF-kB transcription factor in early diet-induced atherogenesis. Abstract. *Circulation* 1995;92:I–628.

Chapter 4

Mechanisms of Regulation of Gene Expression by Estrogen Receptors

Carolyn L. Smith, PhD
and Orla M. Conneely, PhD

Estrogens regulate processes associated with the growth and differentiation of mammary, reproductive, and bone tissues and the sexual differentiation of brain and sexual behavior. In addition, the lower incidence of coronary atherosclerosis in premenopausal women is associated with estrogen action, and the identification of estrogen receptors in human coronary arteries suggests that this effect is mediated, at least in part, by estrogen regulated transcription.[1]

Generally, estrogens are believed to effect their physiological roles via interaction with an intracellular receptor. In its simplest form, this pathway consists of estrogen (ligand) diffusing across the plasma membrane and binding to the estrogen receptor (ER) whereupon this steroid-protein complex binds to DNA and facilitates the transcription of target genes. The resulting mRNA is translated into protein, which in turn alters cellular function and thereby produces an estrogenic response. Although this pathway has been accepted widely for the last 15 years, the use of molecular biological techniques has substantially expanded our appreciation of this process as well as revealed alternative mechanisms by which ER may be regulated and estrogen-like responses achieved.

The ER belongs to a gene superfamily of ligand-activated transcription factors, which includes receptors for steroids (eg, glucocorticoids, progestins, androgens) as well as nonsteroidal ligands such as thyroid hormone, vitamin D, and retinoids. Estrogen action has been studied in a variety of experimental and biological systems and the cloning of ER cDNAs from many species (human, chicken, rat, mouse, rainbow trout and *Xenopus*) has contributed substan-

From: Forte TM, (ed). *Hormonal, Metabolic, and Cellular Influences on Cardiovascular Disease in Women*. Armonk, NY: Futura Publishing Company, Inc.; © 1997.

tially to studies of the receptor's structure, particularly with respect to its function as a transcription factor. Comparison of the deduced primary structures of these ERs cDNAs enabled the sequence to be divided on the basis of homology into six regions, designated A–F. Mutagenesis and deletion of these cDNAs combined with functional analysis of the expressed protein has allowed specific functions to be assigned to distinct portions of the receptor molecule (Figure 1) and has provided a basis for our understanding of the ability of ER to modulate the transcription of estrogen-responsive genes.

Ligand-Dependent Activation of the Estrogen Receptor

Overview

The process of ligand-regulated, steroid receptor-mediated biological activity has been studied from the perspective of many members of the steroid receptor family (eg, glucocorticoid and progesterone receptors) and our overall understanding of steroid receptor-dependent transcription is a compilation of this work. Non-protein-bound estrogens enter the cell by passive diffusion and are bound by the ER with high affinity. Receptors subsequently undergo a conformational change, dissociate from an inhibitory heteroligo-

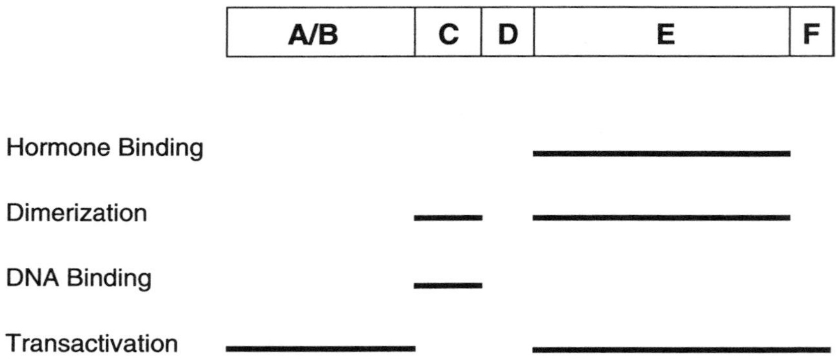

FIGURE 1. *The domain structure of the estrogen receptor. The primary amino acid sequence is divided into six domains (A–F) based on sequence homology between the human and chicken ERs. Domains required for ligand binding, DNA binding, dimerization and activation functions are indicated.*

meric complex of heat shock and other proteins[2-5] and then dimerize and bind to a specific DNA sequence, referred to as an estrogen response element (ERE).[6,7] Once bound to DNA, the ERs interact with the basal transcription machinery to alter gene transcription.[8] This hormone-dependent activation process is accompanied by phosphorylation of the ER whose contribution to ER function is, at present, poorly understood (see below).

Ligand Binding

The ligand binding domain is located within the carboxyl-terminal portion of the ER (domain E) and this region alone (amino acids 302–595) when expressed in yeast is sufficient for high-affinity estradiol binding (K_d, 1.0 nM) with appropriate ligand binding specificity comparable in magnitude to that of native receptor expressed in MCF-7 (breast cancer) cells (K_d, 0.36 nM).[9] In the context of the mouse ER, deletion analysis has defined the carboxyl terminal boundary of sequence required for ligand binding; receptor fragments consisting of amino acids 121–538 retain good hormone binding affinity whereas a slightly smaller deletion mutant (121–507) exhibits no ligand binding activity.[10] Thus, the region between amino acids 507 and 538 is critical for ligand binding. It is not, however, sufficient because a slightly larger, corresponding region of human ER sequence (amino acids 510–551) is incapable of estrogen binding.[9]

Through the use of covalently attaching ER affinity ligands, specific amino acids within the E domain have been identified that contribute to ligand binding. Both the estrogen agonist, ketononestrol aziridine, and the antiestrogen, tamoxifen aziridine, affinity labeled cysteine 530,[11] an amino acid located within the region necessary for ligand binding (see above). Interestingly, when this residue is mutated to alanine, tamoxifen aziridine affinity labeled cysteine 381, suggesting that it is in close proximity to cysteine 530 within the context of the three-dimensional structure of the ligand binding domain.[12] Mutation of amino acids adjacent to cysteine 530 (lysine 529, lysine 531, and asparagine 532) also indicates that this region is critical for appropriate estrogen, but not antiestrogen binding affinity thus suggesting that these amino acids contribute to the ability of receptor to discriminate between estrogen and antiestrogen ligands.[13]

Limited protease digestion experiments indicate that upon hormone binding, the ligand binding domain undergoes a conforma-

tional change and likely folds into a more compact structure, the
nature of which is dependent upon the class of bound ligand (estrogen versus antiestrogen).[14] This change in domain structure precedes the dissociation of heat shock proteins from receptor and is a
prerequisite for *trans*-activation.[5,14] The conformation assumed by
estrogen-activated receptor is postulated to favor ER interactions
with the transcriptional machinery or coactivators and thereby promote transcription initiation by the general transcriptional appara-
tus.[14] It is possible that the antagonist-specific alteration in ligand
binding domain conformation may not facilitate appropriate interactions with other components of a productive transcription complex and therefore provide at least a partial basis for the inability of
antiestrogens to efficiently activate gene expression.

DNA Binding

The DNA binding domain (domain C) is the most highly conserved between all members of the steroid receptor superfamily
(reviewed by Freedman[15]). This relatively cysteine rich sequence
specifies a structural motif proposed to form two type II zinc fin-
gers. Each finger encompasses four cysteine residues, which co-
ordinately bind a single zinc atom, and it is this region in the
context of the surrounding sequence that recognizes the DNA sequence (ERE) to which the receptor will bind as a homodimer.
The ERE from the *Xenopus* vitellogenin A2 gene is considered to
represent the consensus response element (GGTCAnnnTGACC),
but variations of this sequence such as T_GTCActaTGT_CC from
the rat prolactin gene also will serve as functional EREs.[16] These
cis-acting enhancer elements are typically found within the 5'-
regulatory regions of estrogen-responsive genes and confer
steroid-sensitivity regardless of orientation and position with respect to their target gene promoters.[16-18] More recently, EREs
have also been located overlapping a translational initiation site[19]
and within the first coding exon of target genes.[20]

Activation Functions

There are two activation functions (AFs) within the ER sequence; one located in the A/B domain (AF1), which is constitutively
active, and the second (AF2) located in the carboxyl terminal portion
of the receptor (domain E).[21,22] The latter activation function over-

laps the ligand binding domain, and its ability to activate target gene expression is dependent upon estrogen binding.[23] Both deletion and point mutation analysis have been used to characterize the sequences required for AF2 function that are thought to reside primarily within the E domain.[16] For instance, a mouse ER mutant in which amino acids 553–599 (F domain) have been deleted is still capable of activating gene expression in a hormone-dependent manner.[24] Further deletion (removal of amino acids 539–599) rendered a molecule still capable of estrogen and DNA binding but effectively eliminated AF2 activity, thus indicating that amino acids 539–552 are important for AF2 function. The F domain, although not required for AF2 activity, does modulate the ability of estradiol to stimulate gene transcription and antiestrogens to inhibit estrogen-activated gene expression.[25]

Depending on the cell and promoter context, the overall ER transcriptional activity may be derived primarily from AF1, AF2, or a synergistic combination thereof.[21] The specific sequences important for AF1 function also vary. Under conditions where AF1 enhances transcription independently of AF2, a contiguous, hydrophobic, and proline-rich 99 sequence (amino acids 51–149) within the A/B domain is able to activate gene expression.[26] In contexts where AF1 synergizes with AF2, the amino acids responsible for transcriptional activation map to two unlinked subregions (amino acids 51–93 and 102–149) located within the same region as the independently acting AF1 domain.[26] It is possible that distinct regions within the A/B domain are used for AF1 function under different transcriptional contexts because the other transcription factors and/or cofactors with which the ER must interact also would be expected to vary by promoter and cell type.

Phosphorylation

In an unstimulated or basal state, the ER is phosphorylated at a relatively low level. Estrogens, in addition to altering the ligand binding domain conformation, also increase the phosphorylation state of endogenous ER in MCF-7, rat, and mouse uterine cells[27–29] as well as ER transiently expressed in Sf9 (insect) and COS (green monkey kidney) cells.[30,31] Although the precise role of phosphorylation with respect to receptor's transcriptional activation function is not clear, mutant mouse ERs defective in either estrogen or DNA binding are phosphorylated at reduced levels relative to wild-type receptors[32] providing a correlation between this posttranslational modification and receptor function. Serine 167, identified by radiolabeling and amino acid sequence analysis, has been reported to be the major estrogen-induced phosphorylation site of human ER 30 whereas other research groups indicated Ser104 and/or 106 and Ser118 as major estrogen-inducible phosphate acceptor sites.[31,33,34] Mutation of these amino acids from serine to alanine reduced the overall estrogen-dependent phosphorylation of ER as well as its ability to activate the transcription of various synthetic target genes, suggesting that enhanced site-specific receptor phosphorylation may directly influence gene expression.[31,33] The reason for these contrasting data is not known, but a possible explanation may be cell-specific utilization of multiple potential phosphorylation sites. Indeed, the observation that the antiestrogens 4-hydroxytamoxifen and ICI 164,384 also increase overall ER phosphorylation[27,31,33] indicates that the relation between phosphorylation and transcriptional activation is complex.

Ligand-Independent Activation

General

As noted above, phosphorylation events are associated closely with ER activation. Indeed, all of the steroid receptors studied to date, including the ER, are phosphoproteins, and increases in overall receptor phosphorylation, as well as increased phosphorylation of specific amino acid residues, have been demonstrated after exposure of cells to the receptor's cognate ligand.[35] Current models of ligand-dependent steroid receptor activation include multiple phosphorylation steps[35-37] and it has been demonstrated that agents, either synthetic or naturally occurring, capable of altering cellular phosphorylation pathways can activate several members of the steroid receptor superfamily in the apparent absence of ligand.[38-40]

Estrogen Receptor

Several laboratories have examined the ability of ER to be activated in a ligand-independent fashion. Cho and Katzenellebogen[41] used protein kinase A (PKA) pathway activators (cholera toxin that ADP-ribosylates G_s, allowing it to persistently activate adenylate cyclase) and 3-isobutyl-1-methylxanthine (IBMX; a phosphodiesterase inhibitor) as well as activators of protein kinase C (PKC) pathways

(12-O-tetradecanoylphorbol 13-acetate; TPA) to treat MCF-7 and CHO (Chinese hamster ovary) cells, and in neither case was an increase in ER-dependent reporter gene expression observed in the absence of estradiol. The human ER, however, has been ligand-independently activated by okadaic acid (an inhibitor of protein phosphatases 1 and 2A) in CV_1 cells (green monkey kidney), and rat ER is transcriptionally activated by cholera toxin and IBMX or 8-bromo-adenosine 3':5'cyclic phosphate -(cAMP) in primary rat uterine cell cultures.[27,40] The discrepancy in the ability of phosphorylating agents to modulate ER activity in the absence of estradiol may reflect promoter or cell-type specific differences, which also have been noted to influence basal[42] and ligand-stimulated ER-dependent transcription.[43] Indeed, the ability of TPA to synergize with estradiol in the activation of ER-dependent transcription varies with these two parameters.[41]

Although the use of pharmacological modulators of intracellular signal transduction pathways demonstrates the potential of ER to be activated in the absence of ligand, naturally occurring substances should be able to mimic this effect for it to be physiologically relevant. Two classes of agents, neurotransmitters and growth factors, have proven themselves able to stimulate ER-dependent transcription under essentially estrogen-free conditions. The catecholaminergic neurotransmitter, dopamine, was first shown to stimulate ER-dependent gene expression in the absence of estradiol in CV_1 cells,[40] presumably via a signal transduction pathway initiated at a dopamine membrane receptor. Dopaminergic activation of ER is not restricted to a single cell type as evidenced by receptor-dependent gene expression in HeLa (human cervical carcinoma), SK-N-SH (human neuroblastoma), and PC-12 (rat adrenal pheochromacytoma) cells[44,45] (also C. L. Smith, personal observation). In addition to its effects on ER function, dopamine also activates progesterone and vitamin D receptor-dependent transcription,[40] and this suggests that this mechanism of receptor activation may have broad implications for regulating receptor function under a variety of physiological situations.

Dopamine receptors belong to the G-protein linked, serpentine receptor family. At present there are five known dopamine receptor genes that encode for at least 15 distinct receptor forms.[46] Historically, these receptors have been grouped into two subtypes based on the ability of dopamine to either stimulate (D_1 subtype) or inhibit (D_2 subtype) adenylate cyclase activity after receptor stimulation.[47] Synthetic dopamine receptor agonists can be used to distinguish these two receptor subclasses. The D_1 specific receptor agonist, SCH 38393, activated ER-dependent transcription whereas the D2 specific agonist, quinpirole, was unable to support receptor activation. This, taken together with the ability of dopamine to increase in vitro cAMP production in both HeLa and CV_1 cells, would suggest that a receptor of the D_1 subtype is responsible for ER activation.[44] The initial classification of dopamine receptor subtypes subsequently has been shown to be an oversimplification, and D_1 subtype receptor activation has also been associated with a number of intracellular effector systems in addition to adenylate cyclase, such as phospholipase C^{48} and PKC.[49] The specific intracellular signal transduction pathway(s) responsible for dopaminergic activation of steroid receptors is the subject of ongoing investigations in this laboratory.

The ability of peptide growth factors such as epidermal growth factor (EGF) and insulin-like growth factor-I (IGF-I) to mimic a classic estrogen response (increased progesterone synthesis) in uterine and breast cancer cells was an indication that growth factor receptor and ER signal transduction pathways "cross-talk".[50–53] The list of biological responses that can be mediated by both growth factors and estrogens continues to increase and now includes induction of the iron-binding glycoprotein, lactoferrin,[54] uterine growth stimulation,[54] pituitary cell growth,[55] neurite outgrowth and morphological differentiation of neuroblastoma cells,[56] and heregulin stimulation of MCF-7 tumor volume in athymic mice.[57]

Direct evidence for peptide growth factor activation of ER-dependent gene expression has been obtained in multiple cell types, suggesting widespread use of this mode of receptor activation. Transforming growth factor-α (TGF-α) or EGF stimulation of HeLa, Ishikawa (endometrial), and BG-1 (ovarian) cells, transiently transfected with ER-responsive target genes, results in dose-dependent activation of ER in an estrogen-independent manner.[58,59] Furthermore, ER-mediated activation of a synthetic target gene has been observed after IGF-I treatment of primary rat uterine cell cultures,[27] the rat pituitary tumor cell line, GH3,[55] and a neuroblastoma cell line, SK-ER3.[56]

Heregulin, TGF-α, and EGF bind to members of the erb B family of tyrosine kinase receptors, whereas IGF-I binds to the type I IGF receptor, which also possesses tyrosine kinase activity.[60,61] Multiple intracellular signaling pathways initiated by phospholipase C, phosphoinositide 3-kinase, ras, or JAK/STAT can be activated from these receptors.[62,63] As yet, however, the nature of the interaction between the ER and the signal transduction pathway(s) that originates from these plasma membrane, growth factor receptors is not understood, nor is it known if the ER is cytoplasmic or nuclear when it is ligand-independently activated.

Estrogen Receptor Domains Required for Ligand-Independent Activation

In contrast to the relatively detailed maps of ER regions associated with ligand binding and ligand-dependent activation functions, structural information regarding ER regions associated with ligand-independent activation have been derived primarily from gross deletion studies. For example, a deletion mutant consisting of the amino terminus and DNA binding domain of mouse ER (amino acids 1–339) is activated by EGF whereas amino-terminal-deleted receptors (amino acids 121–599) are transcriptionally silent.[58] The ER regions necessary for dopaminergic activation are even less well understood, although a point mutation within the E domain (glycine[400] → valine[400]) abolished ligand-independent activation and implicated the carboxyl terminus in dopaminergic activation,[44] data consistent with that obtained for the chicken progesterone receptor.[40] Modulation of receptor-dependent gene transcription by cholera toxin and IBMX also does not appear to require the amino terminus of ER because deletion of the A/B (AF-1) domain did not block this effect.[41] The reason for the discrepancy between ER regions required for growth factor and dopamine/cAMP mediated activation is not clear. It is possible that more than one type of signal transduction pathway is able to communicate with the ER and that different pathways interact with AF1 and/or AF2 domains.

Mechanism of Ligand-Independent Activation

Little is understood of the nature of the intracellular signal transduction pathway(s) that transmit information from the plasma membrane to the ER. Epidermal growth factor increased the DNA binding activity of mouse uterine ER in vivo and the production of heterogeneous forms of nuclear receptor, indicating that the signal transduction pathway(s) initiated by this peptide is able to influence directly the biochemical properties of ER.[64] Ligand-independent activation has been thought to be associated with phosphorylation processes, but the nature of phosphorylation events associated with ligand-independent activation are at present unknown. It has been postulated that activation of receptor-dependent transcription results from the activation of protein kinases or the inhibition of protein phosphatases resulting in phosphorylation of target(s), which may include the steroid receptor itself, another transcription factor with which the steroid receptor interacts or a cofactor (eg, coactivator) necessary for steroid receptor function. Little progress has been made in this regard, but it has been demonstrated that treatment with cholera toxin and IBMX, TPA, or IGF-I results in an overall increase in ER phosphorylation,[27,33] and heregulin stimulates ER tyrosine phosphorylation.[57] Whether or not these phosphorylation events are necessary or sufficient for ligand-independent activation is unknown. Furthermore, as no ligand-independent phosphorylation sites have been mapped, the interesting possibility of a mutually exclusive ligand-dependent and/or ligand-independent phosphorylation site(s) still remains.

Ligand Influences on Ligand-Independent Activation

Cells in vivo are exposed simultaneously to external stimuli able to initiate intracellular signaling pathways as well as ligands, either agonists or antagonists, able to enter the cell and bind directly to receptor. It is therefore important to consider how different classes of signals impinge upon receptor function. Under conditions where neither TPA nor cholera toxin and IBMX alone were able to increase ER-dependent transcription, the addition of either of these compounds in the presence of estradiol produced a synergistic increase in reporter gene transcription, suggesting that these two signaling pathways may converge on the liganded ER and alter its activity.[41] Similarly, EGF or TGF-α in combination with estradiol also synergistically activated ER-dependent transcription.[58] In contrast, concurrent activation of human ER with estradiol and dopamine was not synergistic, although the resulting gene expression was greater than that induced by either compound alone.[44]

In addition to agonistic ligands, synthetic antihormone compounds have been developed that are bound by ER with high affinity but are unable to effectively activate the receptor to stimulate gene transcription.[42,43] The triphenylethylene-derived antagonist 4-hydroxytamoxifen (4HT), acts as a partial agonist/antagonist of ER activity[65] and is believed to block the ligand-activated transcriptional activation function (AF-2), while leaving the amino-terminal transactivation function (AF-1) able to initiate gene transcription in a promoter context-dependent and cell-specific fashion.[23,43] However, recent experiments indicate that some ligand-independent ER activation pathways overcome the antagonistic properties of 4HT and render the compound a potent agonist. For example, in transient transfection experiments, 4HT was not only unable to attenuate ER activation by dopaminergic but the resulting level of gene induction was greater than that produced by either compound alone suggesting ligand-independent activation differs mechanistically from the steroid dependent process.[44] Similarly, treatment of MCF-7 cells with PKA activators or delivering constitutively active forms of PKA by DNA transfection techniques shifts the agonist/antagonist balance of this antiestrogen and overcomes its antagonist properties.[66]

In contrast to 4HT, the type II antiestrogens ICI 164,384 and ICI 182,780 exert no agonist activity and are thus classified as "pure".[67] Several mechanisms by which ICI 164,384 blocks ER-dependent gene transcription have been proposed, including reduced steady-state levels of ER expression, increased receptor turnover, and impaired dimerization and DNA binding.[42,68-70] Because these antiestrogens lack agonist activity and they effectively block estrogen-stimulated ER transcriptional activity, they also have been used to establish the ER dependent nature of the ligand-independent pathways discussed above. Indeed, ICI 164,384 and ICI 182,780 block target gene transcription activated by dopamine, EGF, IGF-I, insulin, and heregulin signal transduction pathways as well asestrogen-activated receptor function.[27,44,55-59] Thus, these ICI anti-estrogens act as antagonists with respect to both ligand-dependent and -independent activation pathways, which suggests that type II or "pure" antiestrogens are the compounds of choice when no ER activity is desired.

Perspectives

Estrogens contribute to a wide variety of physiological processes in both health and disease. Molecular biological techniques have contributed substantially to our understanding of the structure and function of the ER and are developed sufficiently in many instances to enable their use in investigations of receptor involvement in estrogen responses in vivo. For instance, antibodies and DNA sequence information can be exploited to identify ER within target tissues and assays exist for the measurement of receptor functions such as ligand binding, DNA binding, and trans-activation. Taken together with the ability to identify genes whose expression is estrogen and ER dependent, it is also possible to examine the downstream mediators of estrogen action.

In addition to estrogen-regulated ER activity, it is now apparent that other agents such as growth factors and neurotransmitters may also contribute to ER-dependent biological responses either in the presence or absence of the estrogen ligand via pathway "cross-talk" from plasma membrane receptors. It is possible that ligand-dependent and -independent signals may act together under certain biological contexts to increase ER activity or alter target gene specificity. However, these pathways may also act independently, and the relative contributions of both pathways to ER activation should therefore be considered when evaluating receptor function in vivo.

References

1. Losordo DW, Kearney M, Kim EA, et al. Variable expression of the estrogen receptor in normal and atherosclerotic coronary arteries of premenopausal women. *Circulation* 1994;89:1501–1510.
2. Pratt WB. Transformation of glucocorticoid and progesterone receptors to the DNA-binding state. *J Cell Biochem* 1987;35:51–68.
3. Denis M, Poellinger L, Wikstrom A, et al. Requirement of hormone for thermal conversion of the glucocorticoid receptor to a DNA-binding state. *Nature* 1988;333:686–688.
4. Bagchi MK, Tsai SY, Tsai M-J, et al. Identification of a functional intermediate in receptor activation in progesterone-dependent cell-free transcription. *Nature* 1990;345:547–550.
5. Allan GF, Leng XH, Tsai SY, et al. Hormone and antihormone induce distinct conformational changes which are central to steroid receptor activation. *J Biol Chem* 1992;267:19513–19520.
6. Kumar V, Chambon P. The estrogen receptor binds tightly to its response element as a ligand-induced homodimer. *Cell* 1988;55:145–156.
7. Tsai SY, Carlstedt-Duke J, Weigel NL, et al. Molecular interactions of steroid hormone receptor with its enhancer element: Evidence for receptor dimer formation. *Cell* 1988;55:361–369.
8. Tsai M-J, O'Malley BW. Molecular mechanisms of action of steroid/thyroid receptor superfamily members. *Annu Rev Biochem* 1994;63:451–486.
9. Wooge CH, Nilsson GM, Heierson A, et al. Structural requirements for high affinity ligand binding by estrogen receptors: A comparative analysis of truncated and full length estrogen receptors expressed in bacteria, yeast, and mammalian cells. *Mol Endocrinol* 1992;6:861–869.
10. Fawell SE, Lees JA, Parker MG. A proposed consensus steroid-binding sequence-a reply. *Mol Endocrinol* 1989;3:1002–1005.
11. Harlow KW, Smith DN, Katzenellenbogen JA, et al. Identification of Cysteine 530 as the covalent attachment site of an affinity-labeling estrogen (Ketononestrol Aziridine) and antiestrogen (Tamoxifen Aziridine) in the human estrogen receptor. *J Biol Chem* 1989;264: 17476–17485.
12. Reese JC, Wooge CH, Katzenellenbogen BS. Identification of two cysteines closely positioned in the ligand-binding pocket of the human estrogen receptor: Roles in ligand binding and transcriptional activation. *Mol Endocrinol* 1992;6:2160–2166.
13. Pakdel F, Katzenellenbogen BS. Human estrogen receptor mutants with altered estrogen and antiestrogen ligand discrimination. *J Biol Chem* 1992;267:3429–3437.

14. Beekman JM, Allan GF, Tsai SY, et al. Transcriptional activation by the estrogen receptor requires a conformational change in the ligand binding domain. *Mol Endocrinol* 1993;7:1266–1274.
15. Freedman LP. Anatomy of the steroid receptor zinc finger region. *Endocr Rev* 1992;13:129–145.
16. Green S, Chambon P. The oestrogen receptor: From perception to mechanism. In: Parker MG, ed. *Nuclear Hormone Receptors* San Diego: Academic Press Ltd; 1991:15–38.
17. Chandler VL, Maler BA, Yamamoto KR. DNA sequences bound specifically by glucocorticoid receptor *in vitro* render a heterologous promoter hormone responsive *in vivo*. *Cell* 1983;33:489–499.
18. Klein-Hitpass L, Schorpp M, Wagner U, et al. An estrogen-responsive element derived from the 5'-flanking region of the Xenopus vitellogenin A2 gene functions in transfected human cells. *Cell* 1986;46:1053–1061.
19. Kraus WL, Montano MM, Katzenellenbogen BS. Cloning of the rat progesterone receptor gene 5'-region and identification of two functionally distinct promoters. *Mol Endocrinol* 1993;7:1603–1616.
20. Lee JH, Kim J, Shapiro DJ. Regulation of *Xenopus laevis* estrogen receptor gene expression is mediated by an estrogen response element in the protein coding region. *DNA Cell Biol* 1995;14:419–430.
21. Tora L, White JH, Brou C, et al. The human estrogen receptor has two independent nonacidic transcriptional activation functions. *Cell* 1989; 59:477–487.
22. Kumar V, Green S, Stack G, et al. Functional domains of the human estrogen receptor. *Cell* 1987;51:941–951.
23. Webster NJG, Green S, Jin J, et al. The hormone-binding domains of the estrogen and glucocorticoid receptors contain an inducible transcription activation function. *Cell* 1988;54:199–207.
24. Lees JA, Fawell SE, Parker MG. Identification of two transactivation domain in the mouse oestrogen receptor. *Nucleic Acids Res* 1989; 17:5477–5487.
25. Montano MM, Müller V, Trobaugh A, et al. The carboxy-terminal F domain of the human estrogen receptor: Role in the transcriptional activity of the receptor and the effectiveness of antiestrogens as estrogen antagonists. *Mol Endocrinol* 1995;9:814–825.
26. Metzger D, Ali S, Bornert JM, et al. Characterization of the amino-terminal transcriptional activation function of the human estrogen receptor in animal and yeast cells. *J Biol Chem* 1995;270:9535–9542.
27. Aronica SM, Katzenellenbogen BS. Stimulation of estrogen receptor-mediated transcription and alteration in the phosphorylation state of the rat uterine estrogen receptor by estrogen, cyclic adenosine monophosphate, and insulin-like growth factor-1. *Mol Endocrinol* 1993;7:743–752.
28. Washburn TF, Hocutt A, Brautigan DL, et al. Uterine estrogen receptor in vivo: Phosphorylation of nuclear specific forms on serine residues. *Mol Endocrinol* 1991;5:235–242.
29. Denton RR, Koszewski NJ, Notides AC. Estrogen receptor phosphorylation. *J Biol Chem* 1992;267:7263–7268.
30. Arnold SF, Obourn JD, Jaffe H, et al. Serine 167 is the major estradiol-induced phosphorylation site on the human estrogen receptor. *Mol Endocrinol* 1994;8:1208–1214.
31. Ali S, Metzger D, Bornert JM, et al. Modulation of transcriptional activation by ligand-dependent phosphorylation of the human oestrogen receptor A/B region. *EMBO J* 1993;12:1153–1160.

32. Lahooti H, White R, Danielian PS, et al. Characterization of ligand-dependent phosphorylation of the estrogen receptor. *Mol Endocrinol* 1994;8:182–188.
33. Goff PL, Montano MM, Schodin DJ, et al. Phosphorylation of human estrogen receptor: Identification of hormone-regulated sites and examination of their influence on transcriptional activity. *J Biol Chem* 1994;269:4458–4466.
34. Joel PB, Traish AM, Lannigan DA. Estradiol and phorbol ester cause phosphorylation of serine 118 in the human estrogen receptor. *Mol Endocrinol* 1995;9:1041–1052.
35. Orti E, Bodwell JE, Munck A. Phosphorylation of steroid hormone receptors. *Endocr Rev* 1992;13:105–128.
36. Bagchi MK, Tsai SY, Tsai M-J, et al. Ligand and DNA-dependent phosphorylation of human progesterone receptor in vitro. *Proc Natl Acad Sci USA* 1992;89:2664–2668.
37. Weigel NL, Carter TH, Schrader WT, et al. Chicken progesterone receptor is phosphorylated by a DNA-dependent protein kinase during in vitro transcription assays. *Mol Endocrinol* 1992;6:8–14.
38. Denner LA, Weigel NL, Maxwell BL, et al. Regulation of progesterone receptor-mediated transcription by phosphorylation. *Science* 1990;250:1740–1743.
39. Power RF, Lydon JP, Conneely OM, et al. Dopamine activation of an orphan member of the steroid receptor superfamily. *Science* 1991; 252:1546–1548.
40. Power RF, Mani SK, Codina J, et al. Dopaminergic and ligand-independent activation of steroid hormone receptors. *Science* 1991;254:1636–1639.
41. Cho H, Katzenellenbogen BS. Synergistic activation of estrogen receptor-mediated transcription by estradiol and protein kinase activators. *Mol Endocrinol* 1993;7:441–452.
42. Reese JC, Katzenellenbogen BS. Examination of the DNA-binding ability of estrogen receptor in whole cells: Implications for hormone-independent transactivation and the actions of antiestrogens. *Mol Cell Biol* 1992;12:4531–4538.
43. Berry M, Metzger D, Chambon P. Role of the two activating domains of the oestrogen receptor in the cell-type and promoter-context dependent agonistic activity of the anti-oestrogen 4-hydroytamonifen. *EMBO J* 1990;9:2811–2812.
44. Smith CL, Conneely OM, O'Malley BW. Modulation of the ligand-independent activation of the human estrogen receptor by hormone and antihormone. *Proc Natl Acad Sci USA* 1993;90:6120–6124.
45. Smith CL, Conneely OM, O'Malley BW. Oestrogen receptor activation in the absence of ligand. *Biochem Soc Trans* 1995;23:935–939.
46. Jackson DM, Westlind-Danielsson A. Dopamine receptors: Molecular biology, biochemistry and behavioural aspects. *Pharmacol Ther* 1994; 64:291–369.
47. Kebabian JW, Caine DB. Multiple receptors for dopamine. *Nature* 1979;277:93–96.
48. Felder CC, Blecher M, Jose PA. Dopamine-1-mediated stimulation of phospholipase C activity in rat renal cortical membranes. *J Biol Chem* 1989;264:8739–8745.
49. Kansra V, Chen C, Lokhandwala MF. Dopamine causes stimulation of protein kinase C in rat renal proximal tubules by activating dopamine D1 receptors. *Eur J Pharmacol* 1995;289:391–394.

50. Sumida C, Lecerf F, Pasqualini JR. Control of progesterone receptors in fetal uterine cells in culture: Effects of estradiol, progestins, antiestrogens and growth factors. *Endocrinology* 1988;122:3–11.
51. Sumida C, Pasqualini JR. Antiestrogens antagonize the stimulatory effect of epidermal growth factor on the induction of progesterone receptor in fetal uterine cells in culture. *Endocrinology* 1989;124:591–597.
52. Katzenellenbogen BS, Norman MJ. Multihormonal regulation of the progesterone receptor in MCF-7 human breast cancer cells: Interrelationships among insulin/insulin-like growth factor-I, serum, and estrogen. *Endocrinology* 1990;126:891–898.
53. Aronica SM, Katzenellenbogen BS. Progesterone receptor regulation in uterine cells: stimulation by estrogen, cyclic adenosine 3',5'-monophosphate, and insulin-like growth factor I and suppression by antiestrogens and protein kinase inhibitors. *Endocrinology* 1991; 128:2045–2052.
54. Nelson KG, Takahashi T, Bossert NL, et al. Epidermal growth factor replaces estrogen in the stimulation of female genital-tract growth and differentiation. *Proc Natl Acad Sci USA* 1991;88:21–25.
55. Newton CJ, Buric R, Trapp T, et al. The unliganded estrogen receptor (ER) transduces growth factor signals. *J Steroid Biochem Mol Biol* 1994;48:481–486.
56. Ma ZQ, Santagati S, Patrone C, et al. Insulin-like growth factors activate estrogen receptor to control the growth and differentiation of the human neuroblastoma cell line SK-ER3. *Mol Endocrinol* 1994;8:910–918.
57. Pietras RJ, Arboleda J, Reese DM, et al. HER-2 tyrosine kinase pathway targets estrogen receptor and promotes hormone-independent growth in human breast cancer cells. *Oncogene* 1995;10:2435–2446.
58. Ignar-Trowbridge DM, Teng CT, Ross KA, et al. Peptide growth factors elicit estrogen receptor-dependent transcriptional activation of an estrogen-responsive element. *Mol Endocrinol* 1993;7:992–998.
59. Smith CL, Conneely OM, O'Malley BW. Estrogen receptor activation by ligand-dependent and ligand-independent pathways. In: Moudgil VK, ed. *Steroid Receptors in Health and Disease* Boston: Birkhauser; 1993: 333–356.
60. Earp HS, Dawson TL, Li X, et al. Heterodimerization and functional interaction between EGF receptor family members: A new signaling paradigm with implications for breast cancer research. *Breast Cancer Res Treat* 1995;35:115–132.
61. Schmid C. Insulin-like growth factors. *Cell Biol Int* 1995;19:445–457.
62. Kumar V, Bustin SA, McKay IA. Transforming growth factor alpha. *Cell Biol Int* 1995;19:373–388.
63. Boonstra J, Rijken P, Humbel B, et al. The epidermal growth factor. *Cell Biol Int* 1995;19:413–430.
64. Ignar-Trowbridge DM, Nelson KG, Bidwell MC, et al. Coupling of dual signaling pathways: Epidermal growth factor action involves the estrogen receptor. *Proc Natl Acad Sci USA* 1992;89:4658–4662.
65. Jordan VC. Biochemical pharmacology of antiestrogen action. *Pharmacol Rev* 1984;36:245–276.
66. Fujimoto N, Katzenellenbogen BS. Alteration in the agonist/antagonist balance of antiestrogens by activation of protein kinase A signaling pathways in breast cancer cells: Antiestrogen selectively and promoter dependence. *Mol Endocrinol* 1994;8:296–304.

67. Wakeling AE, Bowler J. Novel antioestrogens without partial agonist activity. *J Steroid Biochem* 1988;31:645–653.
68. Fawell SE, White R, Hoare S, et al. Inhibition of estrogen receptor-DNA binding by the "pure" antiestrogen ICI 164,384 appears to be mediated by impaired receptor dimerization. *Proc Natl Acad Sci USA* 1990; 87:6883–6887.
69. Dauvois S, Danielian S, Parker MG. Antiestrogen ICI 164,384 reduces cellular estrogen receptor content by increasing its turnover. *Proc Natl Acad Sci USA* 1992;89:4037–4041.
70. Gibson MK, Nemmers LA, Beckman WC Jr, et al. The mechanism of ICI 164,384 antiestrogenicity involves rapid loss of estrogen receptor in uterine tissue. *Endocrinology* 1991;129:2000–2010.

Chapter 5

Cardiovascular Estrogen Receptors Regulate Vascular Smooth Muscle Cell Proliferation

Ioakim Spyridopoulos, MD and
Douglas W. Losordo, MD

Epidemiological data indicate that premenopausal women are at lower risk of coronary heart disease than are men of similar age.[1-5] The increased incidence of atherosclerosis in women who undergo premature menopause has also been well described.[6-11] Finally, there is increasing evidence that treatment with replacement estrogen after menopause will reduce cardiovascular mortality.[12-14]

Animal studies have provided further evidence of estrogen's effects on the vascular system. Estrogen treatment prevented collagen and elastin accumulation in the aortic wall in normotensive[15] and thickening of the aorta in hypertensive rats[16] and similarly suppressed atherosclerosis in primate coronary arteries.[17] Alternatively, progesterone (Pr) administered alone resulted in an increase in fatty streak formation in castrated baboons, whereas animals receiving estradiol (E_2) and Pr together had the fewest lesions.[18] Thus, in an intact animal preparation, there have been multiple studies suggesting an effect of sex steroids on vascular biology, specifically alluding to an anti-proliferative effect of estrogen and raising the question of a synergistic effect of progesterone. These studies lend experimental support to the hypothesis, brought forward by epidemiological studies, that female sex hormones are protective against coronary atherosclerosis. What these studies do not address, however, is the mechanism(s) whereby the presence of estrogen is translated into an effect on the biology of the arterial wall.

Endogenous and exogenous estrogens have been observed to alter the levels of serum lipids[7,12,19] and lipid metabolism in hu-

From: Forte TM, (ed). *Hormonal, Metabolic, and Cellular Influences on Cardiovascular Disease in Women.* Armonk, NY: Futura Publishing Company, Inc.; © 1997.

mans.[20,21] In experimental animals fed an atherogenic diet, administration of estrogen inhibited[22-24] or reversed[25] atheroma formation, associated with reversion of lipid levels toward normal. Thus, well-established experimental animal data have demonstrated an atheroprotective effect of estrogen. These studies also demonstrate that estrogen administration results in a more normal lipid profile in animals fed a high-cholesterol diet. Furthermore, these studies are corroborated by human evidence demonstrating a favorable alteration in lipid levels in the presence of endogenous or exogenously administered estrogen, as well as changes in lipid metabolism, which would explain these alterations in lipoprotein profiles.

Early human clinical data suggested that progesterone tended to mitigate the beneficial effect of estrogen on serum lipids.[19,21] More recent studies, however, have demonstrated no significant attenuation of the salutary effects on serum lipid profiles induced by estrogen replacement in postmenopausal women.[14,26]

The experimental animal and human data provide a partial explanation for the salutary effect of estrogen on the incidence of coronary atherosclerosis. The changes in serum lipids noted in human patients, however, fail to account fully for the discrepancy in the incidence of coronary disease between men and premenopausal women.[13,27]

Direct Effects of Estrogen on Vascular Tissue

A direct effect of estrogen on the arterial wall is suggested by animal and human experimental data. Vasodilation in response to estrogen administration was first noted in the rabbit ear artery[28] and later in human umbilical[29] and primate coronary arteries.[30] Gender differences in the contractile response of the aorta in rats have been shown,[31] as has estrogen dependent sexual dimorphism of rat VSMC. Recently, acute administration of estradiol has been shown to attenuate abnormal coronary vasomotor responses in postmenopausal women.[32,33] Although this experimental evidence furthers the suggestion of a direct estrogen effect on vascular tissue, neither a systemic effect nor a nonreceptor mediated effect of estrogen are excluded by these studies.

Examination of vascular smooth muscle cells in culture, however, has provided further data suggesting a direct estrogen effect on vascular tissue. Nichols et al.[34] demonstrated decreased protein synthesis in rat vascular smooth muscle cells in culture when they are exposed to estrogen. Isolating vascular tissue from the systemic effects of sex steroid administration in this study, therefore, provided evidence of a direct effect of E_2 on cells of the artery wall.

Vascular Tissues Express Functional Estrogen Receptor

Estrogen, as is the case with all steroids, acts by binding to a specific receptor. Establishing a direct, genomically mediated mechanism of E_2 action on the vessel wall therefore requires demonstration of estrogen receptor (ER) in the target tissue. ER has been demonstrated in canine peripheral[35] and coronary[36] arteries, in cultured rat aortic VSMC[37] and in human vascular endothelial cells.[38] Smooth muscle cells at low passage in culture have been shown to retain the estrogen receptor expression of the parent tissue.[39] Finally, an association between E_2 stimulation (in these ER containing tissues) and physiological effect has been demonstrated.[36,40,41] The actual function of the ER, however, and the cellular mechanisms that translate E_2-ER interaction into physiological effect on the arterial wall remain to be defined.

The ER belongs to the nuclear receptor superfamily, a class of ligand activated transcription factors that includes 30 receptors, including steroid hormone and thyroid hormone receptors, as well as vitamin D3 and retinoic acid receptors. Classical steroid hormone receptors form homodimers and recognize short palindromic DNA sequences (steroid response elements) often located upstream from their target genes.[42–44] Recent evidence, however, has challenged the assumption that all nuclear receptors act via a single unique palindromic DNA sequence.[45]

Early studies suggested that the unbound ER was located in the cytoplasm and that after binding its ligand the receptor translocated to the nucleus due to an increase in the receptor's affinity for chromatin.[46] More recent work, however, has demonstrated both occupied and unoccupied ER residing in the nucleus.[47,48] ER probably interacts with DNA, chromosomal proteins, and a nuclear chromatin scaffolding structure that may regulate translation and transcriptional activity.[49–52]

Clones of the 2.2-kb ER cDNA have been sequenced from the human breast cancer cell line MCF-7 demonstrating an open reading frame of 1,785 nucleotides sufficient to encode ER.[53] The mRNA codes for a 66 kd protein with strong structural homology to glucocorticoid receptor as well as to the v-erb-A protein of the oncogenic avian erythroblastosis virus. Conservation of the cysteine-rich and hydrophobic regions in these sequences supports the assertion that they are important functional domains, although the complete significance of this homology has not been clarified.

Steroid receptor monomers become quickly bound to the abundant 90-kd heat shock protein (HSP 90) dimer. Binding of cognate hormone to receptor releases the HSP 90 molecule in its dimered form. The receptor, now in its activated state is capable of both homodimerization and DNA binding. In addition to HSP 90, the 27-kd heat shock protein has been shown to be transcriptionally induced by estrogen. The function of this latter protein is uncertain but is known to be phosphorylated to several forms. A relation between estrogen receptor activation, HSP 27 phosphorylation and platelet activity has been suggested.[54] HSP 90, on the other hand, has been shown to participate directly in the signal transduction pathway for steroid receptors.[55]

Much of what has been learned regarding the biological and biochemical effects of the E_2-ER interaction has been derived from study of human breast cancer cells. In these in vitro model systems, E_2 induces a number of enzymes involved in nucleic acid synthesis.[56,57] DNA synthesis by scavenger and de novo pathways is also stimulated.[58] E_2 regulates thymidine kinase and dihydrofolate at the mRNA and translational levels, although the genes that are regulated in this process have not been identified.[57,59,60]

In fact, the exact mechanisms of regulation of cell proliferation by E_2 remain to be clarified. Several hypotheses have been explored regarding the E_2-proliferation link that are useful to consider as a framework for examining the E_2-ER role in arterial wall biology. All of these putative mechanisms have been developed in an attempt to understand the role of estrogen as a synergist or catalyst of proliferative activity, a role directly opposite of that envisioned for E_2 in atherosclerosis. Still it is helpful to consider these same types of actions, if acting in reverse, as theoretical possibilities for E_2 action on human vascular smooth muscle cell (hVSMC) biology. A direct positive mechanism would have E_2 directly triggering the proliferation of target cells. A direct mitogenic effect of E_2 has been shown, for example, in the prepubertal rat uterus.[61] In an indirect-positive model, E_2 induces the production of growth factors, which then result in target cell division.[62] In this model, the growth factors are produced by cells other than the target cells whereas in an autocrine mechanism the target cells themselves elucidate the second messenger.[63]

Recently estrogens have been shown to mediate growth arrest and differentiation in a neuroblastoma cell line.[64] This study demonstrated the involvement of activated ER in metabolic changes leading cells toward a differentiated/nonproliferating state.

Many eukaryotic genes are under the control of multiple hormones, and steroid response elements can be found in multiple copies or tightly clustered with other *cis*-acting DNA elements.[65] Synergism between the estrogen receptor and progesterone receptor has been demonstrated in vitro, but this effect does not appear to result from cooperative binding to their respective response elements.[65] In addition, certain progestins can exhibit estrogenic potential and this effect does appear to be mediated by the estrogen receptor as evidenced by its inhibition by anti-estrogens.[66] Important E_2-Pr interactions have been reported by several investigators.[67-71] The exact nature of this interaction remains to be well characterized.

Thus epidemiological and experimental evidence point to a significant effect of estrogen on vascular biology and suggest the possibility of a direct estrogen effect on cells of the arterial wall.

Although part of the atheroprotective effect of E_2 is mediated by amelioration of serum lipid patterns, a portion of E_2's beneficial effect is not explained by changes in lipids. We theorized that a direct effect of E_2 on the arterial wall was also possible. To exert a direct genomic effect, however, expression of a functional ER would be required. Accordingly, we performed a series of investigations to identify such a receptor in hVSMC[72.]

Estrogen Receptor Expression in Human Vascular Smooth Muscle Cells

Cultures of hVSMC were grown by the explant outgrowth technique as previously reported. This technique has been used successfully in our laboratory to derive cultures of hVSMC from normal arteries as well as from atherosclerotic plaque obtained by directional atherectomy.[73] The identity of the cells in culture is confirmed by staining with antibody to smooth muscle α-actin.

Assay for ER in this system was performed by adapting a technique previously established for receptor assay in breast carcinoma tissue to the assay of ER in hVSMC culture.[37,74] Briefly, hVSMC in their second passage were exposed to tritiated estrogen in concentrations from 1 to 40 nM, alone or in the presence of a 200-fold concentration excess of unlabeled diethylstilbesterol. Cells were incubated for 30 minutes at 37°C and then placed on ice. After washing the cells in PBS, E_2-ER binding was solubilized by the addition of ethanol and bound radioactivity was assayed by liquid scintillation counting.

As shown in Figure 1, characteristic saturation plots were generated from these studies. The binding of receptors was saturable in the concentration range studied, similar to results obtained of ER binding in VSMC culture of other species.[37] The binding curve on the bottom of Figure 1 indicates specific binding of the radiolabeled ligand to estrogen receptor in hVSMC. The binding curve demonstrated here could not be caused by nonspecific interaction of labeled steroid, as this is controlled by the series of experiments performed in the presence of 200-fold excess unlabeled DES. From this same data, the precise quantity of estrogen receptors is calculated to equal 1.16×10^{-13} M/10^6 hVSMC. These data also represent a high-affinity estrogen receptor as is indicated by the calculated Kd of 8×10^{-9}.

These data represent the first verification of high-affinity estrogen receptors in hVSMC and since have been confirmed by others.[75]

Estradiol Dependent Binding of hVSMC ER to an Estrogen-Responsive Element in Vitro

Steroid responsive elements are inducible regulatory DNA sequences that interact with their receptors and modulate transcription of target genes. The "estrogen-responsive element"(ERE) has been shown to bind the ER only when the latter is induced by its ligand. Previous studies have demonstrated a 13-bp palindrome (5'-GGTCACAGTGACC-3') that is the minimal DNA sequence sufficient for significant estrogen induction and specific binding of ER.[76,77] The interaction of hormone-bound ER with the ERE has been shown to alter the transcriptional efficiency of ERE containing genes. Efficient binding of ligand-induced ER to the ERE is therefore a useful measure of the functional integrity of putative receptors.

We examined the ability of ERs from hVSMC to bind ERE using gel mobility assays. This assay is based on the fact that protein-bound DNA migrates more slowly through a polyacrylamide gel than unbound DNA. In the presence of estrogen, the estrogen receptor should form a complex with the estrogen-response element. By labeling the response element with ^{32}P, the complexes can be identified by their altered electrophoretic mobility.

Confluent 100-mm plates of cultured hVSMC were incubated in 10% charcoal stripped FBS in phenol red free M199 for 48

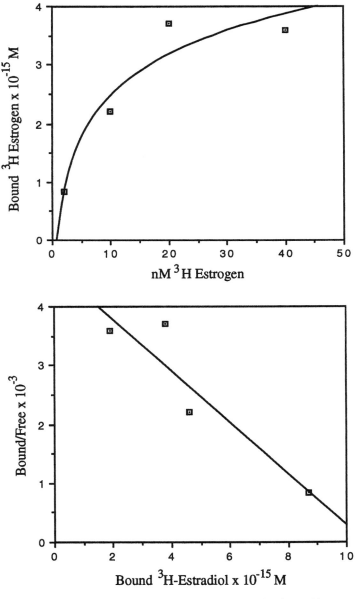

FIGURE 1. *Binding curves generated by incubation of cultured hVSMC with* ³H-estradiol. **Top:** *Specifically bound labeled estradiol (calculated by subtracting binding that occurred in the presence of unlabeled 1,000-fold excess estradiol from* ³H-estradiol *binding in cells incubated with only labeled hormone) is plotted against concentration of labeled estradiol. The equation generating the rectangular hyperbola curve is* $Y = A*X/(B+X)$ *where* $A = Bmax$ *and* $B = Kd$ **Bottom:** *Scatchard plot of* ³H-*estradiol binding in hVSMC.*

hours after which some of the cells were exposed to estradiol (10^{-7} M) for 1 hour. Cells then were lysed by freezing at $-80°C$ in 0.1 mL of buffer containing 20 mM Tris-HCl, 2 mM DTT, 0.4 M KCl, and 20% glycerol. Cells were thawed over ice and centrifuged for 20 minutes at 4°C. The supernatant was used as the crude whole-cell extract. Previously published sequences for the estrogen-response element (ERE)[78] were synthesized commercially and dimerized at room temperature to form a double stranded oligonucleotide probe. The 37-bp probe containing the ERE was end labeled with ^{32}P in a reaction catalyzed by T4 polynucleotide kinase according to the manufacturers guidelines. (Promega, Madison, WI). Whole-cell extracts from hVSMC that had been incubated in the presence or absence of estradiol were incubated with binding buffer for 10 minutes [final buffer concentrations (in mM) were 1 $MgCl_2$, 0.5 EDTA, 0.5 DTT, 50 NaCl, and 10 Tris-HCl plus 0.05 mg/mL poly(dI-dC)]. The labeled oligonucleotide then was added, and the mixture incubated at room temperature for 20 minutes. Reactions were terminated by adding a gel loading buffer containing 250 mM Tris-HCl, 40% glycerol, 0.2% bromphenol blue, and 0.2% xylene cyanol. Controls included addition of excess unlabeled oligonucleotide probe, exclusion of estradiol, exclusion of cell extract, and exclusion of labeled oligonucleotide. Reactions were run on a 5% nondenaturing acrylamide gel. The gel was pre-run for 30 minutes at 20 mA at 4°C and then run at 30 mA at 4°C until the bromphenol dye was approximately half-way down the gel. The gel then was vacuum dried and exposed to autoradiography film overnight at $-80°C$.

As shown in Figure 2 specific and ligand-dependent binding of hVSMC ER to its cognate response element is demonstrated. Only the combination of extract from E_2 exposed cells and labeled ERE probe produces the "shifted" band corresponding to the DNA-receptor complex.

Confirmation of the presence and functional integrity of ER in hVSMC suggests that a direct effect of E_2 on human arteries is a possibility. If the atheroprotective effect of estrogen is mediated, in part, by direct action on the arterial wall, we reasoned, it is possible that the occurrence of coronary atherosclerosis in female patients may be precipitated by one of two events: the loss of circulating ligand (estrogen) or absolute or relative lack of (estrogen) receptor expression by target cells in the arterial wall. The first of these two situations occurs when female patients reach menopause, and this is associated with an increase in the incidence of coronary disease. The latter possibility, however, has not been previously investigated.

WCE	+	+	+	+	-
E₂	+	+	-	+	
LABEL	+	-	+	+	+
XS UN-LAB	-	-	-	+	-

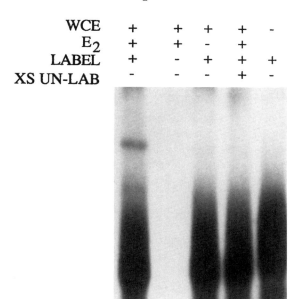

FIGURE 2. *Gel mobility assay. Band in left lane corresponds to complex of estrogen receptor and labeled estrogen response element. Controls included exclusion of labeled oligonucleotide probe, exclusion of estradiol (rendering receptor "inactive"), addition of excess unlabeled oligonucleotide (which competes for binding to the estrogen receptor preventing binding of labeled probe), and exclusion of cell extract. All controls are appropriately negative, indicated by the absence of the band seen in lane 1. E₂, estradiol; label, labeled oligonucleotide probe; WCE, whole-cell extract; XS UNLAB, excess unlabeled oligonucleotide probe.*

Demonstration of Decreased Estrogen-Receptor Expression in Atherosclerotic Coronary Arteries

Accordingly, an investigation was performed to test the hypothesis that premature atherosclerosis in female patients may be mediated by a failure of target cells in the vessel wall to adequately express estrogen receptor, therefore abrogating the possibility of atheroprotection by circulating estrogen. To test this hypothesis, we examined coronary artery specimens from female patients. We surveyed the autopsy records of St. Elizabeth's Hospital for the past 10 years to identify pre- and postmenopausal female patients with nor-

mal and atherosclerotic coronary arteries. Our intention was to identify as many premenopausal subjects as possible, because the testing of our hypothesis would be based largely on our examination
of these tissues. The distribution of subjects identified in our
search of the records is shown in Table 1 and included 18 premenopausal and 22 postmenopausal females. The coronary arteries of these patients were classified as normal in 21 subjects and
atherosclerotic in 19 subjects, based on the histological examination of the specimens.

Evaluation of estrogen-receptor expression in these coronary artery specimens was performed using a monoclonal antibody to the
estrogen receptor (H222spγ, Abbott Labs, Abbott Park, IL). Although this technique was designed for use on fresh tissue, modifications in the preparations of specimens have permitted detection
of estrogen receptor in formalin-fixed, paraffin imbedded tissue.[79]
To ensure the reliability of this technique, positive control tissue
consisting of a breast carcinoma, previously shown by radioligand
binding assays to express high levels of estrogen receptor, was used
in all of the immunohistochemical staining runs on the coronary
specimens. Examples of coronary artery specimens from premenopausal females with normal and atherosclerotic arteries are shown
in Figures 3 and 4, respectively.

Estrogen-receptor expression in the coronary arteries of all subjects studied is shown in Table 2. Of 21 normal arteries studied, 15
of these showed evidence of estrogen receptor expression, whereas
in 19 atherosclerotic arteries, 13 showed no evidence of estrogen
receptor expression when assayed immunohistochemically. Contin-
gency table analysis revealed that the differences between these
groups were statistically significant with $P = 0.0117$.

Interestingly, when the results of the immunohistochemical
staining for ER expression in the coronary arteries of postmeno-

TABLE 1

	n	Age
Premenopausal	18	31.6 ± 1.9
Normal	12	31.2 ± 2.1
Atherosclerotic	6	32.6 ± 4.3
Postmenopausal	22	71.8 ± 2.3
Normal	9	75.1 ± 5.0
Atherosclerotic	13	69.4 ± 1.7

Values are means ± SE. *P* is nonsignificant for both groups.

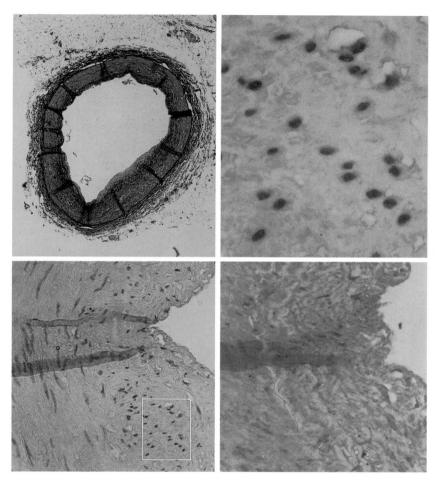

FIGURE 3. *Left, top:* Elastic-trichrome stain reveals minimal intimal thickening in this coronary artery specimen from a premenopausal female who died from noncardiac causes. *Left, bottom:* Immunohistochemical staining for estrogen receptor, coronary artery: Low-power(×100) view of the same artery after staining with monoclonal antibody to estrogen receptor. Blue staining of cell nuclei indicates positive staining for estrogen receptor. Artifact is due to folding of specimen during processing for histology. Area enclosed in white border is shown at high power above right. *Right, top:* High power (×330) view of same section of premenopausal coronary artery demonstrating immunologic evidence of estrogen receptor, indicated by intense blue-black staining of nuclei. *Right, bottom:* Adjacent section of same artery stained with antibody to smooth muscle α-actin to confirm presence of vascular smooth muscle cells in the region of the artery also positive for estrogen receptor expression.

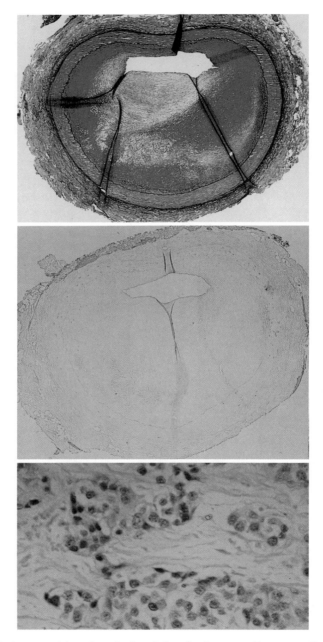

FIGURE 4. *Immunohistochemical staining for Estrogen Receptor.* **Top:** *Elastic trichrome stain of severely atherosclerotic artery from a premenopausal female reveals extensive disease.* **Middle:** *Immunohistochemical staining for estrogen receptor, coronary artery; photomicrographs (×100) of same coronary artery stained with antibody for estrogen receptor demonstrates no evidence of estrogen receptor protein.* **Bottom:** *Immunohistochemical staining for estrogen receptor; breast carcinoma: positive control tissue demonstrating positive staining for the presence of estrogen receptor.*

TABLE 2

	All patients		Premenopausal		Postmenopausal	
	Normal	Athero	Normal	Athero	Normal	Athero
Estrogen receptors						
+	15	6	10	1	5	4
−	6	13	2	5	4	8

Differences between normal and atherosclerotic coronary arteries are: all patients, $P = 0.0117$; premenopausal patients, $P = 0.0062$; postmenopausal patients, $P =$ nonsignificant.

pausal subjects were analyzed separately (Table 2, right panel), the impact of estrogen receptor expression was no longer evident. In nine normal coronary arteries of postmenopausal female patients, estrogen receptor expression was evident in five and was absent in four. In the atherosclerotic arteries, only 4 out of 12 arteries showed evidence of estrogen receptor expression. The differences in ER expression between these groups did not achieve statistical significance.

When the results of ER staining of coronary arteries of premenopausal females were analyzed separately, however, the association between estrogen receptor expression and absence of coronary atherosclerosis was again evident and apparently was responsible for the statistical association noted in the total population studied. In 12 normal arteries, estrogen-receptor expression was shown immunohistochemically in 10 patients, whereas, in 6 atherosclerotic arteries, 5 showed no evidence of estrogen receptor expression. The differences were highly statistically significant with $P = 0.0062$.

These results demonstrate a strong association between estrogen receptor expression and the absence of coronary atherosclerosis in premenopausal women. The absence of this relation in postmenopausal women could be explained by the estrogen-deficient state of the subjects, making the presence of the receptor alone insufficient to exert an atheroprotective effect. This data provide further evidence suggesting a direct action of estrogen in protecting arteries from atherosclerosis. Still, the mere association of estrogen receptor expression and the absence of coronary atherosclerosis in premenopausal women does not establish a cause and effect relation, nor does it provide any information regarding the functionality of the receptor.

Antiproliferative Effect of Estrogen on Human Vascular Smooth Muscle Cells

After establishing ER expression in hVSMC, establishing that ER derived from hVSMC are functionally intact, and demonstrating a relation between ER expression and the absence of atherosclerosis in human arteries, our next goal was to provide further evidence of transcriptional regulation of these receptors. The goal of the next series of preliminary experiments, therefore, was to observe hVSMC in culture for different patterns of behavior in response to varying concentrations of estrogen in the cell culture medium. In this series of experiments, we evaluated the effect of estrogen on proliferative activity as determined by thymidine incorporation.

The experimental design of these studies can be outlined as follows. Human VSMC in their second passage were subcultured and grown in standard medium for 48 hours. After 48 hours, the medium was supplemented with serum containing varying concentrations of estradiol: 10% pooled serum from human male donors (estrogen concentration = 40 pg/mL ≈ 1.5×10^{-10} M), 10% pooled serum from human female donors (estrogen concentration = 270 pg/mL ≈ 10^{-9} M, progesterone concentration 18.5 ng/mL ≈ 5×10^{-8} M), 10% pooled serum from male donors with the addition of estradiol in concentrations ranging from 10^{-10} M to 10^{-7} M. The strategy for utilizing human serum in these studies was to evaluate the effect of estrogen upon hVSMC behavior in a growth medium that contains all of the elements of human serum.

Forty-eight hours after subculture, cells were supplemented with serum containing varying concentrations of estradiol. Twenty-four hours after the addition of the supplemented serum, tritiated thymidine was added to the culture medium of each well (3 μCi/ well), and liquid scintillation counting was performed at 2, 4, 24, and 48 hours. All assays were performed in triplicate.

The results of these assays are shown in Figure 5. In hVSMC cultures, the cells that were grown in medium supplemented by male serum (far left column) demonstrated significantly greater thymidine incorporation than those cells from the same population grown in medium supplemented by serum from female patients (second column). Furthermore, the proliferative effect of male serum on hVSMC in culture was mitigated in part by the addition of estradiol to the culture medium (middle column). This effect is not altered by the addition of varying concentrations of progesterone to the culture medium (right columns).

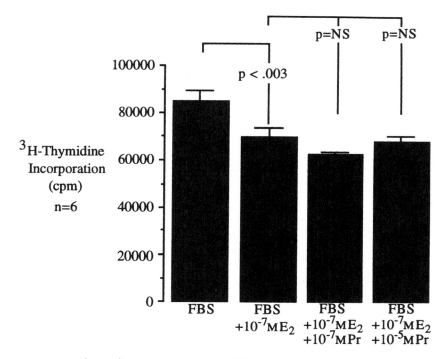

FIGURE 5. *Thymidine incorporation of hVSMC in culture. Thymidine incorporation of cultured hVSMC in fetal bovine serum (FBS) (dextran-charcoal treated to remove all steroid hormones) before and after supplementation with estradiol (10^{-7} M) in the presence or absence of progesterone. After 24 hours, tritiated thymidine was added to the cell cultures and assay for thymidine incorporation was performed by liquid scintillation counting 48 hours later. Thymidine incorporation was significantly greater when cells were incubated in hormone-free FBS and was diminished by the addition of estradiol. The antiproliferative effect of estradiol on human vascular smooth muscle cells is not altered by the addition of progesterone.*

The inhibitory effect of estradiol on proliferative activity of hVSMC in culture is further supported by a dose-response relation with higher doses of estradiol resulting in incremental inhibition of proliferative activity. The design of these experiments was identical to that described above. Cultures of hVSMC derived from the same artery or grown under identical conditions in defined media until serum with varying concentrations of estradiol was added. Tritiated thymidine was added to the culture medium, and thymidine incorporation was assayed after 48 hours. As shown in Figure

6, male serum, with the lowest estradiol concentration, induced the greatest proliferative activity of cultured hVSMC. With the addition of 10^{-9} M, estradiol the proliferative activity of the cells was diminished significantly. A further decrease in proliferative activity was demonstrated when the estradiol concentration was increased further to 10^{-7} M.

Antiproliferative Effect of Estrogen is Mediated by Estrogen Receptor

Tamoxifen is known widely as an "anti-estrogen" for its role in treating estrogen-sensitive breast carcinoma. Tamoxifen does bind to the estrogen receptor and will inhibit the effects of estrogen, when it is present in significant concentrations, in tissues which express a functional estrogen receptor. Tamoxifen is also, however, a partial

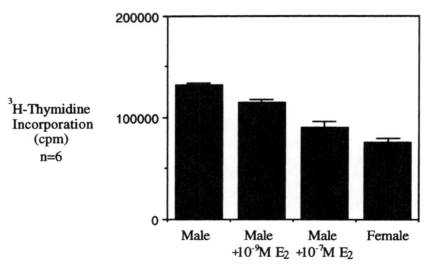

FIGURE 6. *Estradiol dose-response relation. Thymidine incorporation of cultured hVSMC incubated in serum from males(estradiol concentrations 10^{-10} M), before and after the addition of supplemental estradiol. Thymidine incorporation of the same hVSMC (derived from the same donor tissue) incubated with serum from premenopausal females (estradiol concentration 10^{-9} M) is shown for comparison. Decremental thymidine incorporation is seen with incremental concentrations of estradiol added to the male serum.*

antagonist in its own right that will mimic, to some extent, the effects of estrogen upon estrogen-receptor positive tissue. In fact, recent clinical data suggest that tamoxifen may be atheroprotective in post-menopausal women.[80]

To examine the question of whether the antiproliferative effect of E_2 on hVSMC is mediated by a ligand-receptor interaction, studies were performed examining the effect of the pure estrogen receptor antagonist (ERA) ICI 182780 (generously supplied by Dr. Alan Wakeling, Zeneca Pharmaceuticals), to determine whether the antiproliferative effect of E_2 on hVSMC is mediated by ER.

In studies using dextran, charcoal-stripped FBS (Figure 7), the pure ERA mitigated the antiproliferative effect of E_2 when it was added to the culture medium before the E_2 containing culture medium.

Further evidence of a functional role of the estrogen receptor in hVSMC biology is provided by the observation that individual

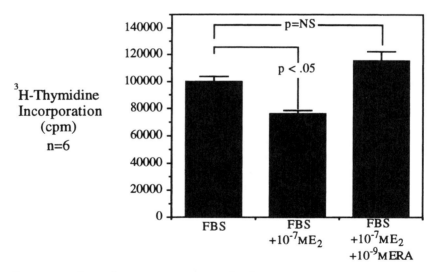

FIGURE 7. *Thymidine incorporation of cultured hVSMC in FBS (dextran-charcoal treated to remove all steroid hormones) before and after supplementation with estradiol (10^{-7} M), with and without pretreatment with the pure estrogen-receptor antagonist ICI 182780. A significant reduction in proliferative activity is seen after estradiol supplementation. When these cells are pretreated with estrogen-receptor antagonist, the growth inhibitory effect of estradiol is blunted significantly. These findings are consistent with a receptor mediated effect of estradiol on hVSMC proliferation.*

hVSMC expressing high levels of estrogen receptor show diminished proliferative activity whereas cells with low levels of ER expression show evidence of entering the cell cycle.

Double labeling studies were performed using autoradiographic detection of estrogen receptor expression in individual cells combined with immunohistochemical detection of bromodeoxyuridine (BrdU) incorporation as an index of proliferative activity. The purpose here was twofold. First the autoradiographic technique would permit detection of estrogen receptor expression among individual cells within the culture population. Previous evaluations of human breast cancer cell culture populations have indicated that only a percentage of cells, even in a population of cells known to express high levels of estrogen receptor, are expressing estrogen receptor at significant levels. Second, as noted above, it would provide the opportunity to disclose any relation between estrogen-receptor expression and proliferative activity within individual cells.

Figure 8 shows an example of the application of this technique to hVSMC in culture. Of the two hVSMC in this field, one is stained positively for BrdU incorporation (the nucleus is stained red) whereas the other cell shows staining only with the counterstain. Interestingly, autoradiographic detection of the labeled estradiol is noted only over the cell nucleus that is negative for BrdU incorporation.

Thus, there is a dissociation of estrogen receptor expression and evidence of proliferation. The hVSMC that is expressing estrogen receptor shows no evidence of proliferative activity in this case. Although these studies are ongoing in our laboratory, this is evidence of a possible relation between estrogen receptor expression and proliferative activity of hVSMC in culture.

There are five observations that can be made from this data. First, serum containing high levels of estradiol induces significantly less proliferative activity of hVSMC than does serum with low levels of estradiol. Second, the enhanced proliferation that is associated with low [E_2] serum is reduced by the addition of estradiol to this same serum. Third, there is a dose-response relation between increasing concentrations of estradiol present in culture medium and decreasing proliferative activity of hVSMC. Fourth, addition of specific estrogen-receptor antagonists to the culture medium before estradiol-containing serum blunts the antiproliferative effects of estradiol, suggesting that the antiproliferative effect of estradiol is a receptor-mediated phenomenon. Finally, in individual hVSMC, there is an apparent inverse relation between estrogen-receptor expression and evidence of proliferative activity. These data support the notion that the effect of E_2 is mediated not only by the concen-

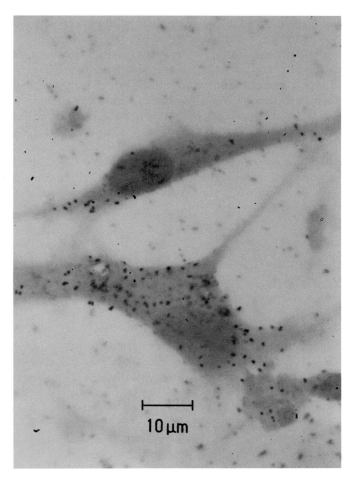

FIGURE 8. *Double labeling of cultured hVSMC for BrdU incorporation and ER expression. Cell in upper left is stained positive for BrdU incorporation (red staining of nucleus) but shows little evidence of ^3H estradiol binding. Cell in lower right is negative for BrdU incorporation but does demonstrate significant autoradiographic evidence of ^3H estradiol binding, manifest as black grains surrounding nucleus, suggesting the presence of ER.*

tration of the ligand present, but also may be significantly effected by the level of expression of ER. Our preliminary data examining postmortem coronary arteries suggested, in fact, that diminished ER expression was associated with the development of coronary atherosclerosis in premenopausal females.

A principal finding of these studies is that of a clearly identified direct estrogen effect upon hVSMC behavior. By changing the concentration of estrogen in the cell culture medium, thymidine incorporation was altered consistently and significantly. The absence of other cell types that could mediate the E_2 effect supports the notion that this effect is the result of direct interaction of estrogen with ER on the hVSMC. To ensure that the suppression of thymidine uptake by addition of E_2 to the culture medium was not a toxic effect, sample wells of all treated cells were subcultured after 72 hours and returned to a standard defined culture medium. Cell viability was shown to be equal in all treatment groups at this time point (data not shown). This indicates that E_2 is suppressive, rather than toxic to hVSMC.

Differential Display Identifies Estrogen-Regulated Genes in Human Vascular Smooth Muscle Cells

The differential display of mRNA using the polymerase chain reaction is a recently described technique[81,82] used to identify and isolate genes that are expressed differentially in various cells under altered conditions. This technique uses a set of oligonucleotide primers, one of which is anchored to the polyadenylate tail of the mRNA whereas the other is short and arbitrary in sequence. The second primer is designed to anneal at different positions relative to the first primer. A reverse transcription reaction then results in the production of a subpopulation of complementary DNAs defined by these primers. The cDNAs then are amplified by polymerase chain reaction and resolved on a DNA sequencing gel.

This technique is suited ideally to cell culture because the cells in culture, when they are derived from a single source, are genetically identical; differences in mRNA expression therefore can be ascribed to precise changes made in the culture medium, in this case, focusing on changes in the estrogen content of the culture medium. Our laboratory has begun using this technique to define the differences in gene expression that result when hVSMC are exposed to estrogen in culture. Results of one of the initial studies performed in our laboratory are shown in Figure 9. In this experiment, hVSMC from a single explant source were grown to 80% confluency in 100-mm culture plates. Cells were grown in hormone-free standard culture media. When the cells reached the appropriate level of con-

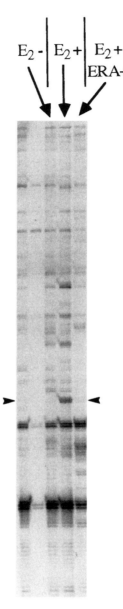

FIGURE 9. *Differential display polymerase chain reaction. Portion of a sequencing gel resolving amplified cDNA fragments after reverse transcription of total RNA. Arrow indicates a cDNA tag that is seen only in the cells exposed to the high levels (2×10^{-9} M) of estrogen present in pooled serum of premenopausal females. This band is absent when cells pretreated with an estrogen receptor antagonist are exposed to the same female serum and also is absent when the same female serum is dextran charcoal stripped before being added to the cultured hVSMC. Cells exposed to male serum or charcoal stripped serum also do not display this band.*

fluency, the media was changed so that one plate of the cells was exposed to a culture medium supplemented by 10% charcoal stripped fetal bovine serum (estradiol content $< 10^{-11}$ M) one plate was grown in medium supplemented by 10% charcoal stripped fetal bovine serum with estradiol added to a level of 10^{-7} M).

As is shown in Figure 10 there is a great degree of similarity in the amplified cDNA sequences defined on this gel. The arrow denotes a band that is present only in the lane corresponding to mRNA derived from hVSMC exposed to estradiol supplemented medium. This band is absent from lanes corresponding to cells exposed to estrogen-free medium. The differences in the cDNA defined on the sequencing gel correspond to differences in mRNA expression by hVSMC when exposed to estrogen.

Our laboratory has confirmed the expression of functional estrogen receptors in human vascular smooth muscle cells. Further evidence suggests a link between diminished ER expression and a propensity to coronary atherosclerosis.

Evidence from our laboratory also has documented an antiproliferative effect of estrogen in the form of human female serum, as exogenous estrogen added to human male serum or added to charcoal-stripped fetal calf serum in defined culture media. The antiproliferative effect of estrogen appears to be unaltered by the presence of progesterone. Evidence for a receptor-mediated action of estrogen on hVSMC is provided by the response of these cells to pretreatment with a pure estrogen-receptor antagonist (ICI 182780) before addition of estradiol (either endogenously contained in the serum of premenopausal females or exogenously added to male serum or charcoal-stripped fetal bovine serum). These findings suggest that both the estrogen content of the serum and the nature of the hVSMC themselves are critical in the translation of E_2 effects on hVSMC biology.

Evidence from our laboratory also has disclosed a differential in mRNA expression in hVSMC growing in the presence or absence of estrogen. Characterization of the changes in mRNA expression that are associated with E_2-ER binding and decreased proliferation will result in a clearer understanding of the mechanisms by which estrogen exerts a *direct* atheroprotective effect.

Coronary heart disease is the leading cause of death among postmenopausal women. This is in stark contrast to the relative freedom from coronary disease that is enjoyed by most premenopausal women. Elucidation of the effect of estrogen on vascular smooth muscle will provide important insights into the atherosclerotic disease process itself, as well as providing the opportunity to understand how best to extend the protection enjoyed by premenopausal women into women in older age groups as well as into the male population.

References

1. Levy H, Boas EP. Coronary artery disease in women. *JAMA* 1936;107:97.
2. Glendy RE, Levine SA, White PD. Coronary disease in youth: Comparison of 100 patients under 40 with 300 persons past 80. *JAMA* 1937; 109:1775–1778.
3. Master AM, Dack S, Jaffe HL. Age, sex and hypertension in myocardial infarction due to coronary occlusion. *Arch Intern Med* 1939;64:767.
4. Clawson BJ. The incidence of types of heart disease among 30, 265 autopsies, with special reference to age and sex. *Am Heart J* 1941;22:607.
5. Underdahl LO, Smith HL. Coronary artery disease in women under the age of 40. *Proc Staff Meet Mayo Clin* 1947;22:479.
6. Rivan AU, Dimitroff SP. The incidence and severity of atherosclerosis in estrogen-treated males, and in females with a hypoestrogenic or a hyperestrogenic state. *Circulation* 1954;9:533–539.
7. Oliver MF, Boyd GS. Effect of bilateral ovariectomy on coronary-artery disease and serum-lipid levels. *Lancet* 1959;2:690–694.
8. Robinson RW, Higano N, Cohen WD. Increased incidence of coronary heart disease in women castrated prior to the menopause. *Arch Intern Med* 1959;104:908–913.
9. Wuest JH, Dry TJ, Edwards JE. The degree of coronary atherosclerosis in bilaterally oophorectomized women. *Circulation* 1953;7:801–808.
10. Ritterband AB, Jaffe IA, Densen PM, et al. Gonadal function and the development of coronary heart disease. *Circulation* 1963;27:237–251.
11. Novack ER, William TJ. Autopsy comparison of cardiovascular changes in castrated and normal women. *Am J Obstet Gynecol* 1966;80:863–872.
12. Matthews KA, Meilahn E, Kuller LH, et al. Menopause and risk factors for coronary heart disease. *N Engl J Med* 1989;321:641–646.
13. Gruchow HW, Anderson AJ, Barboriak JJ, et al. Postmenopausal use of estrogen and occlusion of coronary arteries. *Am Heart J* 1988;115: 954–963.
14. Nabulsi AA, Folsom AR, White A, et al. Association of hormone-replacement therapy with various cardiovascular risk factors in postmenopausal women. *N Engl J Med* 1993;328:1069–1075.
15. Fischer GM, Swain ML. Effect of sex hormone on blood pressure and vascular connective tissue in castrated and noncastrated male rats. *Am J Physiol* 1977;232:H617–H621.
16. Wolinsky H. Effects of estrogen and progestogen treatment on the response of the aorta of male rates to hypertension. Morphological and chemical studies. *Circ Res* 1972;30:341–349.
17. Williams JK, Adams MR, Klopfenstein HS. Estrogen modulates responses of atherosclerotic coronary arteries. *Circulation* 1990;81: 1680–1687.
18. Kushwaha RS, Lewis DS, Carey KD, et al. Effects of estrogen and progesterone on plasma lipoproteins and experimental atherosclerosis in the baboon (Papio sp.). *Arterioscl Thromb* 1991;11:23–31.

19. Knopp RH. Cardiovascular effects of endogenous and exogenous sex hormones over a woman's lifetime. *Am J Obstet Gynecol* 1988;158: 1630–1643.
20. Tikkanen MJ, Nikkilä EA, Kuusi T, et al. High density lipoprotein$_2$ and hepatic lipase: Reciprocal changes produced by estrogen and norgestrel. *J Clin Endocrinol Metab* 1982;54:1113–1117.
21. Tikkanen MJ, Kuusi T, Nikkilä EA, et al. Variation of postheparin plasma hepatic lipase by menstrual cycle. *Metabolism* 1986;35:99–104.
22. Pick R, Stamler J, Rodbard S, et al. The inhibition of coronary atherosclerosis by estrogen in cholesterol-fed chicks. *Circulation* 1952;6: 276–280.
23. Stamler J, Pick R, Katz LN. Prevention of coronary atherosclerosis by estrogen-androgen administration in the cholesterol-fed chick. *Circ Res* 1953;1:94–98.
24. Adams MR, Kaplan JR, Koritnik DR, et al. Pregnancy-associated inhibition of coronary artery atherosclerosis in monkeys: evidence of a relationship with endogenous estrogen. *Arteriosclerosis* 1987;7:378–383.
25. Pick R, Stamler J, Rodbard S, et al. Estrogen-induced regression of coronary atherosclerosis in cholesterol-fed chicks. *Circulation* 1952;6: 858–861.
26. Barrett-Connor E, Wingard DL, Criqui MH. Postmenopausal estrogen use and heart disease risk factors in the 1980s. *JAMA* 1989;261:2095–2100.
27. Bush TL, Barrett-Connor E, Cowan LD. Cardiovascular mortality and noncontraceptive estrogen use in women: Results from the Lipid Research Clinics' Program Follow-up Study. *Circulation* 1987;75:1002–1009.
28. Reynolds SRM, Foster FI. Peripheral vascular action of estrogen, observed in the ear of the rabbit. *J Pharmacol Exp Ther* 1940;68:173–184.
29. Silva de Sá MF, Meirelles RS. Vasodilation effect of estrogen on the human umbilical artery. *Gynecol Invest* 1977;8:307–313.
30. Williams JK, Adams MR, Herrington DM, et al. Short-term administration of estrogen and vascular responses of atherosclerotic coronary arteries. *J Am Coll Cardiol* 1993;20:452–457.
31. Maddox YT, Falcon JG, Ridinger M, et al. Endothelium-dependent gender differences in the response of the rat aorta. *J Pharmacol Exp Ther* 1987;240:392–395.
32. Reis SE, Gloth ST, Blumenthal RS, et al. Ethinyl estradiol acutely attenuates abnormal coronary vasomotor responses to acetylcholine in postmenopausal women. *Circulation* 1994;89:52–60.
33. Gilligan DM, Badar DM, Panza JA, et al. Acute vascular effects of estrogen in postmenopausal women. *Circulation* 1994;90:786–791.
34. Nichols NR, Olsson CA, Funder JW. Steriod effects on protein synthesis in cultured smooth muscle cells from rat aorta. *Endocrinology* 1983; 113:1096–1101.
35. Horwitz KB, Horwitz LD. Canine vascular tissues are targets for androgens, estrogens, progestins, and glucocorticoids. *J Clin Invest* 1982; 69:750–758.
36. Harder DR, Coulson PB. Estrogen receptors and effects of estrogen on membrane electrical properties of coronary vascular smooth muscle. *J Cell Physiol* 1979;100:375–382.
37. Nakao J, Chang W-C, Murota S-I, et al. Estradiol-binding sites in rat aortic smooth muscle cells in culture. *Am Heart J* 1981;–13767:12336–13364.

38. Colburn P, Buonassisi V. Estrogen-binding sites in endothelial cell cultures. *Science* 1978;201:817–819.
39. Ricciardelli C, Horsfall DJ, Skinner JM, et al. Development and characterization of primary cultures of smooth muscle cells from the fibromuscular stroma of the guinea pig prostate. *In Vitro Cell Dev Biol* 1989;25:1016–1024
40. Elam MB, Lipscomb GE, Chesney CM, et al. Effect of synthetic estrogen on platelet aggregation and vascular release of PGI_2-like material in the rabbit. *Prostaglandins* 1980;20:1039–1051
41. Kakar SS, Sellers JC, Devor DC, et al. Angiotensin II type-1 receptor subtype cDNAs: Differential tissue expression and hormonal regulation. *Biochem Biophys Res Commun* 1992;183:1090–1096.
42. Green S. Promiscuous liaisons. *Nature* 1993;361:590–591.
43. Green S, Chambon P. Nuclear receptors enhance our understanding of transcription regulation. *Trends Genet* 1988;4:309–314.
44. Luisi BF, Xu WX, Otwinowski Z, et al. Crystallographic analysis of the interaction of the glucocorticoid receptor with DNA. *Nature* 1991; 352:497–505.
45. Carlberg C, Bendik I, Wyss A, et al. Two nuclear signalling pathways for vitamin D. *Nature* 1993;361:657–660.
46. Jensen EV, Desombre ER. Mechanism of action of the female sex hormones. *Annu Rev Biochem* 1972;41:203–230.
47. King WJ, Greene GL. Monoclonal antibodies localize estrogen receptor in the nuclei of target cells. *Nature* 1984;307:745–747.
48. Welshons WV, Lieberman ME, Gorski J. Nuclear localization of unoccupied estrogen receptors. *Nature* 1984;307:747–749.
49. Spelsberg TC, Webster RA, Pikler GM. Chromosomal proteins regulate steroid binding to chromatin. *Nature* 1976;262:65–67.
50. Barrack ER, Coffey DS. The specific binding of estrogen and androgens to the nuclear matrix of sex hormone responsive tissues. *J Biol Chem* 1980;255:7265–7275.
51. Pardoll DM, Vogelstein B, Coffey DS. A fixed site of DNA replication in eucaryotic cells. *Cell* 1980;19:527–530.
52. Robinson SI, Nelkin BD, Vogelstein B. The ovalbumin gene is associated with the nuclear matrix of chicken oviduct cells. *Cell* 1985;28:99–106.
53. Walter P, Green S, Greene G, et al. Cloning of the human estrogen receptor cDNA. *Proc Natl Acad Sci USA* 1985;82:7889–7893.
54. Mendelsohn ME, Zhu Y, O'Neill S. The 29-kDa proteins phosphorylated in thrombin-activated human platelets are forms of the estrogen receptor-related 27-kDa heat shock protein. Abstract. *Proc Natl Acad Sci USA* 1991;88:11212–11216.
55. Picard D, Khursheed B, Garabedian MJ, et al. Reduced levels of hsp90 compromise steroid receptor action in vivo. *Nature* 1990;348 (6297):166–168.
56. Aitken SC, Lippman ME. Hormonal regulation of *de novo* pyrimidine synthesis and utilization in human breast cancer cells in tissue culture. *Cancer Res* 1983;43:4681–4690.
57. Aitken SC, Lippman ME. Effect of estrogens and antiestrogens on growth-regulatory enzymes in human breast cancer cells in tissue culture. *Cancer Res* 1985;45:1611–1620.
58. Dickson RB, Lippman ME. Control of human breast cancer by estrogen, growth factors, and oncogenes. In: Lippmann ME, Dickson RB, eds.

Breast Cancer: Cellular and Molecular Biology. Norwell, MA: Kluwer Academic Publishers; 1988:119–165.

59. Cowan K, Levine R, Aitken S, et al. Dihydrofolate reductase gene amplification and possible rearrangement in estrogen-responsive methotrexate resistant human breast cancer cells. *J Biol Chem* 1982;257: 15079–15086.

60. Kasid A, Davidson N, Gelmann E, et al. Transcriptional control of thymidine kinase gene expression by estrogens and antiestrogens in MCF-7 human breast cancer cells. *J Biol Chem* 1986;261:5562–5567.

61. Stack G, Gorski J. Direct mitogenic effect of estrogen on the prepuberal rat uterus: Studies on isolated nuclei. *Endocrinology* 1984;115:1141–1150.

62. Sirbasku DA. Estrogen inductin of growth factors specific for hormone-responsive mammary, pituitary, and kidney tumor cells. *Proc Natl Acad Sci USA* 1978;75:3786–3790.

63. Sporn MB, Todaro GJ. Autocrine secretion and malignant transformation of cells. *N Engl J Med* 1980;303:878–882.

64. Ma ZQ, Spreafico E, Pollio G, et al. Activated estrogen receptor mediates growth arrest and differentiation of a neuroblastoma cell line. *Proc Natl Acad Sci USA* 1993;90:3740–3744.

65. Bradshaw MS, Tsai SY, Leng XH, et al. Studies on the mechanism of functional cooperativity between progesterone and estrogen receptors. *J Biol Chem* 1991;266:16684–16690.

66. Jeng MH, Parker CJ, Jordan VC. Estrogenic potential of progestine in oral contraceptives to stimulate human breast cancer cell proliferation. *Cancer Res* 1992;52:6539–6546.

67. Coibion M, Kiss R, Jossa V, et al. In vitro influence of estradiol or progesterone one the thymidine labeling indices of human benign breast tumors. *Anticancer Res* 1989;9:475–482.

68. Scheven BA, Damen CA, Hamilton NJ, et al. Stimulatory effects of estrogen and progesterone on proliferation and differentiation of normal human osteoblast-like cells in vitro. *Biochem Biophys Res Commun* 1992;186:54–60.

69. Caronti B, Palladini G, Bevilacqua MG, et al. Effects of 17 beta-estradiol, progesterone and tamoxifen on in vitro proliferation of human pituitary adenomas: Correlation with specific cellular receptors. *Tumour Biol* 1993;14:59–68.

70. Michna H, Nishino Y, Neef G, et al. Progesterone antagonists: Tumor-inhibiting potential and mechanism of action. *J Steriod Biochem Mol Biol* 1992;41:339–348.

71. Okulicz WC, Balsamo M, Tast J. Progesterone regulation of endometrial estrogen receptor and cell proliferation during the late proliferative and secretory phase in artificial menstrual cycles in the rhesus monkey. *Biol Reprod* 1993;49:24–32.

72. Losordo DW, Kearney M, Kim EA, et al. Variable expression of the estrogen receptor in normal and atherosclerotic coronary arteries of premenopausal women. *Circulation* 1994;89:1501–1510.

73. Pickering JG, Weir L, Rosenfield K, et al. Smooth muscle cell outgrowth from human atherosclerotic plaque: Implications for the assessment of lesion biology. *J Am Coll Cardiol* 1992;20:1430–1439.

74. Horwitz KB, Costlow ME, McGuire WL. MCF–7: A human breast cancer cell line with estrogen, androgen, progesterone, and glucocorticoid receptors. *Steroids* 1975;26:785–795.

75. Karas RH, Patterson BL, Mendelsohn ME. Human vascular smooth muscle cells contain functional estrogen receptor. *Circulation* 1994; 89:1943–1950.
76. Klein-Hitpass L, Kaling M, Ryffel GU. Synergism of closely adjacent estrogen-responsive elements increases their regulatory potential. *J Mol Biol* 1988;201:537–544.
77. Klein-Hitpass L, Ryffel GU, Heitlinger E, et al. A 13 bp palidrome is a functional estrogen responsive element and interacts specifically with estrogen receptor. *Nucleic Acids Res* 1988;16:647–663.
78. Kumar V, Chambon P. The estrogen receptor binds tightly to its responsive element as a ligand-induced homodimer. *Cell* 1988;55:145–156.
79. Hiort O, Kwan PWL, DeLellis RA. Immunohistochemistry of estrogen receptor protein in paraffin sections: Effects of enzymatic pretreatment and cobalt chloride intensification. *Am J Clin Pathol* 1988;90:559–563.
80. Rutqvist LE, Mattsson A. Cardiac and thromboembolic morbidity among postmenopausal women with early-stage breast cancer in a randomized trial of adjuvant tamoxifen. *J Natl Cancer Inst* 1993;85:1398–1406.
81. Liang P, Pardee AB. Differential display of eukaryotic messenger RNA by means of the polymerase chain reaction. *Science* 1992;257:967–971.
82. Liang P, Averboukh L, Pardee AB. Distribution and cloning of eukaryotic mRNAs by means of differential display: Refinements and optimization. *Nucleic Acids Res* 1993;21:3269–3275.

Chapter 6

Effects of Sex Hormones on Responses to Endothelium-Derived Factors in Coronary Arteries

Virginia M. Miller PhD,
Dustan A. Barber RPh, PhD
and Gary C. Sieck PhD

Epidemiological studies provide indirect evidence for estrogen or estrogen status to be protective against the development of cardiovascular disease in women.[1-3] However, there are few definitive studies identifying the mechanism by which estrogen, in particular, and sex steroid hormones, in general, affect the function of the vasculature. Receptors for the sex steroids have been identified in the vasculature.[4-6] Therefore, sex steroid hormones have the potential to affect all components of the vascular wall including release and uptake of transmitter from autonomic neurons, production and release of antithrombogenic, mitogenic or vasoactive factors from the endothelium, and responses of the smooth muscle to both neurotransmitters and endothelium-derived factors. This chapter will focus on how gender and estrogen might affect responses of the vascular smooth muscle to four products of endothelial cells: eicosanoids, nitric oxide (NO), C-type natriuretic factor, and endothelin-1. Interest in these endothelium-derived factors is prompted by their ability to alter platelet aggregation, vasomotion, and smooth muscle proliferation.[7-19] Therefore, any modulation in production or response to these factors by estrogen and/or other sex steroid hormones has the potential to influence thrombosis, vasospasm and proliferative occlusive vascular disease.

From: Forte TM, (ed). *Hormonal, Metabolic, and Cellular Influences on Cardiovascular Disease in Women.* Armonk, NY: Futura Publishing Company, Inc.; © 1997.

AORTA FROM ESTROGEN TREATED AND UNTREATED RABBITS

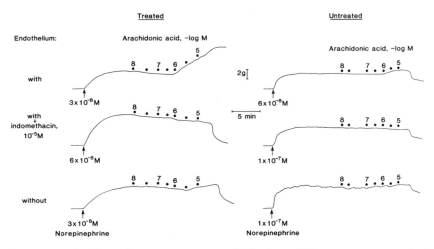

FIGURE 1. *Tracing of responses to arachidonic acid in aortas suspended for the meausrement of isometric force in organ chambers. Aortas were derived from estrogen-treated (left panels) and untreated (right panels) rabbits. Contractions to arachidonic acid were greater in aortas from estrogen-treated rabbits. Contractions were reduced by indomethacin (10^{-5} M; middle traces) and by removal of the endothelium (bottom traces). Each aorta was contracted with a concentration of norepinephrine that produced between 25% and 40% of maximal contraction. Reproduced with premission from Reference 28.*

Vascular Smooth Muscle and Endothelium-Derived Products

Eicosanoids

Arachidonic acid is a component of the cellular membrane that can be metabolized by at least three enzymatic pathways in both endothelial cells and vascular smooth muscle: cyclooxygenase, lipooxygenase, and cytochrome P450.[20-24] Addition of exogenous arachidonic acid causes contraction of aortas isolated from ovariectomized female rabbits.[25] These contractions, which are increased by treatment of animals with estrogen, are probably due to metabolism of arachidonic acid in the endothelium by cyclooxygenase because contractions are reduced both by removal of the endothelium and by incubation of the rings with an inhibitor of cyclooxygenase, indomethacin (Figure 1). It is not known whether these contractions are due to differences in production of the various end products of arachidonic acid metabolism such as thromboxane, prostacyclin, or prostaglandins because these metabolites were not measured. An alternative explanation for increased contractions to arachidonic acid is that the sensitivity of the smooth muscle to one or more of the products was altered by the estrogen-treatment. For example, exogenous administration of prostacyclin caused contraction in rings without endothelium (the smooth muscle alone) from estrogen-treated rabbits rather than relaxation as is typically seen with prostacyclin in other blood vessels.[26] These results suggest that estrogen may modify intracellular signaling pathways associated with prostacyclin-mediated relaxation, such as adenylate cyclase and/or adenosine 3′:5′-cyclic phosphate (cAMP).

One caveat of such experiments is that metabolism of exogenously applied arachidonic acid or prostacyclin may not be representative of the metabolism or actions of endogenous activation. However, the ability of indomethacin to modify stimulation of receptor-mediated processes in isolated blood vessels provides indirect evidence that estrogen-treatment modifies production and sensitivity of the smooth muscle to end products of cyclooxygenase. For example, treatment of rabbits with estrogen increases contractions of aortic rings with endothelium to the neurotransmitter norepinephrine. Moreover, indomethacin reduces the sensitivity to norepinephrine of rings with but not without endothelium from estrogen-treated rabbits.[25] These results suggest that estrogens could modulate responses to adrenergic neuronal stimulation indirectly by affecting adrenergic-coupled metabolism of arachidonic acid in endothelial cells.

Another endogenous substance that may stimulate metabolism of arachidonic acid through cyclooxygenase is the platelet-derived substance, adenosine diphosphate.[27] Adenosine diphosphate causes direct relaxation of smooth muscle of femoral arteries from estrogen-treated rabbits; these relaxations are increased by indomethacin.[28] Therefore, estrogens may influence retention of platelet aggregates indirectly through changes in the response of the vessel wall to platelet-derived factors. It is attractive to speculate that estrogen may contribute to vasospastic or thrombotic events in coronary arteries through modulation of metabolism of arachidonic acid. However, extrapolation of effects of hormones on systemic arteries, such as the aorta and femoral artery, to those of the coronary circulation should be made with caution as cell-specific differentiation will direct hormone-directed genomic events. Interpretation of the results also is limited by the conditions of hormone replacement (dose and duration) as no systematic studies on concentration effect or time effect of hormone replacement on metabolism of arachidonic acid or other metabolic pathways are available at this time.

Nitric Oxide

In addition to eicosanoids, NO also is released from endothelial cells by neurotransmitters and platelet-derived substances.[27,29] Endothelium-dependent relaxations to the α_2-adrenergic agonist BHT 920 are increased in canine coronary arteries from ovariectomized dogs treated with estrogen compared with those from dogs without hormonal treatment or those treated with progesterone alone (Figure 2)[30] In ovariectomized dogs treated with a combination of estrogen and

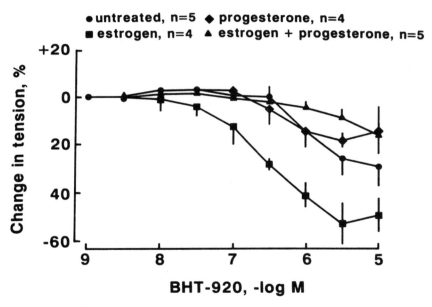

FIGURE 2. *Relaxations to an α_2-adrenergic agonist, BHT-920 in coronary arteries with endothelium from hormone-treated dogs. Rings cut from the arteries were suspended in organ chamboers for the measurement of isometric force. All experiments were conducted in the presence of indomethacin (10^{-5} M); data are shown as mean $\pm$ SEM and are expressed as a percent change in tension from a submaximal contraction to prostaglandin $F_{2\alpha}$. Relaxations in rings from estrogen-treated dogs were significantly greater than those in other groups (analysis of variance of areas under the curves, $P < 0.05$). Reproduced with permission from Reference 30.*

progesterone, relaxations to BHT 920 are not different from those of untreated, ovariectomized animals, suggesting that progesterone antagonized the effects of estrogen.[30] Because these experiments were conducted in the presence of indomethacin, it is unlikely that cyclooxygenase products contributed to the relaxations. Relaxations to α_2-adrenergic agonists in coronary arteries are inhibited by analogs of L-arginine, therefore, NO is likely the primary mediator of response to α_2-adrenergic agonists. One possible mechanism by which estrogen could influence endothelium-dependent relaxations is by alterations in sensitivity of the smooth muscle to NO. However, relaxations of rings without endothelium to NO were not different among coronary arteries

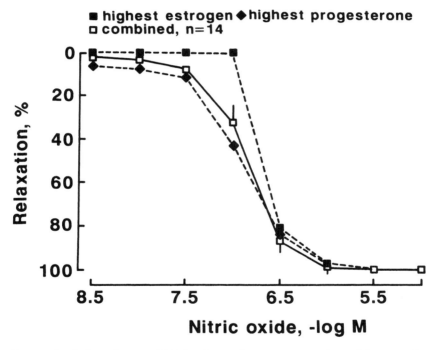

FIGURE 3. *Relaxations to NO in rings of coronary arteries without endothelium from hormone-treated dogs described in Figure 2. Rings cut from the arteries were suspended in organ chambers for the measurement of isometric force. All experiments were conducted in the presence of indomethacin (10^{-5} M); data for the combined responses are shown as mean ± SEM and expressed as a percent change in tension from a submaximal contraction to prostaglandin $F_{2\alpha}$. Response of individual dogs with either the highest serum estrogen or progesterone concentrations are shown (-/-/-).*

from dogs of the different hormone-treatment groups. In fact, relaxations to NO in the animal with the highest circulating level of estrogen were to the right of the mean response-curve of all the animals (Figure 3). This shift in the curve is opposite of what would be predicted if increases in sensitivity of the smooth muscle to NO were to account for increased relaxations to BHT-920.

These results suggest that intracellular mechanisms proposed for NO such as activation of soluble guanylate cyclase or potassium channels[31,32] may not be affected by estrogen treatment. The mechanisms by which sex steroid hormones may modulate endothelium-dependent relaxations to NO including those initiated by α_2-adrenergic agonists are not clear. It remains controversial whether estrogens regulate production of NO synthase by transcriptional regulation of the enzyme[33,34] or activity of the enzyme through regulation of oxygen-derived free radicals, cofactor availability, or receptor-coupled processes including guanine nucleotide regulatory proteins.[35–37]

C-Type Natriuretic Peptide

C-type natriuretic factor (CNP) is a 22 amino-acid peptide and represents the most highly conserved member of the natriuretic peptides, which include atrial (ANP) and brain (BNP) natriuretic pep-

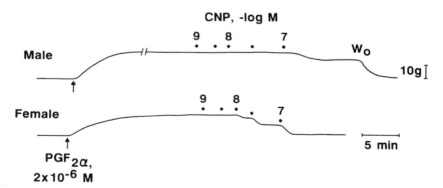

FIGURE 4. *Tracing of responses to CNP in rings of coronary arteries without endothelium from gonadally intact, sexually mature male (upper trace) or female (lower trace) pigs. Rings cut from the right coronary artery were suspended in organ chambers for the measurement of isometric force. CNP caused greater relaxation of arteries from female pigs compared to male pigs. Abbreviations: PGF 2α, prostaglandin $F_{2\alpha}$, Wo, washout.*

tides.[38] CNP is synthesized and secreted by endothelial cells and may act as a paracrine hormone to reduce vascular tone and inhibit proliferation of vascular smooth muscle.[16,17,19] Actions of CNP are associated with binding to an ANP-B receptor with subsequent activation of particulate guanylate cyclase (a component of the ANP-B receptor) and accumulation of cyclic quanosine monosphosphate (cGMP).[39,40] In addition, CNP may also hyperpolarize vascular smooth muscle via activation of potassium channels as has been observed for natriuretic peptides in other cell types.[41,42] Relaxations to CNP in coronary arterial smooth muscle from sexually mature, gonadally intact female pigs are greater than in male pigs (Figure 4). This may be related to differences in types or activity of phosphodiesterases. This conclusion is supported by the observation that accumulation of cGMP in response to a maximal concentration of CNP was greater in coronary arterial smooth muscle from female pigs compared with male pigs; a difference that was eliminated by incubation of the tissue with the phosphodiesterase inhibitor isomethylbutylxanthine (IBMX; Figure 5).

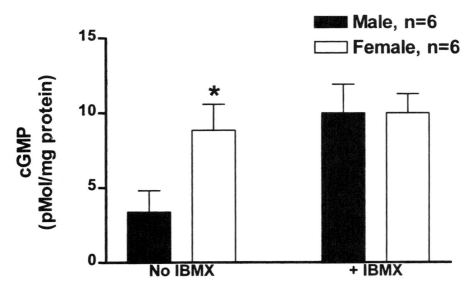

FIGURE 5. *Changes in cGMP 30 seconds after addition of a maximal concentration of CNP (10^{-7} M) to isolated rings of porcine coronary arteries without endothelium from gonadally intact, sexually mature pigs. Data are shown as the mean ± SEM of accumulation of cGMP per milligram portein in the absence and presence of the phosphodiesterase inhibitor isomethylbutylxanthine (IBMX; 10^{-4} M). *Statistical significance between male and female by Student's t-test for unpaired observations. $P < 0.05$.*

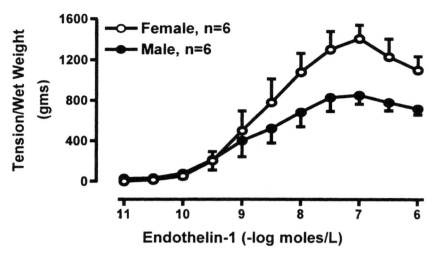

FIGURE 6. *Concentration-response curves to endothelin-1 in rings of coronary arteries without endothelium from gonadally intact, sexually mature pigs. Rings were suspended in organ chambers for the measurement of isometric force. Data are shown as mean ± SEM of contractions expressed as gram of tension/grams of wet weight of tissue. Maximal contractions (at 10^{-7} M) in rings from female coronary arteries were significantly greater than those from males (one-way analysis of variance, $P < 0.05$).*

When analyzed by gender, neither inhibitor of ATP-sensitive potassium channels, high-conductance calcium-activated potassium channels, or low-conductance calcium-activated potassium channels was effective in significantly inhibiting the relaxations to CNP (unpublished observations). These results suggest gender differences in relaxations to CNP may be receptor-coupled and that potassium channel activation may be secondary to stimulation of cGMP. Whether or not and how production of CNP in endothelial cells might be regulated by sex steroid hormones is not known.

Endothelin-1

Endothelin-1 is a 27 amino-acid peptide, which, unlike NO and CNP, causes contraction and acts synergistically with other growth factors to promote cellular proliferation.[18,43-45] Contractions to endothelin-1 are significantly greater in coronary arteries from sexually mature, gonadally intact female pigs than male pigs (Figure 6).

TRITON-X PREPARATION

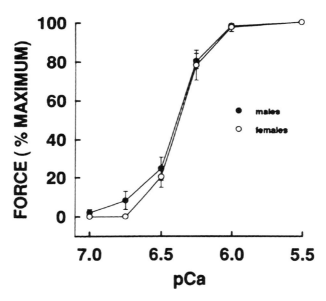

FIGURE 7. *Force-calcium relation in coronary arterial strips from gonadally intact, sexually mature pigs permeabilized with triton X (1% solution for 20 minutes). Data are shown as mean ± SEM; n = 4.*

These differences could be due to either regulation of receptors for endothelin-1 or receptor-coupled events leading to contraction. There are at least two populations of receptors causing contractions to endothelins: endothelin-A and endothelin-B receptors.[44,46–50] From receptor-binding experiments, two populations of endothelin receptors were identified in coronary arteries of male and female pigs. However, differences in number or affinity of endothelin receptors could not account entirely for the differences in contractile response to the peptide. Gender-related differences in contractile responses to endothelin-1 were evaluated in strips of porcine coronary arteries permeabilized with Triton-X. This procedure disrupts both the sarcolemma and the sarcoplasmic reticulum and allows direct manipulation of myoplasmic calcium. There were no differences in the calcium-dependent increases in force between smooth muscle from male and female pigs (Figure 7). These results indicate that there is not an intrinsic gender difference in calcium-sensitivity of the contractile proteins and that differences in contractions to endothelin-1 may be due to differences in regulation of intracellular calcium stores.

Summary

A potential mechanism by which estrogens and other sex steroid hormones affect development of thrombosis, vasospasm, and occlusive vascular disease could be related to regulation of the response of the smooth muscle to endothelium-derived factors thereby affecting responses to aggregating platelets, tone, and proliferation of the underlying smooth muscle. Responses to at least three endothelium-derived factors are modulated by estrogen-status and/or gender: eicosanoids, CNP, and endothelin-1. Possible intracellular pathways affected by estrogens include activation of cAMP, regulation of phosphodiesterases, and regulation of intracellular calcium stores. It remains to be determined whether sex steroid hormones act nongenomically through direct biochemical interactions with the second messenger pathways or by genomic regulation of protein synthesis.

References

1. Stampfner MJ, Colditz GA, Willett WC, et al. Postmenopausal estrogen therapy and cardiovascular disease: Ten-year follow-up from the Nurses' Health Study. *N Engl J Med* 1991;325:756–762.
2. Castelli WP. Cardiovascular disease in women. *Am J Obstet Gynecol* 1988;6:1553–1560.
3. Colditz GA, Willett WC, Stampfner MJ, et al. Menopause and the rule of coronary heart disease in women. *Am J Cardiol* 1993;316:1185.
4. Losordo DW, Kearney M, Kim EA, et al. Variable expression of the estrogen receptor in normal and atherosclerotic coronary arteries of premenopausal women. *Circulation* 1994;89:1501–1510.
5. Harder DR, Coulson PB. Estrogen receptors and effects of estrogen on membrane electrical properties of coronary vascular smooth muscle. *J Cell Physiol* 1979;100:375–382.
6. Lin AL, Shain SA. Estrogen-mediated cytoplasmic and nuclear distribution of rat cardiovascular estrogen receptors. *Arteriosclerosis* 1985; 5:668–677.
7. Garg UC, Hassid A. Nitric oxide-generating vasodilators and 8-bromo-cyclic guanosine monophosphate inhibit mitogenesis and proliferation of cultured rat vascular smooth muscle cells. *J Clin Invest* 1989;83:1774–1777.

8. Bush HL, Graber JN, Jakubowski JH, et al. Favorable balance of pros-tacyclin and thromboxane H_2 improves early patency of human in situ vein grafts. *J Vasc Surg* 1984;1:149–159.
9. Shimokawa H, Flavahan NA, Lorenz RR, et al. Prostacyclin releases endothelium-derived relaxing factor and potentiates its action in coro-nary arteries of the pig. *Br J Pharmacol* 1988;95:1197–1203.
10. Vallance P, Collier J, Moncada S. Effects of endothelium-derived nitric oxide on peripheral arteriolar tone in man. *Lancet* 1989;2:997–1000.
11. Thiemermann C, May GR, Page CP, et al. Endothelin-1 inhibits platelet aggregation *in vivo*: A study with [111]indium-labelled platelets. *Br J Phar-macol* 1990;99:303–308.
12. Alheid U, Frolich JC, Forstermann U. Endothelium-derived relaxing fac-tor from cultured human endothelial cells inhibits aggregation of hu-man platelets. *Thromb Res* 1987;47:561–571.
13. Macdonald PS, Read MA, Dusting GJ. Synergistic inhibition of platelet aggregation by endothelium-derived relaxing factor and prostacyclin. *Thromb Res* 1988;49:437–449.
14. Berti F, Rossoni G, DellaBella D, et al. Nitric oxide and prostacyclin influence coronary vasomotor tone in perfused rabbit heart and mod-ulate endothelin-1 activity. *J Cardiovasc Pharmacol* 1993;22:321–326.
15. Dubin D, Pratt RE, Cooke JP, et al. Endothelin, a potent vasoconstrictor, is a vascular smooth muscle mitogen. *J Vasc Med Biol* 1989;1:150–154.
16. Furuya M, Yoshida M, Hayashi Y, et al. C-type natriuretic peptide is a growth inhibitor of rat vascular smooth muscle cells. *Biochem Biophys Res Commun* 1991;177:927–931.
17. Furuya M, Aisaka K, Miyazaki T, et al. C-type natriuretic peptide inhib-its intimal thickening after vascular injury. *Biochem Biophys Res Com-mun* 1993;193:248–253.
18. Miller VM, Komori K, Burnett JC Jr, et al. Differential sensitivity to endothelin in canine arteries and veins. *Am. J. Physiol.* 1989;257:H1127–H1131.
19. Wei C, Aarhus LL, Miller VM, et al. The action of c-type natriuretic peptide in isolated canine arteries and veins. *Am J Physiol* 1993; 264:H71–H73.
20. Gryglewski RJ, Botting RM, Vane JR. Mediators produced by the en-dothelial cell. *Hypertension* 1988;12:530–548.
21. DeMey JG, Vanhoutte PM. Heterogeneous behavior of the canine arte-rial and venous wall. *Circ Res* 1982;51:439–447.
22. Singer HA, Saye JA, Peach MJ. Effects of cytochrome P-450 inhibitors on endothelium-dependent relaxation in rabbit aorta. *Blood Vessels* 1984;21:223–230.
23. Singer HA, Peach MJ. Endothelium-dependent relaxation of rabbit aorta. II. Inhibition of relaxation stimulated by methacholine and A23187 with antagonists of arachidonic acid metabolism. *J Pharmacol Exp Ther* 1983;226(3):796–801.
24. Cao L, Banks RO. Cardiorenal actions of endothelin. I. Effects of con-verting enzyme inhibition. *Life Sci* 1990;46:577–583.
25. Miller VM, Vanhoutte PM. 17β-Estradiol augments endothelium-dependent contractions to arachidonic acid in rabbit aorta. *Am J Physiol* 1990;258:R1502–R1507.
26. Bunting S, Gryglewski R, Moncada S, et al. Arterial walls generate from prostaglandin endoperoxides a substance (prostaglandin X) which re-

laxes strips of mesenteric and coeliac arteries and inhibits platelet aggregation. *Prostaglandins* 1976;12(6):897–913.

27. Houston DS, Shepherd JT, Vanhoutte PM. Adenine nucleotides, serotonin, and endothelium-dependent relaxations to platelets. *Am J Physiol* 1985;248:H389–H395.

28. Miller VM, Gisclard V, Vanhoutte PM. Modulation of endothelium-dependent and vascular smooth muscle responses by oestrogens. *Phlebology* 1988;3:63–69.

29. Cocks TM, Angus JA. Endothelium-dependent relaxation or coronary arteries by noradrenalin and serotonin. *Nature* 1983;305:627–630.

30. Miller VM, Vanhoutte PM. Progesterone and modulation of endothelium-dependent responses in canine coronary arteries. *Am J Physiol* 1991;261:R1022–R1027.

31. Ignarro LJ. Haem-dependent activation of guanylate cyclase and cyclic gmp formation by endogenous nitric oxide: A unique transduction mechanism for transcellular signaling. *Pharmacol Toxicol* 1990;67:1–7.

32. Bolotina VM, Najibi S, Palacino JJ, et al. Nitric oxide directly activates calcium-dependent potassium channels in vascular smooth muscle. *Nature* 1994;368(6474):850–853.

33. Marsden PA, Heng HHQ, Scherer SW, et al. Structure and chromosomal localization of the human constitutive endothelial nitric oxide synthase gene. *J Biol Chem* 1993;268(23):17478–17488.

34. Venema RC, Nishida K, Alexander RW, et al. Organization of the bovine gene encoding the endothelial nitric oxide synthase. *Biochim Biophys Acta* 1994;1218:413–420.

35. Buga GM, Griscavage JM, Rogers NE, et al. Negative feedback regulation of endothelial cell function by nitric oxide. *Circ Res* 1993;73:808–812.

36. Niki E, Nakano M. Estrogens as Antioxidants. *Methods Enzymol* 1990;186:330–333.

37. Bredt DS, Ferris CD, Snyder SH. Nitric oxide synthase regulatory sites. *J Biol Chem* 1992;267:10976–10981.

38. Tawaragi Y, Fuchimura K, Tanaka S, et al. Gene and precursor structures of human C–type natriuretic peptide. *Biochem Biophys Res Commun* 1991;175:645–651.

39. Drewett JG, Garbers DL. The family of guanylyl cyclase receptors and their ligands. *Endocr Rev* 1994;15:135–162.

40. Koller KJ, Lowe DG, Bunnett GL, et al. Selective activation of the B-natriuretic peptide receptor by C-type natriuretic peptide (CNP). *Science* 1991;252:120–123.

41. Wei C, Hu S, Miller VM, et al. Vascular actions of c-type natriuretic peptide in isolated porcine coronary arteries and coronary vascular smooth muscle cells. *Biochem Biophys Res Commun* 1994;205(1):765–771.

42. White RE, Lee AB, Shcherbatko AD, et al. Potassium channel stimulation by natriuretic peptides through cGMP-dependent dephosphorylation. *Nature* 1993;361:263–266.

43. Yanagisawa M, Kurihara H, Kimura S, et al. A novel potent vasoconstrictor peptide produced by vascular endothelial cells. *Nature* 1988;332:411–415.

44. Gray GA, Löffler B, Clozel M. Characterization of endothelin receptors mediating contraction of rabbit saphenous vein. *Am J Physiol* 1994;266:H959–H966.

45. Kohno M, Horio T, Yokokawa K, et al. Endothelin modulates the mitogenic effect of PDGF on glomerular mesangial cells. *Am J Physiol* 1994;266:F894–F900.
46. Eguchi S, Hirata Y, Imai T, et al. Phenotypic changes of endothelin receptor sybtype in cultured rat vascular smooth muscle cells. *Endocrinology* 1994;134:222–228.
47. MacLean MR, McCulloch KM, Baird M. Endothelin ET_A- and ET_B-receptor-mediated vasoconstriction in rat pulmonary arteries and arterioles. *J Cardiovasc Pharmacol* 1994;23:838–845.
48. Teerlink JR, Breu V, Sprecher U, et al. Potent vasoconstriction mediated by endothelin ETB receptors in canine coronary arteries. *Circ Res* 1994;74:105–114.
49. Shetty SS, Okada T, Webb RL, et al. Functionally distinct endothelin b receptors in vascular endothelium and smooth muscle. *Biochem Biophys Res Commun* 1993;191(2):459–464.
50. White DG, Cannon TR, Garratt H, et al. Endothelin ET_A and ET_B Receptors mediate vascular smooth-muscle contraction. *J Cardiovasc Pharmacol* 1993;22:S144–S148.

Chapter 7

Effect of Estrogen in Vascular Smooth Muscle Injury and Restenosis

Marie L. Foegh, MD, DSc
and Peter W. Ramwell, PhD

The continued rise in the use of estrogen in an increasing post-menopausal female population makes investigating the effect of estrogen on the vascular system important. The most recent prospective study on the cardiovascular effects of estrogen replacement therapy (ERT) has confirmed previous retrospective studies.[1] Estrogen studies in both primates that were fed a high-cholesterol diet and in the clinic consistently have shown decreased risk of coronary disease that is not completely explained by changes in the plasma lipoprotein profile. It now is thought that some of the beneficial effects of estrogen are due to a direct effect on the vascular wall exerted through specific estrogen receptors. As early as 1978, Colburn and Buonassisi[2] showed that smooth muscle cells obtained from the rat aorta had estrogen binding sites. The presence of estrogen binding sites in blood vessels since then has been confirmed by other groups, and more recently estrogen binding sites have been identified in coronary arteries.[3,4] Over the years, our laboratories have shown a consistent inhibitory effect of estradiol on arterial smooth muscle cell proliferation in both native and allograft vessels (Table 1).

Smooth Muscle Cells In Vitro

A study in our laboratory using explants of pig coronary arteries showed for the first time that estradiol has a direct and dose-

From: Forte TM, (ed). *Hormonal, Metabolic, and Cellular Influences on Cardiovascular Disease in Women.* Armonk, NY: Futura Publishing Company, Inc.; © 1997.

TABLE 1

Estradiol Mechanisms for Inhibition of Myointimal Hyperplasia

Results/findings	Reference
Inhibition of coronary artery transplant arteriosclerosis (1987)	19
Prevention of endothelial degeneration (1991)	23
Prevention of macrophage appearance in the neointima (1991)	23
Inhibition of smooth muscle cell proliferation of pig coronary artery (1993)	5
Inhibition of arterial neointimal hyperplasia after balloon injury (1994)	15
Inhibition of smooth muscle cell proliferation induced by free radicals (1994)	32
Abolition of class II antigen expression (1995)	20
Specific bindiing to rat coronary artery smooth muscle cells (1995)	4

dependent inhibitory effect on smooth muscle cell proliferation.[5] Other in vitro studies[6,7] using primary smooth muscle cell cultures from rat aorta showed the inhibitory effect of estradiol on cell proliferation to be specific in that an anti-estrogen (ZK 119010, Schering AG, Berlin, Germany) abolished the antiproliferative effect of estradiol[6] (Figure 1). This inhibitory effect of estradiol on smooth muscle cells may be due to a number of factors. For example, the growth arresting gene (GAS-1) is activated in smooth muscle cells in culture after 48 hours exposure to estradiol (D. W. Losordo, unpublished data). Here, we focus on the effect of estradiol on the expression of insulin-like growth factor-I (IGF-I), because this growth factor has been shown by Delafontaine and collaborators[8] to be crucial in smooth muscle cell proliferation. The role of other growth factors like PDGF, FGF, and EGF is very interesting in that they increase IGF-I receptor expression of smooth muscle cells to permit IGF-I to exert its mitogenic effect.

We have confirmed in vascular smooth muscle cells in culture that IGF-I is indeed a mitogen and that the mitogenic effect of IGF-I is specific insofar as IGF-I antibody abolishes the IGF-I-induced mitogenic effect.[6] We suggest that the mechanisms by which estradiol inhibits smooth muscle cell proliferation may be by abrogating the mitogenic effect of IGF-I because estradiol abolishes cell proliferation after smooth muscle cell exposure to IGF-I. The more specific molecular mechanisms by which this inhibition occurs need to be defined. It is interesting that this inhibitory action of estradiol on the IGF-I mitogenic effect is contrary to what occurs in breast cancer

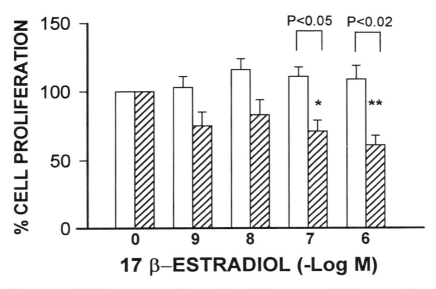

FIGURE 1. *Rabbit aorta smooth muscle cells (passages 4-7) in serum free culture medium show a dose-dependent estradiol inhibition of cell proliferation at 48 hours. The inhibition is significant at doses of 10^{-7} M (P < 0.05) and 10^{-6} M (**P < 0.002). This inhibition is abolished by the specific anti-estrogen ZK 119010. Clear bars, ZK 119010; shaded bars, estradiol.*

cells in culture.[9,10] These contrary effects may be due either to differences in gene regulation or to differences in the secondary messenger signals in vascular smooth muscle cells and immortalized breast cancer cells. In this context, it is important to note that both oral estrogen and the partial estrogen agonist tamoxifen, which is used in treating breast cancer, decrease the circulating IGF-I levels in postmenopausal women.[11,12]

Venous Smooth Muscle Cells

Our experimental work done in rabbit jugular vein grafts in vivo and in venous segments from the human saphenous and dog femoral veins in vitro, has made it clear that smooth muscle cells from different vascular beds respond differently to antiproliferative agents. For example, in male New Zealand white rabbits, we conducted a series of experiments in which the jugular vein was interpositioned in the carotid artery to mimic saphenous vein bypass grafts of coronary artery lesions in patients. The grafts were harvested 3 weeks after the original surgical procedure. It was found that estradiol had no effect on the area of myointimal hyperplasia.[13] In contrast, Angiopeptin, a somatostatin analogue, decreases myointimal hyperplasia in the venous graft in vivo.[14] In vitro, forskolin has an excellent inhibitory effect on smooth muscle cell proliferation of the human saphenous vein, measured as tritiated thymidine incorporation. In contrast, in both human and dog veins, estradiol failed to inhibit thymidine incorporation.[13] We conclude therefore that estradiol does not inhibit venous smooth muscle cell proliferation in vitro or in vivo.

In Vivo Estradiol Inhibition of Myointimal Proliferation

Several publications during the years show estradiol to inhibit experimental arteriosclerosis in animal models including the rabbit. All these studies support the findings that estradiol positively affects the plasma lipoprotein profile and thus inhibits arteriosclerosis. To further explore the beneficial effects of estradiol that are unrelated to changes in lipoprotein profiles, we studied the effect of chronic estradiol treatment and myointimal hyperplasia after intravascular balloon injury in the rabbit. The animals were treated with either placebo or estradiol-17β cypionate. Another group of rabbits was treated with Angiopeptin, the stable somatostatin analogue, to serve as a positive control. At the end of 3 weeks, the rabbits were sacrificed and the aorta and iliac vessels were harvested after perfusion pressure fixation at 80 mmHg. Computerized morphometry was performed on at least three cross-sections from each vessel segment, namely the aorta, common iliac, and external iliac arteries. We found that in all three arteries, treatment with estradiol, as well as with the positive control Angiopeptin, significantly inhibited the myointimal hyperplasia expressed as percentage area of intimal hyperplasia over total vessel area.[15]

In additional experiments, balloon injury of the aorta was performed, and 48 hours later the rabbits were injected with tritiated thymidine, then sacrificed after 24 hours. In vitro scintillation counting of the aorta showed that thymidine incorporation was reduced significantly in the animals receiving estradiol compared with the placebo. In this model, because the endothelium is removed by the embolectomy balloon, the endothelium does not contribute to any possible effect of estradiol.[15] Removal of the endothelium usually promotes smooth muscle cell proliferation.[5]

Because of the protective effect of estrogen treatment, we performed a series of experiments in a rat model in which orthotopic syngeneic aorta transplantation was performed in male and female rats.[16] The combinations are illustrated in Figure 2. The aorta segments were harvested 1 month after the transplantation procedure. The results are shown in Figure 3. Female gender of the blood vessel protected against myointimal proliferation after surgical injury, which includes both ischemic and reperfusion injury. Our finding that female arteries responded with less myointimal hyperplasia than male vessels, independent of a male or female environment, made us consider whether female arteries would respond with the same degree of myointimal hyperplasia to balloon angioplasty as the male. Knowing that in balloon injury the endothelium is removed, we balloon-injured male and female aortas and iliac vessels and harvested those vessels 3 weeks later. As can be seen from Figure 4, there is no significant difference in the degree of myointimal hyperplasia in the male and female vessels. This suggests that the gender difference we discovered in the syngeneic transplant model (see Figure 3) lies in the female endothelium exerting a greater inhibitory

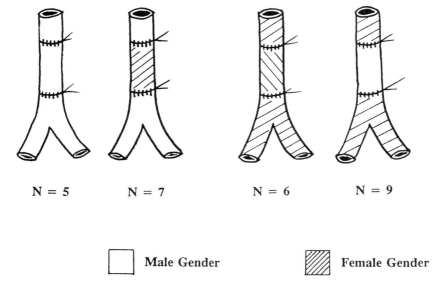

N = 5   N = 7   N = 6   N = 9

☐ Male Gender   ▨ Female Gender

FIGURE 2. *The orthotopic syngeneic aorta transplantation is illustrated here, showing the gender combination and the number of animals in the four possible combinations.*

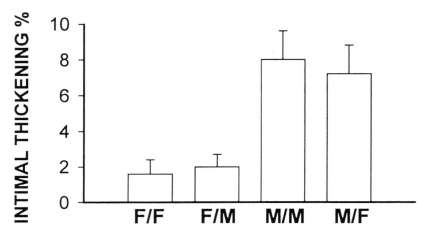

FIGURE 3. *In orthotopic syngeneic aorta transplants, the female gender of the vessel protects against myointimal proliferation. F/F, female donor, female recipient; F/M, female donor, male recepient; M/M, male donor, male recipient; M/F, male donor, female recipient.*

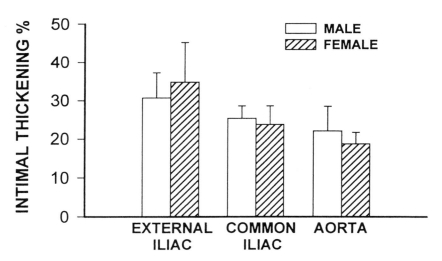

FIGURE 4. *Male and female rabbits underwent balloon angioplasty of the aorta and iliac arteries. The animals were sacrificed 3 weeks later, and the vessels harvested after perfusation fixation. The area of myointimal proliferation and the total vessel area were determined by computerized morphometry. After balloon injury, male and female vessels shown no significant difference in degree of myointimal hyperplasia, expressed as area of myointima over total vessel area × 100%.*

effect on smooth muscle cell neointima formation than in the male. This seems a reasonable possibility because estrogen has been shown to induce nitric oxide (NO) synthase[17] and NO promotes cyclic guanosine monophosphate (cGMP), which is antiproliferative.[18]

In Vivo Immune Injury to Coronary Arteries

In the rabbit transplant model of accelerated coronary artery transplant arteriosclerosis, we demonstrated in 1987 that estrogen inhibits coronary graft myointimal thickening.[19] We later replicated these experiments and obtained similar results.[20] In this transplant model, the rabbits are exposed to chronic estradiol treatment for 6–7 weeks. All donors and recipients are fed a 0.5% cholesterol diet to bring the rabbit cholesterol level closer to that of humans.[21] By this diet the rabbit serum lipoproteins changed as shown in Table 2. The antiproliferative effect of estradiol on transplant arteriosclerosis is similar to that of Angiopeptin, our positive control.[22] The mechanism of estradiol inhibition of transplant arteriosclerosis was shown previously to be associated with preventing the appearance of monocytes/macrophages in the neointima. Furthermore, in the estradiol-treated aorta evaluated by electron microscopy, the endothelium is preserved.[23] In contrast, the aorta transplants from the control animals exhibited degenerative endothelial changes and numerous macrophages in the neointima. We speculate that estradiol may exert its protective effect by promoting nitric oxide synthesis and increasing cGMP.

In a recent study in the rabbit cardiac transplant arteriosclerosis model, we also harvested parts of the ascending aorta belonging to

TABLE 2

Plasma Lipoprotein Levels (mg/dl) in Rabbits on Normal Diet and Rabbits Fed a 0.5% Cholesterol Diet

	Normal diet	Cholesterol diet
Total cholesterol	30 ± 5	396 ± 149
VLDL	13 ± 4	150 ± 67
ILDL	0.3 ± 0.3	88 ± 38
LDL	3.7 ± 2	123 ± 42
HDL	13 ± 3	35 ± 6

Values are means ±

the cardiac graft as well as the native aorta. These vessels were challenged in vitro with IGF-I for 48 hours to determine their responsiveness to this growth factor. We found that IGF-I was a potent mitogen for the cell proliferation in the aorta belonging to the transplanted heart, and further, that chronic estradiol treatment (7 weeks) completely abolished this mitogenic response to IGF-I. These findings suggest that estradiol treatment prevents IGF-I mitogenic effects in both native and transplanted arteries.[20] Estradiol may inhibit IGF-I synthesis or receptor.

The effects of estradiol on IGF-I are also complicated by the fact that IGF-I has six different binding proteins, which, in addition to binding IGF-I, may have effects of their own.[24–26] Thus, some of the effects of estradiol on the IGF-I mitogenic response could be through the binding proteins, particularly binding proteins 3 and 6.[27,28]

Clinical Use of Estrogens

The beneficial experimental effects of estradiol and the known effect of estradiol in preventing cardiovascular disease in women suggest that it might be advantageous to administer estrogen to women undergoing coronary angioplasty,[29] bypass surgery (arterial grafts), and cardiac transplantation or other organ transplants. Recently a study has been published in which women undergoing coronary angioplasty were evaluated for clinical event outcome, depending on whether they were on estrogen replacement therapy. It was found that estrogen replacement therapy indeed decreased the risk of serious clinical events. The events that were decreased by estradiol treatment were death and myocardial infarction but not revascularization. There was no effect on the actual angiographic restenosis of the target coronary lesion but this may be due to the small number of women on estrogen replacement therapy (n=54) in contrast to the nonestrogen treated women (n=223).[30]

At present, there is no information on whether estrogen treatment decreases the reocclusion of a venous bypass graft. On the basis of our in vitro studies with human saphenous vein and the in vivo study of jugular veins interpositioned in the carotid artery in rabbits, one may suspect that there would be no effect of estradiol treatment on reocclusion of vein grafts. In contrast, estradiol may be beneficial for the arterial mammary bypass grafts.

The question of the outcome for female recipients of cardiac transplants compared with male recipients is more complex in that both women and men can receive a graft from either the same or a different gender. Currently there is only one small study available evaluating the effect of gender on both the graft and the recipient. This study showed that the worst outcome was in the male patient receiving a female cardiac transplant, followed by a male patient receiving a male cardiac graft; the best combination was that of a male graft to a female recipient.[31] Unfortunately there is no information on female grafts to female recipients, because most donors are men. This rank order is not in accordance with our findings in our syngeneic grafts, in which an advantage existed for a female vessel compared with a male vessel. In transplantation, the issues are complex, and it is known that female grafts represent a stronger immune challenge than male grafts. Knowing that immune phenomena play a role in development of transplant arteriosclerosis, it is not difficult to accept that a female graft to a male recipient may cause a stronger immunologic response, and thus, in terms of transplant arteriosclerosis, is the least desirable combination. This interference of immunology in the inherited gender differences in myointimal hyperplasia in the presence of endothelium is further confirmed by the fact that a male cardiac graft into a female recipient is the best of the three available combinations. The answer to whether a female-to-female graft is the most beneficial will help confirm this speculation. There is no information on the effect on graft rejection of estradiol treatment in women receiving a transplant. However, experimental data strongly suggest that estradiol treatment will inhibit the development of transplant arteriosclerosis.

References

1. The writing group for the PEPI Trial. Effects of estrogen or estrogen/ progestin regimens on heart disease risk factors in postmenopausal women. The postmenopausal estrogen/progestin interventions (PEPI) trial. *JAMA* 1995;273:199–208.
2. Colburn P, Buonassisi V. Estrogen-binding sites in endothelial cell cultures. *Science* 1978;201:817–819.
3. Losordo DW, Kearney M, Kim EA, et al. Variable expression of the estrogen receptor in normal and atherosclerotic coronary arteries of premenopausal women. *Circulation* 1994;89(4):1501–1510.
4. Bei M, Lavigne MC, Foegh ML, et al. Specific binding of 17β-estradiol to rat coronary artery smooth muscle cells. *J Steroid Biochem Mol Biol* 1996;58:83–88.
5. Vargas R, Wroblewska B, Rego A, et al. Oestradiol inhibits smooth muscle cell proliferation of pig coronary artery. *Br J Pharmacol* 1993; 109:612–617.
6. Lou H, Zhao Y, Delafontaine, P, et al. Estrogen inhibits vascular smooth muscle cell proliferation induced by insulin-like growth factor-I in na-

tive and graft arteries. Submitted. Effects on insulin-like growth factor-I (IGF-I) induced cell proliferation and IGF-I protein expression in native and allograft vessels. *Circulation* In press.

7. Foegh ML, Zhao Y, Lou H, et al. Estrogen and prevention of transplant atherosclerosis. *J Heart Lung Transplant* 1995;14:S170–S172.

8. Delafontaine P, Meng XP, Ku L, et al. Regulation of vascular smooth muscle cell insulin-like growth factor-I receptors by phosphorothioate oligonucleotides: Effects on cell growth and evidence that sense targeting at the ATG site increases receptor expression. *J Biol Chem* 1995; 270:14383–14388.

9. Dickson RB, Lippman ME. Estrogen regulation of growth and polypeptide growth factor secretion in human breast carcinoma. *Endocr Rev* 1986;8:29–43.

10. Davidson NE, Lippman ME. The role of estrogens in growth regulation of breast cancers. *Oncogenesis* 1989;1(suppl 1):89–111.

11. Weissberger AJ, Ho KK, Lazarus L. Contrasting effects of oral and transdermal routes of estrogen replacement therapy on 24-hour growth hormone (GH) secretion, insulin-like growth factor-I, and GH-binding protein in postmenopausal women. *J Clin Endocrinol Metab* 1991;72: 374–381.

12. Huynh HT, Tetenes E, Wallace L, et al. In vivo inhibition of insulin-like growth factor-I gene expression by Tamoxifen. *Cancer Res* 1993;53: 1727–1730.

13. Calcagno D, Bei M, Ross SA, et al. Effects of estrogen on vein grafts. *J Cardiovasc Surg* 1992;33:579–584.

14. Calcagno D, Conte JV, Howell MH, et al. Peptide inhibition of neointimal hyperplasia in vein grafts. *J Vasc Surg* 1991;13:475–479.

15. Foegh ML, Asotra S, Howell MH, et al. Estradiol inhibition of arterial neointimal hyperplasia after balloon injury. *J Vasc Surg* 1994;19: 722–726.

16. Foegh M, Rego A, Lou H, et al. Gender effects on graft myointimal hyperplasia. *Transplant Proc* 1995;27:2070–2072.

17. Weiner CP, Lizasoain I, Baylis SA, et al. Induction of calcium-dependent nitric oxide synthases by sex hormones. *Proc Natl Acad Sci USA* 1994; 91(11):5212–5216.

18. Seki J, Nishio M, Kato Y, et al. FK409, a new nitric-oxide donor, suppresses smooth muscle proliferation in the rat model of balloon angioplasty. *Atherosclerosis* 1995;117:97–106.

19. Foegh ML, Khirabadi BS, Nakanishi T, et al. Estradiol protects against experimental cardiac transplant atherosclerosis. *Transplant Proc* 1987; 19:90–95.

20. Lou H, Kodama T, Zhao F, et al. Inhibition of transplant coronary arteriosclerosis in rabbits by chronic estradiol treatment is associated with abolition of MHC class II antigen expression. *Circulation* 1996;95:3355–3359.

21. Howell MH, Adams MM, Wolfe MS, et al. Angiopeptin inhibition of myointimal hyperplasia after balloon angioplasty of large arteries in hypercholesterolaemic rabbits. *Clin Sci* 1993;85:183–188.

22. Foegh ML, Khirabadi BS, Chambers E, et al. Inhibition of coronary artery transplant atherosclerosis in rabbits with Angiopeptin, an octapeptide. *Atherosclerosis* 1989;78:229–236.

23. Cheng LP, Kuwahara M, Jacobsson J, et al. Inhibition of myointimal hyperplasia and macrophage infiltration by estradiol in aorta allografts. *Transplantation* 1991;259:905–915.

24. Figueroa JA, Sharma J, Jackson JG, et al. Recombinant insulin-like growth factor binding protein-1 inhibits IGF-I, serum, and estrogen-dependent growth of MCF-7 human breast cancer cells. *J Cell Physiol* 1993;157(2):229–236.
25. Mouhieddine OB, Cazals V, Maitre B, et al. Insulin-like growth factor-II (IGF-II), type 2 IGF receptor, and IGF-binding protein-2 gene expression in rat lung alveolar epithelial cells: Relation to proliferation. *Endocrinology* 1994;135(1):83–91.
26. Valentinis B, Bhala A, De Angelis T, et al. The human insulin-like growth factor (IGF) binding protein-3 inhibits the growth of fibroblasts with a targeted disruption of the IGF-I receptor gene. *Mol Endocrinol* 1995; 9(3):361–367.
27. Kleinman D, Karas M, Roberts CT Jr, et al. Modulation of insulin-like growth factor-I (IGF-I) receptors and membrane-associated IGF-binding proteins in endometrial cancer cells by estradiol. *Endocrinology* 1995;136(6):2531–2537.
28. Martin JL, Coverley JA, Pattison ST, et al. Insulin-like growth factor-binding protein-3 production by MCF-7 breast cancer cells: Stimulation by retinoic acid and cyclic adenosine monophosphate and differential effects of estradiol. *Endocrinology* 1995;136(3):1219–1226.
29. Bell MR, Grill DE, Garratt KN, et al. Long-term outcome of women compared with men after successful coronary angioplasty. *Circulation* 1995;91:2876–2881.
30. Abu-Halawa S, Stokes MJ, Lynn P, et al. Estrogen replacement therapy reduces recurrent clinical events after coronary angioplasty in post-menopausal women. Abstract. *Circulation* 1994;90(part 2):I-22.
31. Mehra MR, Ventura HO, Escobar A, et al. Does donor and recipient sex influence the development of cardiac allograft vasculopathy? *Transplant Proc* 1995;27:1926–1929.
32. Cathapermal S, Leong-Son MY, Ramwell PW. The role of estradiol 17β on free radical induced vascular myointimal hyperplasia. Abstract. *J Am Coll Cardiol* (Special Issue), 44th Annual Scientific Session, American College of Cardiology, New Orleans, LA, March 19–22, 1995;72A.

Chapter 8

The Role of Estrogen on Nitric Oxide-Mediated Monocyte Adherence to the Aortic Endothelium

Lauren Nathan, MD, Rajan Singh, PhD,
Shehla Pervin, PhD,
Gautam Chaudhuri, MD, PhD,
and Michael Rosenfeld, PhD

The exact mechanism by which estrogen affords protection against atherogenesis in women is unknown. One of the early events in atherogenesis is the adhesion of monocytes to endothelial cells. As yet, the role of estrogen in modulating this step has not been elucidated. An understanding of factors controlling this crucial step, and specifically how they may be modulated by estradiol is imperative for the design of novel strategies to prevent coronary artery disease.

Estrogens and Atherosclerosis

Women in the reproductive age group are protected from coronary artery disease when compared with men.[1] Similarly, estrogen replacement therapy in postmenopausal women reduces the risk of coronary artery disease relative to the risk in postmenopausal women who do not receive estrogen replacement.[2] This protection is seen also in other animal species. Adams et al.[3] demonstrated less coronary artery lesion formation in oophorectom-

From: Forte TM, (ed). *Hormonal, Metabolic, and Cellular Influences on Cardiovascular Disease in Women*. Armonk, NY: Futura Publishing Company, Inc.; © 1997.

ized subhuman primates receiving estrogen or estrogen plus progesterone as compared with oophorectomized animals receiving placebo. This effect was seen despite comparable lipid levels in all groups.[3] Estradiol administration to rabbits fed a high-cholesterol diet led to decreased aortic accumulation of cholesterol when compared with the control group.[4,5] In these studies, the beneficial effect of estradiol on atherosclerosis could only partly be explained by its effect in lowering serum total cholesterol or VLDL cholesterol. Using quantitative coronary angiography, it was demonstrated that in oophorectomized, adult female cynomolgus macaque monkeys, whose coronary arteries were rendered atherosclerotic, intracoronary infusion of the endothelium-dependent vasodilator, acetylcholine, caused paradoxical constriction of coronary arteries.[6] After estradiol administration, acetylcholine tended to dilate maximally the coronary vessels, and this altered response was not related to plaque extent.[6]

Nitric Oxide

Various substances may be involved in estrogen's protection against atherosclerosis. Nitric oxide (NO) is one such substance that has received attention over the past few years and that has been proposed to play a protective role in atherogenesis. NO, previously referred to as endothelium-derived relaxing factor (EDRF), mediates the vascular relaxation produced by various endothelium-dependent vasodilators such as acetylcholine, and bradykinin.[7] NO is formed in endothelial cells from the guanidino nitrogen of L-arginine by a calcium-dependent oxidative reaction.[8] An arginine-citrulline cycle has been described and the conversion of arginine to citrulline results in the formation of NO.[8] The synthesis of NO in NO-generating cells is inhibited by the arginine analogues, eg, N^G-monomethyl-L-arginine (L-NMA) and N^G-nitro-L-arginine (L-NA).[9,10] Based on data outlined below, NO could be involved in estrogen's modulation of monocyte adhesion to endothelial cells.

Nitric Oxide and Atherosclerosis

There is some evidence suggesting that decreased production of NO may be involved in the pathogenesis of atherosclerosis. In ani-

mal models and in humans, hypercholesterolemia causes endothelial dysfunction that is manifested by an attenuation of endothelium-
dependent vasorelaxation.[11–13] Furthermore, native and oxidized
low-density lipoproteins inactivate NO in vitro.[14] As these lipoproteins accumulate in atherosclerotic plaques,[15–17] it has been speculated that there may be an accelerated inactivation of NO by these
lipoproteins.[13] Thus, decreased NO formation may be associated
with progression of atherosclerotic lesions.

Decreased NO formation also may be associated with the initiation of atherogenesis. Tsao et al.[18] suggested this in a study of
monocyte binding in an ex vivo rabbit model. Briefly, animals were
fed a high-cholesterol diet alone or high-cholesterol diet supplemented with L-arginine, the precursor of NO. After the feeding period, animals were sacrificed, and the aortas harvested. Aortas then
were incubated with a monocyte cell line and adhesion observed. It
was found that the percent binding of monocytes after cholesterol
feeding was reversed to control levels with L-arginine. To lend support to the concept that NO was responsible for the observed decrease in monocyte binding, these investigators also demonstrated,
in a separate arm of the study, that inhibition of NO synthesis in
animals fed a normal diet led to increased monocyte adhesion.[18]
Other investigators have found that NO is involved in monocyte adhesion by demonstrating in vitro that NO itself can prevent adhesion
of monocytes to endothelial cells[19].

Estrogen, Nitric Oxide, and Atherosclerosis

As previously discussed, monocyte adhesion is one of the earliest steps in atherogenesis. Furthermore, several lines of evidence
suggest that estrogen may exert its protective effect at this early
stage via an NO-mediated mechanism. Hayashi et al.[20] demonstrated greater basal release of NO from aortic rings obtained
from female as compared with male rabbits and oophorectomized
female rabbits. In this study, greater contractile responses of aortic rings in females as compared with males were observed after
inhibition of NO synthesis. The presence of estrogen in the females could have accounted for the increased basal release of NO.
It also has been suggested that expression of NO synthase mRNA[21]
and protein[21,22] from endothelial cells is enhanced in the presence
of estradiol. Furthermore, as enumerated above, NO has been
shown to decrease monocyte adhesion to endothelial cells.[18,19]
Thus, increased production of NO, enhanced by estradiol, may

inhibit monocyte adhesion and thereby prevent the early stages of atherogenesis.

Estrogen and Monocyte Adhesion

Based on the above background, we decided to evaluate whether estradiol inhibits monocyte adhesion in an in vivo model and then to evaluate if any inhibition observed is mediated by NO. To address this question, we elected to first evaluate gender differences in monocyte adhesion in rabbits after an atherogenic diet. Adult male and female rabbits were placed on an atherogenic (0.5% cholesterol) diet for 4 weeks, after which they were anesthetized and their aortic trees fixed in vivo via perfusion of paraformaldehye. After the fixation process, the aortic tree was dissected from the animal. A portion of aorta containing the celiac bifurcation was selected for preparation for scanning electron microscopy (SEM). SEM then was used to evaluate monocyte adhesion to endothelial cells in a 13.5 mm² area just distal to the celiac branch point.

Preliminary results from this protocol suggest that the number of adherent monocytes is less in female as compared with male rabbits, despite comparable lipid levels throughout the 4-week feeding period. Given the small number of specimens that have been evaluated thus far, however, it is impossible to draw any firm conclusions from this data. We are in the process of carrying out similar experiments assessing the specific role of estradiol in monocyte adhesion after hypercholesterolemia by performing the above experiments in oophorectomized female rabbits supplemented with placebo or estradiol pellets.

Based on our preliminary data, we have begun to evaluate potential mechanisms by which estrogen could modulate monocyte adhesion in vivo. A large number of surface molecules have been described that have adhesive properties on either endothelial cells or monocytes[23] and that well may be targets of estrogen's protective action. Significant among these molecules are vascular cell adhesion molecule-1 (VCAM-1) and monocyte chemoattractant protein-1 (MCP-1). VCAM-1 holds particular interest with regard to the initiation of macrophage-rich fatty streak lesions because of its functional specificity and pattern of expression.[24] VCAM-1, a member of the immunoglobulin gene superfamily, is a mononuclear leukocyte selective adhesion molecule expressed in cultured human vascular endothelial cells after activation by certain cytokines released locally at the site of atherogenesis, such as interleukin-1 (IL-1) and interferon-γ (IFN-γ).[24,25] This inducible endothelial cell surface molecule mediates intercellular adhesion via interaction with its counter receptor, very late activation antigen-1 (VLA-4), a β1-integrin expressed by monocytes.[26] Recent studies have disclosed that the endothelium that overlies foam cell lesions of aortas in hyperlipidemic rabbits focally and selectively expresses VCAM-1, as detected with the monoclonal antibody (mAb) Rb1/9.[27] Furthermore, a study by Nakai et al.[28] demonstrated that estradiol inhibited expression of VCAM-1 in human umbilical vein endothelial cells stimulated with IL-1β.

MCP-1 is a potent chemoattractant for monocytes and belongs to a novel family of pro-inflammatory proteins also known as chemokines.[29] This protein is also expressed on endothelial cells by cytokines.[30] It also appears to be modulated by estradiol according to a study by Frazier-Jessen and Kovacs[31]; the study demonstrated that estrogen inhibited LPS-stimulated expression of MCP-1 in a murine macrophage cell line. These studies suggest a potential mechanism by which estrogen may be modulating this early step in atherogenesis. We therefore decided to evaluate whether estradiol modulated expression of these factors in our in vivo model.

We have performed preliminary experiments assessing the expression of VCAM-1 protein in the following groups of female rabbits: group 1, oophorectomized and fed normal chow for 6 weeks; group 2, oophorectomized and fed atherogenic diet for 6 weeks; and group 3, oophorectomized/estradiol supplemented and fed an atherogenic diet for 6 weeks. After the 6-week feeding period, animals were sacrificed and sections of aorta taken for Western blot analysis. Preliminary results revealed decreased VCAM-1 protein in abdominal aorta at the level of the celiac bifurcation in group 2, as compared with groups 1 or 3. This suggests modulation of VCAM-1 expression by estradiol, but further analyses will need to be carried out before definitive conclusions can be drawn.

Nitric Oxide and Monocyte Adhesion

Because NO may play an important role in the early stages of atherogenesis, the next aspect we plan to explore is the role of NO in monocyte adhesion in our in vivo model. Our future studies therefore will involve evaluating monocyte adhesion in estradiol and placebo supplemented oophorectomized rabbits in the presence and absence of an inhibitor of NO synthesis. It is hoped that studies such as these will allow us to identify one or more important mechanisms

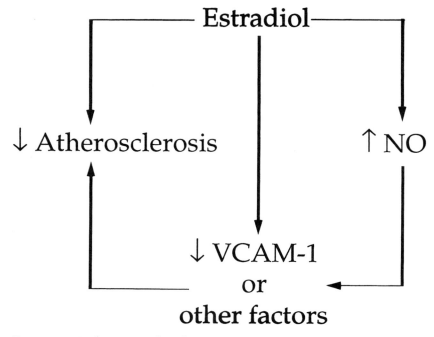

FIGURE 1. *Mechanisms whereby estrogen modulates monocyte adhesion and the early steps in atherosclerosis.*

(as outlined in Figure 1) by which estrogen may be acting to prevent this most prevalent disease process.

References

1. Kannel WB, Hjortland MC, McNamara PM, et al. Menopause and the risk of cardiovascular disease: The Framingham Study. *Ann Int Med* 1976;85:447–452.
2. Stampfer MJ, Colditz BA. Estrogen replacement therapy and coronary heart disease: A quantitative assessment of the epidemiologic evidence. *Prev Med* 1991;20:47–63.
3. Adams MR, Kaplan JR, Manuck SP, et al. Inhibition of coronary artery atherosclerosis by 17βestradiol in ovariectomized monkeys: Lack of an effect of added progesterone. *Arteriosclerosis* 1990;10:1051–1057.
4. Haarbo J, Leth-Espensen P, Stender S, et al. Estrogen monotherapy and combined estrogen-progestogen replacement therapy attenuate aortic accumulation of cholesterol in ovariectomized cholesterol-fed rabbits. *J Clin Invest* 1991;87:1274–1279.

5. Hough JL, Zilversmit DB. Effect of 17βestradiol on aortic cholesterol content and metabolism in cholesterol-fed rabbits. *Arteriosclerosis* 1986; 6:57–63.
6. William JK, Adams MR, Klopfenstein HS. Estrogen modulates responses of atherosclerotic coronary arteries. *Circulation* 1990;81: 1680–1687.
7. Furchgott RF. The role of endothelium in the responses of vascular smooth muscle to drugs. *Ann Rec Pharmacol Toxicol* 1984;24:175–197.
8. Palmer RMJ, Ashton DS, Moncada S. Vascular endothelial cells synthesize nitric oxide from L-arginine. *Nature* 1988;333:664–666.
9. Rees DD, Palmer RMJ, Moncada S. Role of endothelium-derived nitric oxide in the regulation of blood pressure. *Proc Natl Acad Sci USA* 1981;86:3375–3378.
10. Vargas HM, Cuevas JM, Ignarro LJ, et al. Comparison of the inhibitory potencies of N^G-methyl-, N^G-nitro- and N^G-amino-L-arginine on EDRF function in the rat: Evidence for continuous basal EDRF release. *J Pharmacol Exp Therap* 1991;257:1208–1215.
11. Zeiher AM, Drexler H, Wollschlager H, et al. Modulation of coronary vasomotor tone in humans: Progressive endothelial dysfunction with different early stages of coronary atherosclerosis. *Circulation* 1991;83: 391–401.
12. Verbeuren T, Jordaens F, Zonnekeyen L, et al. Endothelium-dependent and endothelium-independent contractions and relaxations in isolated arteries of control and hypercholesterolemic rabbits. *Circ Res* 1986 58:552–564.
13. Galle J, Busse R, Bassange E. Hypercholesterolemia and atherosclerosis change vascular reactivity in rabbits by different mechanisms. *Arterioscler Thromb* 1991;11:1712–1718.
14. Galle J, Mulsch A, Busse R, et al. Effects of native and oxidized low density lipoproteins on formation and inactivation of endothelium-derived relaxing factor. *Arterioscler Thromb* 1991;11:198–203.
15. Yla-Herttuala S, Palinsky W, Rosenfeld ME, et al. Evidence for the presence of oxidatively modified low density lipoprotein in atherosclerotic lesions of rabbit and man. *J Clin Invest* 1989;84:1086–1095.
16. Daugherty A, Zweifel BS, Sobel BE, et al. Isolation of low density lipoprotein from atherosclerotic vascular tissue of Watanabe heritable hyperlipidemic rabbits. *Arteriosclerosis* 1988;8:768–777.
17. Hoff HF, Morton RE. Lipoproteins containing apo-β extracted from human aortas. *Ann NY Acad Sci* 1985;454:183–194.
18. Tsao PS, McEvoy LM, Drexler H, et al. Enhanced endothelial adhesiveness in hypercholesterolemia is attenuated by L-arginine. *Circulation* 1994;89:2176–2182.
19. Bath PMW, Hassal DG, Gladwin AM, et al. Nitric oxide and prostacyclin. Divergence of inhibitory effects on monocyte chemotaxis and adhesion to endothelium in vitro. *Arterioscler Thromb* 1991;11:254–260.
20. Hayashi T, Fukuto JM, Ignarro LJ, et al. Basal release of nitric oxide from aortic rings is greater in female rabbits than in male rabbits: Implications for atherosclerosis. *Proc Natl Acad Sci USA* 1992;89:11259–11263.
21. Schray-Utz V, Zeiher AM, Busse R. Expression of constitutive NO synthase in cultured endothelial cells is enhanced by 17βestradiol. Abstract. *Circulation* 1993;88(pt 2) I-80.

22. Hishikawa K, Nakaki T, Marumo T, et al. Up-regulation of nitric oxide by estradiol in human aortic endothelial cells. *FEBS Lett* 1995;360: 291–293.
23. Beekhuizen H, van Furth R. Monocyte adherence to human vascular endothelium. *J Leukocyte Biol* 1993;54:363–378.
24. Li H, Cybulsky MI, Gimbrone MA, et al. An atherogenic diet rapidly induces VCAM-1, a cytokine-regulatable mononuclear leukocyte adhesion molecule, in rabbit aortic endothelium. *Arterioscler Thromb* 1993; 13:197–204.
25. Bevilacqua MP, Pober JS, Mendrick DL, et al. Identification of an inducible endothelial-leukocyte adhesion molecule. *Proc Natl Acad Sci USA* 1987;84:9238–9242.
26. Elices JF, Osborn L. VCAM-1 on activated endothelium, interacts with the leukocyte integrin VLA-4 at a site distinct from the VLA-4/fibronectin binding site. *Cell* 1990;60:577–584.
27. Cybulsky MI, Gimbrone MA, Jr. Endothelial expression of a mononuclear leukocyte adhesion molecule during atherogenesis. *Science* 1991; 251:788–791.
28. Nakai K, Itoh C, Hotta K, et al. Estradiol-17β regulates the induction of VCAM-1 mRNA expression by interleukin-Iβ in human umbilical vein endothelial cells. *Life Sci* 1994;54:221–227.
29. Rojas A, Delgado R, Glaria L, et al. Monocyte chemotactic protein-1 inhibits the induction of nitric oxide synthase in J774 cells. *Biochem Biophys Res Commun* 1993;196:274–279.
30. Cushing SD, Fogelman AM. Monocytes may amplify their recruitment into inflammatory lesions by inducing monocyte chemotactic protein. *Arterioscler Thromb* 1992;12:78–82.
31. Frazier-Jessen MR, Kovacs EJ. Estrogen modulation of JE/monocyte chemoattractant protein mRNA expression in murine macrophages. *J Immunol* 1995;154:1838–1845.

Chapter 9

Enigma of Vascular Calcification in Osteoporotic Women

Linda L. Demer, MD, PhD,
Kristina Boström, MD, PhD,
Mihaela Balica, MD, and
Karol E. Watson, MD

Two disease processes, atherosclerosis and osteoporosis, are responsible for the vast majority of morbidity and mortality in women. Much of the research on these diseases has occurred in isolation. However, as advances in biomedical research demonstrate more and more that key factors have roles in both processes, it is clear that we can no longer study one disease at a time. Regulatory factors identified in one process soon are found to regulate others, such as nitric oxide (NO), transforming growth factor-β (TGF-β), insulin-like growth factors, and interleukins. The need for an integrated approach is particularly acute in women's health, where systemic hormonal changes add marked time variance to pathophysiological processes. Disease processes and their therapies must be studied and tested in context rather than in isolation.

There is little data to indicate whether osteoporosis prevention and therapy affects vascular calcification. (The terms calcification and ossification used herein refer to the mineralization and bone formation processes, respectively, or to the calcium mineral deposits themselves. Although the latter use has been challenged, it is widely used and accepted by Webster.) Osteoporosis prevention therapies are used widely. More than seven million women in the United States have osteoporosis,[1] and even asymptomatic postmenopausal

This work was supported in part by National Institutes of Health Grants HL-43379 and HL-30568 as well as by the Oberkotter Foundation, the Stein-Oppenheimer Award, and the Streisand Research Fund of the Lincy Foundation.

From: Forte TM, (ed). *Hormonal, Metabolic, and Cellular Influences on Cardiovascular Disease in Women.* Armonk, NY: Futura Publishing Company, Inc.; © 1997.

women are advised across the board to increase their calcium and/ or vitamin D intake to prevent possible osteoporosis.[2] Importantly, it is well known from animal studies that vitamin D and calcium supplements induce vascular calcification. In these animal studies, much higher doses were used than routinely are recommended for humans; however, the calcification occurs extremely rapidly, in <6 weeks. It generally is accepted in biomedical research that short-term high doses or agents administered to animals can be useful models of long-term use in humans, in part because it may not be reasonable or even possible to wait for long-term results of animal studies. Surprisingly, even though postmenopausal women are far more likely to die from cardiovascular disease than hip fracture, to our knowledge, no study of vitamin D and calcium supplements in humans has assessed the effects on coronary or aortic calcification.

Understanding potential relations between osteoporosis and vascular calcification—whether direct or more likely due to common regulatory mechanisms—is essential to prevent adverse consequences for a huge segment of our population. Vascular calcification is widespread. It hardens arteries and raises the risk of heart failure, myocardial ischemia and infarction, systolic hypertension, and complications of cardiovascular procedures. In previous studies, we identified bone developmental and regulatory factors in human calcified arteries, and we developed an in vitro model of vascular calcification using cloned subpopulations of vascular smooth muscle cells. These findings have raised the disturbing hypothesis that agents used to prevent osteoporosis may promote calcification of the vasculature more than that of the skeleton, increasing risk of heart disease, which presents a greater threat to life. Importantly, animal studies indicate that it is not only possible to prevent calcification, but the biological potential for regression and reversal are there.[3]

History of Understanding of Vascular Calcification

Calcification in the coronary arteries and other arteries has been regarded widely as an uncommon, insignificant, end-stage, passive, degenerative process of aging. These terms, which once were applied to atherosclerosis, may be just as inapplicable to vascular calcification. New in vivo imaging methods, ultrafast computed tomography (UFCT), and intravascular ultrasound, have revealed that vascular calcification is extremely common, occurring in 90% of patients with coronary artery disease[4] and in 80% of significant lesions.[5] Recent studies have revealed that vascular calcification is clinically significant, carrying an increased risk of mortality, myocardial infarction, ischemia, systolic hypertension, heart failure, and serious complications of surgery and interventional procedures.[6-13] The new imaging methods also have revealed that vascular calcification is progressive, beginning in the fatty streak stage[14] as early as the second and third decades of life[15,16] and often preceding coronary narrowing.[17] Our studies and those of others are furnishing evidence that vascular and valvular calcification are active, regulated processes involving bone differentiation and regulatory factors.[18-22]

Plaque Rupture and Myocardial Infarction

Coronary calcification is an independent risk factor for cardiac events.[8,23] Coronary calcification is also the single most important risk factor for dissection in coronary angioplasty,[11] a procedure to which hundreds of thousands of patients are subjected every year. Dissection accounts for most of the mortality and morbidity of the procedure. In vivo, during clinical angioplasty, plaque rupture occurs along the interface between calcium deposits and softer plaque elements where solid shear stress is highly concentrated.[11,24] The same mechanism may account for the increased risk of complications of balloon valvuloplasty of calcified valves[25] and spontaneous plaque rupture and would account for the increased risk of myocardial infarction and mortality in patients with coronary calcification.[6,9]

Aortic Calcification

Aortic calcification is also extremely common, and it is more common in older women than men.[9,26,27] It is an independent cardiovascular disease risk factor,[26] and it correlates with myocardial infarction.[9] Accumulation of calcium mineral, not cholesterol, is responsible for aortic rigidity and its adverse cardiovascular consequences[28-31] including ischemia,[32] left ventricular hypertrophy,[13] heart failure[33-36] and stroke.[37]

Ischemia is one consequence of aortic rigidity. Cardiac perfusion depends on diastolic coronary flow, which depends on diastolic aortic pressure and reverse aortic flow. The low compliance in a calcified aorta means less blood volume stored in the aorta at the start of diastole as well as little elastic recoil to drive reverse flow to the coronaries. In patients with little or no aortic compliance, reverse aortic flow and coronary perfusion are impaired significantly.[26,38] The ischemic syndromes reported by such patients have been attributed to insufficient blood flow through the coronary inlets, independent of coronary stenosis. Coronary insufficiency and ischemia also occur, even in the absence of coronary stenosis, in animals with artificially imposed chronic aortic rigidity but not controls.[13] Aortic rigidity results in even greater ischemia, hypoxemia, and ventricular dysfunction in combination with coronary stenosis.[39] These factors may explain the increased risk of myocardial infarction[9] and clinical coronary artery disease[40] associated with aortic calcification.

Heart failure is another consequence of aortic rigidity. The increased outflow impedance in a rigid aorta greatly increases cardiac work.[41] In animal studies, aortic rigidity increases the energy cost to the heart for maintaining adequate flow, doubles the oxygen requirement for a given stroke volume, and limits reserve capacity.[42] In patients, the acute increase in aortic rigidity due to insertion of a noncompliant graft was found to produce left ventricular hypertrophy, systolic hypertension, diastolic hypotension, and decreased coronary flow, resulting in some cases in fatal heart failure attributed to loss of the "Windkessel effect" ie, aortic compliance and elastic recoil.[36] The physiology of the Windkessel effect is comparable with aortic balloon counterpulsation. Heart failure is further compounded by outflow impedance added by aortic valve calcification. Valvular calcification also involves mature bone tissue and bone regulatory proteins.[43,44]

Systolic hypertension and end-organ damage also result from aortic rigidity. Aortic stiffness is a major determinant of systolic blood pressure.[45,46] Isolated systolic hypertension, which results from aortic rigidity, is a significant, independent risk factor for cardiovascular morbidity and mortality.[47-49]

Arrest of Compensatory Enlargement

Early in atherosclerosis, vessel lumen is preserved by compensatory arterial enlargement.[44] Eventually, this process fails and stenosis results. Calcification itself may be the limiting factor.[50] Intravascular ultrasound imaging has revealed that calcified coronary segments are more likely to be stenotic, have less compensatory enlargement relative to plaque area, and are more likely to require treatment.[51] Comparison of angiographic and UFCT results revealed that coronary calcification often occurs in the absence of stenosis, suggesting that it is an early aspect of atherosclerosis. Because autopsy studies indicate that calcification nearly always colocalizes with atherosclerosis, this suggests that calcification precedes failure of compensatory enlargement, contrary to the impression that it is end-stage. In addition, it has been shown that restenosis after angioplasty is due to failure of compensatory enlargement.[52] Thus, if prevention of calcification allowed compensatory enlargement to proceed indefinitely, stenosis and its clinical consequences might never occur.

Location and Distribution of Vascular Calcification

Vascular calcification may occur in either intima or media. Ossification is usually at the base of lesions, in the intima immediately adjacent to the luminal side of the fragmented internal elastic lamina. Because of compensatory enlargement, intimal calcification may appear to be at the outer edge of the artery wall. The most common form of vascular calcification is a sharply delimited, acellular focus of calcified matrix lacking mature bone architecture. It is not known whether these foci are precursors of mature bone. However, they contain hydroxyapatite, matrix vesicles and the bone regulatory protein osteopontin;[18,20,53,54] they also occur as part of normal bone formation.[55] Ossification appears to require microvascular invasion, which may explain its location at the lesion base closer to vasa vasorum ingrowth.

Relation to Cell Death

Vascular calcification often is dismissed as an inadvertent consequence of cellular necrosis. However, association with cell death does not imply lack of regulation or relation to bone formation because both apoptosis and necrosis are regulated aspects of endochondral ossification and intramembranous ossification.[56] One reason vascular calcification has been considered passive may be that it occurs extracellularly, not within cells. However, the same is true for bone mineral formation. What is active and regulated is the secretion of matrix vesicles and the specialized matrix, osteoid containing crystal-regulating phosphoproteins. Each provides a nidus for crystal formation at low calcium/phosphate concentrations, and osteoid regulates crystal growth. Osteoid calcifies ~10 days after secretion, at ~10 μm from the secretory cell. Both matrix vesicles and most components of osteoid have been demonstrated in human atherosclerosis[18,54] and in calcified human valves,[43,57] including collagen I, matrix gla protein, osteonectin, osteocalcin, and bone sialoprotein.[14,21,54,58,59]

Pericytes

Calcifying vascular cells (CVC), a subpopulation of adult aortic medial cells identified by our laboratory to undergo osteoblastic differentiation in vitro, share many features with microvascular pericytes. Pericytes, but not endothelial cells, are derived from the neural crest.[60] They are postulated to be immature mesenchymal progenitor cells[61] located in the subendothelial basement membrane in microvessels. As do CVC, they form calcifying nodules in vitro,[62] and they can differentiate into osteoblasts in the periosteum.[63] The spontaneous calcification of pericytes and CVC in the absence of exogenous stimuli such as β-glycerophosphate or growth factors, probably reflects the similarity of culture conditions with injury. In mature bone, BMP-2 expression appears to be limited to the periosteum at fractures, presumably sites of active bone development.[64] Pericytes are identified uniquely in the microvessels by mAb 3G5,[65] which also uniquely identifies CVC in large arteries.[66] Its epitope is a surface ganglioside, which has not been identified.

Pericyte-Specific Ganglioside

Gangliosides, glycolipids with sialic acid groups, regulate cell proliferation, signaling response to growth factors[67] and cell-cell adhesion.[68,69] Gangliosides vary in the nature and number of sugars and the glycosidic linkages of sialic acids. They are amphiphilic: the hydrophilic region consists of two or more sugars. The hydrophobic region consists of sphingosine and fatty acid, the length, saturation and hydroxylation of which varies. Because of their dual affinity, gangliosides are found in lipid layers, in lipophilic proteins such as LDL, and on glycophilic proteins. The major ganglioside in plasma is GM3, most of which is carried by LDL.[70] Gangliosides GM3 and GM1 are increased twofold in atherosclerotic plaque.[71]

Mechanism of Osteoblastic Differentiation

Osteoblastic differentiation is preceded by proliferation, and it is inversely related to proliferation.[72] An early marker of osteoblastic differentiation is alkaline phosphatase,[73] an ectoenzyme associated with matrix vesicles and required for in vivo calcification.[74] Its mechanism of action remains uncertain. Osteopontin is expressed in quiescent CVC and in immature smooth muscle cells (SMC),[75] but not in quiescent SMC.[66] Expression in SMC requires activation by cell-cycling or growth factors.[76] In the mineralization phase, matrix vesicles are released into the extracellular matrix and serve as the nidus for hydroxyapatite crystal formation. They are ~200 nm diameter proteolipid vesicles associated with bone matrix proteins and enzymatic activities. Their release is promoted by transforming growth factor (TGF)-β.[77]

Relation of Vascular Calcification to Oxidant Stress and Morphogenetic Protein

Oxidant stress may have a role in osteoblastic differentiation. We observed that in vitro calcification of vascular cells is accelerated by the response to prooxidant TGF-β as well as oxysterols.[66] An intriguing analogy is that expression of drosophila decapentaplegic, which is functionally interchangeable with BMP-2, is regulated by dorsal, the homologue of the oxidant-signaling transcription factor NF-kappa B. Our laboratory previously demonstrated expression of the potent osteogenic differentiation factor, bone morphogenetic protein-2 (BMP-2, previously named "BMP-2a") in calcified human atherosclerotic lesions using in situ hybridization.[78]

In Vitro Model of Vascular Calcification

Further elucidation of the cellular and molecular mechanisms of vascular calcification required an in vitro model. We observed that bovine aortic smooth muscle cell primary cultures spontaneously produce occasional cellular nodules after ~2 weeks in culture. Based on the similarity of these nodules to those in bone cell cultures, we tested these nodules for calcium mineral deposits. Both von Kossa and Alizarin red histochemical stains were positive. To exclude histochemical artifact from differential access of solutions to the nodule interior, we confirmed the results in sectioned nodules. We also identified the calcium mineral as the bone mineral, hydroxyapatite, using energy-dispersive x-ray analysis. We found that the phenotype could be enriched by cloning and that the nodules are calcified. Cloned cultures produced nodules at 10-to 100-fold greater density. They were negative for markers of endothelial and inflammatory cells, positive for smooth muscle actin, but more strongly immunoreactive for nonsmooth muscle β-actin than primary SMC cultures. They uniquely expressed a surface ganglioside identified by monoclonal antibody 3G5, a marker for microvascular pericytes. The cells in these nodules had immunocytochemical features typical of microvascular pericytes, but not those of any other cells found in the artery wall. The similarity to pericytes is intriguing given that pericytes are capable of differentiation into osteoblasts.[79]

Human and bovine aortic tissue specimens also showed positive immunostaining with the ganglioside antibody 3G5 in scattered individual cells in the subendothelial space and occasional cells in the media, indicating that the surface ganglioside was also present in vivo. In culture, 3G5-positive cells also could be obtained directly from primary aortic smooth muscle cells without passage through the nodule stage. Subsequent studies have been performed using clones derived directly from primary cultures of medial cells without requiring nodule formation in the primary culture. These cloned CVC's exhibit many osteoblastic features: hydroxyapatite production and expression of alkaline phosphatase, collagen I, osteopontin, osteonectin, and osteocalcin, suggesting that CVC are mesenchymal intimal cells that have committed partially to osteoblastic differentiation, which becomes complete on culturing.[66] Other investigators now independently have localized expression of bone-related proteins in calcified atherosclerosis and successfully have used this in vitro model. These findings suggest that arterial calcification is a regulated process mediated by cells related to microvascular pericytes through a mechanism resembling osteogenesis.

To determine whether factors in atherosclerosis in vivo contribute to this differentiation, we tested the effects of factors known to occur in atherosclerotic plaque: transforming growth factor-β1 (TGF-β1), platelet-derived growth factor (PDGF), interferon-gamma, 1,25 dihydroxyvitamin D and 25-hydroxycholesterol. TGF-β1 and 25-hydroxycholesterol significantly accelerated the formation of calcifying nodules in culture, PDGF had a moderate effect, and vitamin D and interferon-gamma had little or no effect compared with vehicle alone. These results suggest that factors in atherosclerotic lesions, such as TGF-β1 and oxysterols may induce osteoblastic differentiation of artery wall cells.

Possible Connection between Osteoporosis and Vascular Calcification?

Some evidence suggests an association between vascular calcification and osteoporosis.[80,81] Although these studies have not been randomized, double-blind trials, in many cases, the finding was incidental but significant, suggesting an especially strong relation. Nevertheless, it would be very difficult to ascertain causality because of the confounding factor of age, with which each is associated. In addition, it is difficult to assess these correlative studies because measurements of bone density, particularly of the spine, are influenced directly by calcification of the overlying abdominal aorta, which is often necessarily included, though not wanted, in the measurement. We hypothesize that the association may not be causal, but that the two are related in that their regulation is similar. Thus, calcium metabolic status and hormonal status may change both processes. Similarity of regulatory mechanisms could support either calcification would increase in both when procalcification factors are administered or else it is possible that local factors cause one site to be more sensitive or even solely responsive to systemic regulatory factors. The enigma of vascular calcification and osteoporosis may be an open feedback loop as in the case of the single-thermostat, double electric blanket. If the electric circuit to one side of a double blanket were to stop working, the person on that side may dial up the thermostat setting higher and higher, which would turn up the heat on the other side. The first person would remain cold, the other would cook. Thus osteoporotic bone may release systemic regulatory factors indicating need for calcification-promoting processes. Local factors may preclude benefit to the bone, but deposit calcium mineral in the arteries. Evidence suggests that parathyroid hormone (PTH) may be the systemic mediator released as a result of osteoporosis, and causing aortic valve calcification.[82] PTH acts through several mechanisms, one of which is activation of plasminogen, an activator of latent TGF-β in osteoblasts.

Another phenomenon that suggests a common factor or factors linking osteoporosis and vascular calcification is the recent finding that osteoporosis correlates with stroke independently of age.[83] If calcification predisposes to plaque rupture in the carotid and ascending aorta and aortic valve, then this connection could be explained.

Atherosclerotic Matrix Similarities to Bone Matrix

Matrix vesicles and collagen each can serve as a nidus for crystal formation in bone. Collagen type I[58] as well as numerous matrix vesicle-like structures also are found in human intimal thickenings[84] and in human atherosclerotic plaque.[85] These findings suggest that the matrix in atherosclerotic plaque resembles bone matrix, and thus, the combination of bone matrix proteins, matrix vesicles, and collagen I in atherosclerotic matrix, it may be equally permissive for calcium mineralization as bone osteoid itself.

Estrogen Effects on Bone and Smooth Muscle Cells

Based on epidemiological studies, estrogens are associated with lower risk of cardiovascular disease and reduced bone loss in post-menopausal women. Possible mechanisms of protection against vascular disease include favorable changes in the lipoprotein profile and lipoprotein metabolism in the artery wall, inhibition of intimal cell proliferation, alteration of vascular reactivity, LDL-oxidation, and arterial myointimal thickening following vascular injury.[86–89]

Both osteoblasts and vascular smooth muscle cells have functional estrogen receptors.[90,91] Endothelial cells of bone also have functional estrogen receptors.[92] Direct effects of estrogen include osteoblast proliferation and expression of alkaline phosphatase, osteoblast gene expression, and incorporation of growth factors into bone matrix, the last of which provides coupling between resorption and reformation.

Paradox of Estrogen's Protective and Procalcification Effects

A paradox arises from the evidence that estrogen is protective against coronary artery disease. If estrogen also promotes vascular calcification as it does bone calcification by the same mechanisms and if vascular calcification is harmful, then one would not expect this beneficial effect. One possible, though less likely, explanation is that the epidemiological evidence for protection against heart disease may not be fully established. Many studies that indicate benefit of estrogen are for surrogate markers, such as reduction of lipoprotein levels. Many other studies were performed in nonrandomized or nonblinded studies (allowing the possibility of selection bias) that women who take estrogen are also more health conscious in general and have lifestyles that are protective against heart disease. Another possible explanation is that estrogen does not promote vascular calcification, although there is preliminary data supporting a positive effect. Some evidence of a paradoxical effect of estrogen on soft tissue calcification (tumors) has been reported.[93] Finally, it is possible that vascular calcification is actually protective. One may speculate that early stages of calcification increase risk when only part of the artery wall is calcified, providing a high shear stress concentration along a dissection plane, but that extensive, circumferential calcification may harden the artery to the point that it is completely rigid, and protected from rupture. Calcification also may preclude high-risk palliative interventions.

Paradox of Soft Tissue Calcification in the Face of Skeletal Calcium Loss

A second paradox is that, if osteoporosis is due to a systemic problem, an inadequate calcium balance, then it is difficult to explain how calcium deposition and bone formation can be occurring in vascular calcification and osteophytes in the face of this systemic imbalance. Local factors must be responsible for the differences.

Vitamin D and Calcium Supplements

Vitamin D and calcium generally are considered harmless and beneficial supplements. There is even recent evidence that calcium intake is related to reduction of blood pressure. In support of the positive effect on skeletal preservation, in vitro studies have shown that vitamin D and calcium supplements promote calcium mineral deposition. However, in vitro studies also show promotion of calcium mineral deposition in vascular cells. Furthermore, in animals, primarily the rat model, supplemental vitamin D alone or with calcium has been shown to induce marked vascular calcification as well as endothelial dysfunction and impairment of vasodilation.[94-95]

Effects of Vitamin D on Bone

Osteoblasts have receptors for vitamin D. Under some circumstances, vitamin D has promineralization effects, such as induction of osteocalcin through the vitamin D response element in its promoter, and positive effects on osteoblast differentiation and chondroblast maturation. However, because the primary function of vitamin D appears to be maintenance of serum calcium rather than bone calcification, it also can promote bone resorption, in part by promoting osteoclast differentiation. The serum calcium, PTH, and vitamin D receptor levels determine whether vitamin D promotes bone mineralization or resorption. At the levels recommended, it generally is believed that the only effect of vitamin D is to enhance intestinal absorption of calcium. However, dietary vitamin D may be carried into the wall by lipoproteins and accumulate at high levels, where its effects may be entirely different. At high concentration, vitamin D has many effects on a variety of cells and ubiquitous signaling molecules. It induces osteopontin in the epidermis, colony stimulating factors, insulin-like growth factor binding protein, nerve growth factor and interleukins IL-1 and IL-6. Polymorphisms of the vitamin D receptor were recently linked to osteoporosis.[97] This was confirmed by some independent investigators, but refuted by others.

Interactions

There are interrelations between vitamin D and estrogen and other calcium regulatory factors. Epidemiologically, hormone replacement therapy is associated with higher vitamin D levels.[98] The reason for this association remains unclear; it may be the result of potentially greater health consciousness on the part of women choosing to take hormone replacement therapy or it may be a biological effect. Vitamin D receptors have been shown to induce the estrogen receptor in bone marrow cells, and estrogen modulates vitamin D effects, especially on macrophages.[99] An important clue to the mechanism of osteoporosis is that estrogen normally inhibits the IL-6 promoter[100] and that estrogen deficiency is not sufficient to induce osteoporosis, but it requires expression of IL-6 to lead to osteoporosis.[101] Results of in vitro studies of estrogen dose responses must be evaluated in light of evidence that factors released from plastic culture dishes during incubation, as well as the phenol red in many commercial preparations of culture medium, have estrogenic effects.[102] These effects appear to vary significantly with culture conditions and treatment protocols.

Possible Effects of Osteoporosis Prevention Therapies on Vascular Calcification

One of the newer agents for osteoporosis is bisphosphonate. This drug inhibits osteoclastic bone resorption either directly or through effects on osteoblasts. Interestingly, bisphosphonates were previously shown to inhibit atherosclerosis in rabbits.[103] These results have been confirmed by independent investigators. Both vitamin D and estrogen induce TGF-β production in bone cells, and TGF-β has been shown to promote growth of the subpopulation of CVC in the artery wall.

Future Research

Although this discussion is limited to issues of osteoporosis and vascular calcification, one other issue should be mentioned in keeping with the theme of awareness of interactions with other pathophysiological processes. Breast cancer also must be considered in judging whether postmenopausal women should be advised to take calcium regulatory factors and supplements. Calcium and bone regulatory factors, including osteopontin, osteonectin, and matrix gla protein, also are involved in the soft tissue calcification adjacent to breast tumors.[104] It is first necessary to establish whether the associated calcification is protective (by blocking tissue invasion or ingrowth of angiogenic vessels), harmful, or incidental and then to determine the effects of the pharmacotherapeutic agents or supplements.

References

1. Melton, LJ. How many women have osteoporosis now? *J Bone Miner Res* 1995;10:175–177.
2. Smith R. Prevention and treatment of osteoporosis: Common sense and science coincide (Editorial). *J Bone Joint Surg* 1994;76-B:345–347.

3. Wagner WD, St. Clair RW, Clarkson TB, et al. A study of atherosclerosis regression in Macaca mulatta. *Am J Pathol* 1980;100:633–650.
4. Agatston AS, Janowitz WR, Hildner FJ, et al. Quantification of coronary artery calcium using ultrafast computed tomography. *J Am Coll Cardiol* 1990;15:827–832.
5. Honye J, Mahon DJ, Jain A, et al. Morphological effects of coronary balloon angioplasty in vivo assessed by intravascular ultrasound imaging. *Circulation* 1992;85:1012–1025.
6. Beadenkopf WG, Daoud AS, Love BM. Calcification in the coronary arteries and its relationship to arteriosclerosis and myocardial infarction. *Am J Roentgenol* 1964;92:865–871.
7. Baron MG. Significance of coronary artery calcification (Editorial). *Radiology* 1994;192:613–614.
8. Detrano RC, Wong ND, Tang W, et al. Prognostic significance of cardiac cinefluoroscopy for coronary calcific deposits in asymptomatic high risk subjects. *J Am Coll Cardiol* 1994;24:354–358.
9. Mitchell JR, Adams JH. Aortic size and aortic calcification: A necropsy study. *Atherosclerosis* 1977;27:437–446.
10. Pearson AC, Guo R, Orsinelli DA, et al. Transesophageal echocardiographic assessment of the effects of age, gender, and hypertension on thoracic aortic wall size, thickness, and stiffness. *Am Heart J* 1994;128:344–351.
11. Fitzgerald PJ, Ports TA, Yock PG. Contribution of localized calcium deposits to dissection after angioplasty. An observational study using intravascular ultrasound. *Circulation* 1992;86:64–70.
12. Niskanen LK, Suhonen M, Siitonen O, et al. Aortic and lower limb artery calcification in type 2 (non-insulin-dependent) diabetic patients and non-diabetic control subjects A five year follow-up study. *Atherosclerosis* 1990;84:61–71.
13. Ohtsuka S, Kakihana M, Watanabe H, et al. Chronically decreased aortic distensibility causes deterioration of coronary perfusion during increased left ventricular contraction. *J Am Coll Cardiol* 1994;24:1406–1414.
14. Guyton JR, Klemp KF. Transitional features in human atherosclerosis: Intimal thickening, cholesterol clefts, and cell loss in human aortic fatty streaks. *Am J Pathol* 1993;143:1444–1457.
15. Cornhill JF, Herderick EE, Stary HC. Topography of human aortic sudanophilic lesions. *Monogr Atheroscler* 1990;15:13–19.
16. Hoeg JM, Feuerstein IM, Tucker EE. Detection and quantitation of calcific atherosclerosis by ultrafast computed tomography in children and young adults with homozygous familial hypercholesterolemia. *Arterioscler Thromb* 1994;14:1066–1074.
17. Rumberger JA, Schwartz RS, Simons B, et al. Relation of coronary calcium determined by electron beam computed tomography and lumen narrowing determined by autopsy. *Am J Cardiol* 1994;73:1169–1173.
18. Ikeda T, Shirasawa T, Esaki Y, et al. Osteopontin mRNA is expressed by smooth muscle-derived foam cells in human atherosclerotic lesions of the aorta. *J Clin Invest* 1993;92:2814–2820.
19. Giachelli CM, Bae N, Almeida M, et al. Osteopontin is elevated during neointima formation in rat arteries and is a novel component of human atherosclerotic plaques. *J Clin Invest* 1993;92:1686–1696.

20. Fitzpatrick LA, Severson A, Edwards WD, et al. Diffuse calcification in human coronary arteries: Association of osteopontin with atherosclerosis. *J Clin Invest* 1994;94:1597–1604.
21. Shanahan CM, Cary NRB, Metcalfe JC, et al. High expression of genes for calcification-regulating protiens in human atherosclerotic plaques. *J Clin Invest* 1994;93:2393–2402.
22. Otto CM, Kuusisto J, Reichenbach DD, et al. Characterization of the early lesion of "degenerative" valvular aortic stenosis: Histological and immunohistochemical studies. *Circulation* 1994;90:844–853.
23. Kaufmann RB, Sheedy PF II, Maher JE, et al. Quantity of coronary artery calcium detected by electron beam computed tomography in asymptomatic subjects and angiographically studied patients. *Mayo Clin Proc* 1995;70:223–232.
24. Lee RT, Loree HM, Cheng GC, et al. Computational structural analysis based on intravascular ultrasound imaging before in vitro angioplasty: Prediction of plaque fracture locations. *J Am Coll Cardiol* 1993;21:777–782.
25. Zhang HP, Allen JW, Lau FY, et al. Immediate and late outcome of percutaneous balloon mitral valvotomy in patients with significantly calcified valves. *Am Heart J* 1995;129:501–506.
26. Wittman JC, Kok FJ, van Saase JL, et al. Aortic calcification is a predictor of cardiovascular mortality. *Lancet* 1986;2:1120–1122.
27. Elkeles A. A comparative radiological study of calcified atheroma in males and females over 50 years of age. *Lancet* 1957;714–715.
28. Taquet A, Bonithon-Kopp C, Simon A, et al. Relations of cardiovascular risk factors to aortic pulse wave velocity in asymptomatic middle-aged women. *Eur J Epidemiol* 1993;9:298–306.
29. Newman DL, Gosling RG, Bowden NLR. Changes in aortic distensibibility and area ratio with the development of atherosclerosis. *Atherosclerosis* 1971;14:231–240.
30. Nakashima T, Tanikawa J. A study of human aortic distensibility with relation to atherosclerosis and aging. *Angiology* 1971;22:477–490.
31. Demer LL. Effect of calcification on in vivo mechanical response of rabbit arteries to balloon dilation. *Circulation* 1991;83:2083–2093.
32. Simonson E, Nakagawa K. Effect of age on pulse wave velocity and aortic ejection time in healthy men and in men with coronary artery disease. *Circulation* 1960;22:126–129.
33. Bouthier JD, DeLuca N, Safar ME, et al. Cardiac hypertorophy and arterial distensibility in essential hypertension. *Am Heart J* 1985;109:1345–1352.
34. Katz AM. Cardiomyopathy of overload: A major determinant of prognosis in congestive heart failure. *N Engl J Med* 1990;332:100–110.
35. Dart AM, Lascome F, Yeoh JK, et al. Aortic distensibility in patients with isolated hyperchlesterolemia, coronary artery disease, or cardiac transplant. *Lancet* 1991;338:270–273.
36. Maeta H, Hori M. Effects of a lack of aortic "Windkessel" properties on the left ventricle. *Jpn Circ J* 1985;49:232–237.
37. Franklin SS, Weber MA. Measuring hypertensive cardiovascular risk: The vascular overload concept. *Am Heart J* 1994;128:793–803.
38. Bogren HG, Mohiaddin RH, Klipstein RK, et al. The function of the aorta in ischemic heart disease: A magnetic resonance and angiographic study of aortic compliance and blood flow patterns. *Am Heart J* 1989;118:234–247.

39. Watanabe H, Ohtsuka S, Kakihana M, et al. Decreased aortic compliance aggravates subendocardial ischemia in dogs with stenosed coronary artery. *Cardiovasc Res* 1992;26:1212–1208.
40. Stefanadis C, Wooley CF, Bush CA, et al. Aortic distensibility abnormalities in coronary artery disease. *Am J Cardiol* 1987;59:1300–1304.
41. Kim SY, Hinkamp TJ, Jacobs WR, et al. Effect of an inelastic synthetic vascular graft on exercise hemodynamics. *Ann Thorac Surg* 1995; 59:981–989.
42. Kelly RP, Tunin R, Kass DA. Effect of reduced aortic compliance on cardiac efficiency and contractile function of in situ canine left ventricle. *Circ Res* 1992;71:490–502.
43. O'Brien ER, Garvin MR, Stewart DK, et al. Osteopontin is synthesized by macrophage, smooth muscle, and endothelial cells in primary and restenotic human coronary atherosclerotic plaques. *Arterioscler Thromb* 1994;14:1648–1656.
44. Glagov S, Weisenberg E, Zarins CK, et al. Compensatory enlargement of human atherosclerotic coronary arteries. *N Engl J Med* 1987; 316:1371–1375.
45. O'Rourke M. Arterial stiffness, systolic blood pressure, and logical treatment of arterial hypertension. *Hypertension* 1990;15:339–347.
46. Moynahan K, Yoshino MT. Aortic and renal atherosclerotic calcifications seen on computed tomography of the spine: A positive predictor of hypertension. *Invest. Radiol* 1993;28:811–813.
47. Kannel WB, Gordon T. Evaluation of cardiovascular risk in the elderly: The Framingham study. *Bull NY Acad Med* 1978;54:573–591.
48. Kannel WB, Wolf PA, McGee DL, et al. Systolic blood pressure, arterial rigidity and risk of stroke. *Am Med Assoc* 1981;245:1225–1229.
49. Garland C, Barrett-Connor E, Suarez L, et al. Isolated systolic hypertension and mortality after age 60 yrs. *Am J Epidemiol* 1983;118: 365–376.
50. Pickering JG, Ford CM, Novick RJ. Collagen elaboration following balloon angioplasty—evidence for rapid expression and deposition. *J Am Coll Cardiol* 1994;235A.
51. Mintz GS, Painter JA, Pichard AD, et al. Atherosclerosis in angiographically "normal" coronary artery reference segments: An intravascular ultrasound study with clinical correlations. *J Am Coll Cardiol* 1995; 25:1479–1485.
52. Kakuta T, Currier JW, Haudenschild CC, et al. Differences in compensatory vessel enlargement, not intimal formation, account for restenosis after angioplasty in the hypercholesterolemic rabbit model. *Circulation* 1994;89:2809–2815.
53. Yu SY. Calcification processes in atherosclerosis. *Adv Exp Med Biol* 1974;43:403–425.
54. Anderson HC. Calcific disease: A concept. *Arch Pathol Lab Med* 1983; 107:341–348.
55. Gruber HE. Adaptations of Goldner's Masson trichrome stain for the study of undecalcified plastic embedded bone. *Biotech Histochem* 1992;67:30–34.
56. Zimmermann B. Occurrence of osteoblast necroses during ossification of long bone cortices in mouse fetuses. *Cell Tissue Res* 1994;275: 345–353.
57. Kim KM. Calcification of matrix vesicles in human aortic valve and aortic media. *Fed Proc* 1976;35:156–162.

58. Rekhter MD, Zhang K, Narayanan AS, et al. Type I Collagen gene expression in human atherosclerosis. *Am J Pathol* 1993;143:1634–1648.
59. Fleet JC, Hock JM. Identification of osteocalcin in mRNA in nonosteiod tissue of rats and humans by reverse transcription-polymerase chain reaction. *J Bone Miner Res* 1994;9:1565–1573.
60. LeLievre CS, LeDouarin NM. Mesenchymal derivatives of the neural crest. Analysis of chimaeric quail and chick embryos. *J Embryol Exp Morphol* 34:125–154, 1975.
61. Rhodin JAG. Ultrastructure of mammalian venous capillaries, venules, and small connecting veins. *J Ultrastruct Res* 1968;25:452–500.
62. Schor AM, Allen TD, Canfield AE, et al. Pericytes derived from the retinal microvasculature undergo calcification in vitro. *J Cell Sci* 1990;97:449–461.
63. Brighton CT, Hunt RM. Histochemical localization of calcium in the fracture callus with potassium pyroantimonate. Possible role of chondrocyte mitochondrial calcium in callus calcification. *J Bone Joint Surg* 1986;68:703–715.
64. Nakase T, Nomura S, Yoshikawa H, et al. Transient and localized expression of bone morphogenetic protein 4 messenger RNA during fracture healing. *J Bone Miner Res* 1994;9:651–659.
65. Nayak RC, Attawia MA, Cahill CJ, et al. Expression of a monoclonal antibody (3G5) defined ganglioside antigen in renal cortex. *Kidney Int* 1992;41:1638–1645.
66. Watson KE, Boström K, Ravindranath R, et al TGF-β1 and 25-hydroxy-cholesterol stimulate osteoblast-like vascular cells to calcify. *J Clin Invest* 1994;93:2106–2113.
67. Raines EW, Lane TF, Iruela-Arispe ML, et al. The extracellular glycoprotein SPARC interacts with platelet-derived growth factor (PDGF)-AB and -BB and inhibits the binding of PDGF to its receptors. *Proc Natl Acad Sci USA* 1992;89:1281–1285.
68. Chatterjee S. Lactosylceramide stimulates aortic smooth muscle cell proliferation. *Biochem Biophys Res Commun* 1991;181:554–561.
69. Cheresh DA, Harper JR, Shulz G, et al. Localization of the gangliosides GD2 and GD3 in adhesion plaques and on the surface of human melanoma cells. *Proc Natl Acad Sci USA* 1984;81:5767–5771.
70. Senn H, Orth M, Fitzke E, et al. Gangliosides in normal human serum: Concentration, pattern and transport by lipoproteins. *Eur J Biochem* 1989;181:657–662.
71. Mukhin DN, Prokazova NV, Bergelson LD, et al. Galglioside content and composition of cells from normal and atherosclerotic human aorta. *Atherosclerosis* 1989;78:39–45.
72. Stein GS, Lian JB. Molecular mechanisms mediating proliferation/differentiation interrelationships during progressive development of the osteoblast phenotype. *Endocr Rev* 1993;14:424–442.
73. Marie PJ, Hott M, Lomri A. Regulation of endosteal bone formation and osteoblasts in rodent vertebrae. Review. *Cells Materials* 1994; 4:143–154.
74. Beertsen W, van den Bos T. Alkaline phosphatase induces the mineralization of sheets of collagen implanted subcutaneously in the rat. *J Clin Invest* 1992;89:1974–1980.
75. Giachelli C, Bae N, Lombardi D, et al. Molecular cloning and characterization of 2B7, a rat mRNA which distinguishes smooth muscle cell

phenotypes in vitro and is identical to osteopontin (secreted phospho-protein I, 2aR). *Biochem Biophys Res Commun* 1991;177:867–873.
76. Gadeau AP, Campan M, Millet D, et al. Osteopontin overexpression is associated with arterial smooth muscle cell proliferation in vitro. *Arterioscler Thromb* 1993;13:120–125.
77. Bonewald LF, Schwartz Z, Swain LD, et al. Stimulation of matrix vesicle enzyme activity in osteoblast-like cells by 1,25(OH)2D3 and transforming growth factor beta (TGF beta). *Bone Miner* 1992;17:139–144.
78. Bostrom K, Watson KE, Horn S, et al. Bone morphogenetic protein expression in human atherosclerotic lesions. *J Clin Invest* 1993;91:1800–1809.
79. Brighton CT, Lorich DG, Kupcha R, et al. The pericyte as a possible osteoblast progenitor cell. *Clin Orthopaed Relat Res* 1992;275:287–299.
80. Boukhris R, Becker KL. Calcification of the aorta and osteoporosis. *JAMA* 1972;219(10):1307–1311.
81. Dent CE, Engelbrecht HE, Godfrey RC. Osteoporosis of lumbar vertebrae and calcification of abdominal aorta in women living in Durban. *Br Med* 1968;4:76–79.
82. Ouchi Y, Akishita M, de Souza AC, et al. Age-related loss of bone mass and aortic/aortic valve calcification—reevaluation of recommended dietary allowance of calcium in the elderly. *Ann NY Acad Sci* 1993;676:297–307.
83. Browner WS, Pressman AR, Nevitt MC, et al. Association between low bone density and stroke in elderly women. The study of osteoporotic fractures. *Stroke* 1993;24:940–946.
84. Tirziu D, Dobrian A, Tasca C, et al. Intimal thickenings of human aorta contain modified reassembled lipoproteins. *Atherosclerosis* 1995;112:101–114.
85. Guyton JR, Klemp KF. Development of the atherosclerotic core region. Chemical and ultrastructural analysis of microdissected atherosclerotic lesions from human aorta. *Arterioscler Thromb* 1994;14:1305–1314.
86. Varga R, Wroblewska B, Rego A, et al. Oestradiol inhibits smooth muscle cell proliferation of pig coronary artery. *Br J Pharmacol* 1993;109:612–617.
87. Salas E, López MG, Villarroya M, et al. Endothelium-independent relaxation by 17-alpha-estradiol of pig coronary arteries. *Eur J Pharmacol* 1994;258:47–55.
88. Rifici VA, Khachadurian AK. The inhibition of low-density lipoprotein oxidation by 17-β estradiol. *Metabolism* 1992;41:1110–1114.
89. Foegh ML, Asotra S, Howell MH, et al. Estradiol inhibition of arterial neointimal hyperplasia after balloon injury. *J Vasc Surg* 1994;19:722–726.
90. Ikegami A, Inoue S, Hosoi T, et al. Immunohistochemical detection and northern blot analysis of estrogen receptor in osteoblastic cells. *J Bone Miner Res* 1993;8:1103–1109.
91. Karas RH, Patterson BL, Mendelsohn ME. Human vascular smooth muscle cells contain functional estrogen receptor *Circulation* 1994;89:1943–1950.
92. Brandi ML, Crescioli C, Tanini A, et al. Bone endothelial cells as estrogen targets. *Calcif Tissue Int* 1993;53:312–317.
93. Van Hook DM, Meilstrup JW. Women's health case of the day. Regressing arterial calcifications in breast. *Am J Roentgenol* 1994;162:1459–1460.

94. Kitagawa S, Yamaguchi Y, Kunitomo M, et al. Impairment of endo-thelium-dependent relaxation in aorta from rats with arteriosclerosis induced by excess vitamin D and a high-cholesterol diet. *Jpn J Pharmacol* 1992;59:339–347.

95. Shinozuka K, Kitagawa S, Kunitomo M, et al. Release of endogenous ATP from the caudal artery in rats with arteriosclerosis. *Eur J Pharmacol* 1994;292:115–118.

96. Porta R, Conz A, Conto A, et al. Comparable beneficial effects of defi-brotide and nifedipine in calcium induced atherosclerosis. *Life Sci* 1994;54:799–812.

97. Morrison NA, Qi JC, Tokita A, et al. Prediction of bone density from vitamin D receptor alleles. *Nature* 1994;367:284–287.

98. van Hoof HJ, van der Mooren MJ, Swinkels LM, et al. Hormone re-placement therapy increases serum 1,25-dihydroxyvitamin D: A 2-year prospective study. *Calcif Tissue Int* 1994;55:417–419.

99. Abu-Amer Y, Bar-Shavit Z. Modulation of vitamin D increased H2O2 production and MAC-2 expression in the bone marrow-derived mac-rophages by estrogen. *Calcif Tissue Int* 1994;55:29–32.

100. Pottratz ST, Bellido T, Mocharla H, et al. 17 beta-Estradiol inhibits expression of human interleukin-6 promoter-reporter constructs by a receptor-dependent mechanism. *J. Clin Invest* 1994;93:944–950.

101. Poli V, Balena R, Fattori E, et al. Interleukin-6 deficient mice are pro-tected from bone loss caused by estrogen depletion. *EMBO J* 1994; 13:1189–1196.

102. Berthois Y, Katzenellenbogen JA, Katzenellenbogen BS, et al. Phenol red in tissue culture media is a weak estrogen. Implications concerning the study of estrogen-responsive cells in culture. *Proc Natl Acad Sci USA* 1986;83:2496–2500.

103. Kramsch DM, Aspen AJ, Rozler LJ. Atherosclerosis: Prevention by agents not affecting abnormal levels of blood lipids. *Science* 1981; 213:1511–1512.

104. Hirota S, Ito A, Nagoshi J, et al. Expression of bone matrix protein messenger ribonucleic acids in human breast cancers. Possible in-volvement of osteopontin in development of calcifying foci. *Lab Invest* 1995;72:64–69.

Chapter 10

Effect of Estrogens on Arterial LDL Metabolism

Janice D. Wagner, DVM, PhD, Li Zhang, MD, and Michael R. Adams, DVM

Although coronary heart disease (CHD) is more prevalent in men than women, it is the leading cause of death in both pre- and postmenopausal women in Western societies. The available data suggest that both natural and surgical menopause are associated with accelerated development of coronary artery atherosclerosis.[1] There is extensive evidence that estrogen replacement therapy reduces the risk of CHD in postmenopausal women by ~50%.[2,3] Although the above findings suggest beneficial effects of ovarian hormones and exogenous estrogens, the mechanisms for these beneficial effects are largely unknown.

Risk of CHD and atherosclerosis is associated epidemiologically with increased concentrations of total plasma cholesterol (TPC) and low-density lipoprotein (LDL) cholesterol and decreased concentrations of high-density lipoprotein cholesterol (HDL-C).[4] Some of the beneficial effects of estrogen therapy may be related to estrogen-induced changes in plasma lipoproteins. The effects of exogenous mammalian estrogens on plasma lipoproteins vary with dose, route of administration, and preparation of estrogen used, but generally cause a decrease in TPC and LDL cholesterol and an increase in HDL-C and triglycerides.[1,5] However, only 25% to 50% of the beneficial effects of estrogen on CHD are believed to be due to changes in plasma HDL and LDL cholesterol.[3] This suggests that estrogen use is protective largely through mechanisms other than theoretically "anti-atherogenic" effects on plasma lipid concentrations. Es-

These studies were supported in part by grants from the National Center for Research Resources (K01 RR-00072) and from the National Heart, Lung, and Blood Institute (P01 HL-45666).

From: Forte TM, (ed). *Hormonal, Metabolic, and Cellular Influences on Cardiovascular Disease in Women.* Armonk, NY: Futura Publishing Company, Inc.; © 1997.

trogens may retard atherogenesis by interacting directly with the arterial wall, by affecting such things as the size and composition of lipoprotein particles to decrease their atherogenicity, or by modifying plasma components other than lipoproteins.[3]

Although there is overwhelming evidence that estrogen monotherapy markedly reduces risk of CHD in postmenopausal women, the effects of estrogen/progestin or estrogen/androgen regimens on CHD risk are less clear. The addition of a progestational steroid may or may not affect lipoprotein concentrations depending on the type of progestin and the estrogen-to-progestin dose ratio.[1,5,6] The fact that some estrogen/androgen combinations[7,8] and oral contraceptives (OC)[9,10] may lower plasma HDL-C concentrations has led to concerns that they may increase cardiovascular risk. However, there is no evidence that OC increase cardiovascular risk, unless these women also smoke.[9,10]

The initiation and progression of coronary artery atherosclerosis and related cardiovascular diseases are exceedingly difficult to study prospectively in human subjects because atherosclerosis develops slowly during a period of many years. Also, although CHD is the leading cause of morbidity and mortality in American women, clinical events occur relatively infrequently in the population as a whole. Therefore, in the studies described here, we have used cynomolgus monkeys (*Macaca fascicularis*), a well-characterized animal model, to study effects of sex hormone deficiency, sex hormone replacement therapy, and OC treatment on the pathogenesis of atherosclerosis.[11]

Characteristics of the Model

Studies from our group have focused on surgically postmenopausal (ie, estrogen-deficient) animals fed a moderately atherogenic diet that mimics the nutrient composition of the average American diet. These studies have shown that male and ovariectomized monkeys do not differ with respect to coronary artery atherosclerosis (CAA), whereas premenopausal females develop one-half the CAA of their ovariectomized counterparts.[11] Subsequent studies investigated the influence of sex hormone replacement therapy in ovariectomized monkeys. In this model, physiological replacement of estrogen or estrogen/progesterone (via Silastic implants) inhibited progression of coronary artery atherosclerosis by ~50%, while having little effect on plasma lipid concentrations.[12] One mechanism for this beneficial effect on atherosclerosis progression may be estrogen's direct effects at the level of the arterial wall.

In our laboratory, we have sought to determine the cellular mechanisms for the beneficial effects of estrogens and progestins on atherogenesis. To study the effects of hormone treatment on arterial, hepatic, and whole-body lipoprotein metabolism, we used LDL coupled to radiolabeled tyramine cellobiose (TC). The labeled TC-LDL, originally described by Pittman et al.,[13] allows quantification of the accumulation of products of LDL degradation and undegraded LDL in arterial and other tissue samples. Furthermore, by using differentially labeled LDL, ie, ^{125}I-TC-LDL and ^{131}I-LDL, it is possible to calculate separately the amount of undegraded and degraded LDL.[14,15] Thus, in the following studies described below, labeled LDLs [^{125}I-labeled tyramine cellobiose (^{125}I-TC) and ^{131}I] were injected via indwelling catheters before necropsy, allowing determination of plasma decay of labeled LDL as well as LDL metabolism (ie, rates of LDL degradation, amount of undegraded LDL, and total accumulation of ^{125}I-TC representing both degraded and undegraded LDL) in various arteries and tissues.

In contrast to investigations of coronary artery atherosclerosis in which we studied monkeys after ~2 years of consuming an atherogenic diet, in most of the studies described here, we used monkeys fed an atherogenic diet for only 12–18 weeks. The brevity of the atherogenic stimulus provided stimulation of the early events of atherogenesis but was not sufficient for development of treatment differences in extent of atherosclerosis, which would affect the amount of LDL taken up by the artery.[16,17]

Study 1: Parenteral Estradiol and Progesterone

Our first study was designed to investigate pathogenetic mechanisms that might be involved in the long-term study described above, in which parenteral estrogen or estrogen and progesterone decreased CAA independently of plasma lipids and lipoproteins.[12] We used ovariectomized female monkeys that had eaten a moderately atherogenic diet for only 18 weeks. During that time, one group (n=9) received estradiol-17β and cyclic progesterone replacement therapy in physiological concentrations via subcutaneous Silastic implants, whereas the controls (n=8) received no treatment. LDL were isolated from each monkey, labeled, and re-injected 24 hours

before necropsy, after which the uptake and metabolism of the LDL
was determined in various arteries and tissues.

Hormone replacement therapy significantly decreased the accumulation and degradation of LDL in coronary arteries[18] as well as
other arteries[19] (Figure 1). Hormone replacement decreased the rate
of arterial LDL degradation by an average of 78% and total arterial
LDL accumulation by ~60%. These changes in arterial LDL metabolism were independent of changes in plasma lipid, lipoprotein, or
apoprotein concentrations and occurred without changes in indices
of endothelial injury (ie, leukocyte adhesion and endothelial cell
turnover rate) or changes in hepatic or whole-body LDL metabolism.

The brevity of the atherogenic stimulus caused minimal changes
in arterial morphology (small accumulations of subendothelial foam
cells) and indices of endothelial cell injury. The intima was thickest
in the aorta, and leukocyte adhesion and endothelial cell turnover
rates were greatest in the carotid bifurcation and thoracic aorta.

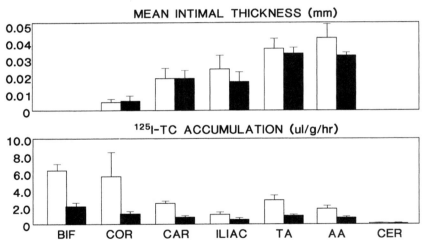

FIGURE 1. *Effect of hormone treatment on mean intimal thickness and* [125]*I-
labeled tyramine cellobiose (*[125]*I-TC) accumulation for control animals
(open bars) and hormone treatment group (filled bars) with the carotid
bifurcation (BIF), coronary arteries (COR), common carotid (CAR) and
iliac arteries, thoracic (TA) and abdominal aortas (AA), and cerebral arteries (CER). Repeated measures analyses for intimal thickness; effect of
treatment, P = 0.67; site, P < 0.0001; and treatment by site interaction,
P = 0.61. Repeated measures analysis for* [125]*I-TC accumulation; effect of
treatment, P = 0.02; site, P < 0.0001; and treatment by site interaction,
P = 0.48. Reproduced with permission from Reference 19.*

There also were regional differences among arterial sites in all indices of LDL metabolism we studied. Accumulation of LDL, LDL degradation rate, and the concentration of undegraded LDL were greatest in the coronary arteries and carotid bifurcations compared with the aorta, iliac, and common carotid arteries, and least in cerebral arteries (Figure 1). Interestingly, the arteries that had the greatest LDL accumulation (coronary arteries) had the least intimal thickening, suggesting differences in inherent LDL metabolism among arterial sites. Sex hormone deficiency caused the same percent increase in arterial LDL degradation and accumulation in all arterial sites, but the absolute amount of the increase was greatest for the coronary arteries. Thus, it is possible that with the onset of menopause (surgical or natural), coronary arteries may be among the first arterial sites to increase the metabolism and accumulation of LDL, contributing to the development of clinically significant atherosclerosis.

As was found in the long-term study, there was no significant effect of hormone therapy on plasma lipid, lipoprotein, or apoprotein concentrations. The minimal effect of the hormones on plasma lipoprotein concentrations is consistent with reports in women given parenteral estrogen replacement therapy.[5] The lack of effect of hormone therapy on hepatic and whole-body LDL removal [ie, fractional catabolic rate (FCR)] also may be due to the parenteral route of administration or our use of physiological concentrations of natural estrogens rather than pharmacological doses of synthetic estrogens.

Although lipoprotein concentrations were not affected, there were changes in the size of both LDL and HDL particles. HDL subfraction size heterogeneity was analyzed by gradient gel electrophoresis. Animals receiving hormone treatment had a significantly greater amount of protein in the HDL_{2b} subfraction and less in the HDL_{3b} subfraction compared with controls. However, the combined HDL_2 and HDL_3 subfractions for controls (61% and 39%, respectively) and treatment group (65% and 35%, respectively) were not different. The increase in amount of protein in the HDL_{2b} subfraction is most likely due to an estrogen-induced inhibition of hepatic lipase.[20]

There was also a decrease in LDL size as determined by LDL molecular weight. Furthermore, this was the only variable that was consistently correlated with LDL degradation and accumulation, which suggests that sex hormone deficiency results in larger LDL particles that are more atherogenic. This is consistent with other studies in nonhuman primates, where LDL size also was associated highly with coronary artery atherosclerosis.[21]

Study 2: Oral Conjugated Equine Estrogens With or Without Medroxyprogesterone Acetate

To further investigate mechanisms involved in the beneficial effects of hormone replacement therapy, we decided to study whether arterial LDL metabolism is affected by hormone treatment after only 12 weeks of atherogenic stimulus. Earlier studies had used animals fed atherogenic diets for 16 or 18 weeks. In this study, ovariectomized monkeys were treated with oral conjugated equine estrogens (CEE) with or without medroxyprogesterone acetate (MPA). Monkeys were randomized to four treatment groups of 10 animals each based on equivalent TPC and HDL concentrations: no treatment (ovariectomized controls) or the following hormones added to the diet: CEE (Premarin, Wyeth-Ayerst, Princeton, NJ) at a dose equivalent to 0.625 mg/day for women, 2.5 mg MPA (Cycrin, Wyeth-Ayerst), or combined CEE/MPA, at above doses and treated for 12 weeks.[22]

A detailed analysis of LDL composition and distribution was done in a subset of five animals of each group.[23] There were no differences among treatment groups in total plasma, LDL, or HDL cholesterol concentrations. However, significant differences in LDL size and composition were found. To further characterize changes in LDL size, LDLs were isolated by combined ultracentrifugation and size exclusion chromatography. In these animals, CEE treatment resulted in smaller LDLs that were relatively enriched in protein and triglyceride and poor in cholesteryl ester and apolipoprotein (apo) E. LDLs were further subfractionated by density gradient centrifugation into three density ranges ($d = 1.015-1.025$, $1.025-1.035$, and $1.035-1.045$). Significant chemical compositional changes were seen primarily in the lighter subfractions, where there was an increase in triglyceride and a decrease in cholesteryl ester. The plasma LDL from the CEE group in general had a lower apo E/B molar ratio than the other groups; however, the difference was statistically significant only in relation to the MPA group. This change was found to be due primarily to changes in the denser subfractions. There also was a 30% decrease in whole plasma apo E concentrations in CEE-treated monkeys compared with controls, but with only five animals per group, this was not statistically significant.

LDL particle size also may affect the interaction between proteoglycans and LDLs, which subsequently may affect arterial LDL metabolism. Thus, we compared the binding of LDL (from the different treatment groups) with arterial proteoglycans, in an in vitro binding assay. However, no differences were found among the groups in the percentage of LDLC in the proteoglycan complex.[22]

Forty-eight hours before necropsy, LDL isolated from pooled plasma from control animals were labeled with ^{131}I and with ^{125}I-TC and injected intravenously as described above.[22] There was a 40% increase in whole-body FCR with CEE treatment, but this did not reach statistical significance. However, there was a significant increase in the accumulation of hepatic LDL due primarily (>90%) to degradation products. The MPA groups, with or without CEE, showed no increase in LDL FCR; however, hepatic LDL accumulation in the CEE/MPA group was intermediate to either treatment alone.

Although there was an increase in hepatic LDL receptor activity with CEE, interestingly, there was a 50% decrease in total hepatic cholesterol content, due primarily to a decrease in cholesteryl ester. The decrease in hepatic cholesteryl ester may in turn lead to reduced hepatic cholesteryl secretion in apo B-containing lipoproteins and also may explain partially the decrease in LDL size.

In an attempt to explain the decreased hepatic cholesterol, total cellular ribonucleic acid (RNA) was purified from liver and 7α-hydroxylase messenger RNA (mRNA) content measured by DNA-excess solution hybridization.[23] mRNA abundance of 7α-hydroxylase (the rate-limiting step for bile synthesis) was increased in all treatment groups from 50% to 130%.[24] This finding is similar to studies in baboons,[25] where estrogen treatment alone or with progesterone resulted in a 2.7-fold increase in 7α-hydroxylase activity. These results also are consistent with studies of women,[26] where CEE treatment increased cholesterol secretion in the bile. The above studies suggest that estrogen treatment results in an increased secretion of hepatic cholesterol into the bile acid biosynthetic pathway.

Whereas significant differences were found in hepatic cholesterol metabolism in this short-term study, the results of arterial LDL metabolism studies revealed no effect of treatment (CEE alone or with MPA) on coronary artery LDL degradation (Figure 2) or any other index of arterial LDL metabolism for the coronary arteries or other arterial sites as well.[22] The lack of effect of treatment suggests that the 12 weeks of atherogenic stimulus may have been too short to induce sufficient atherogenic changes in the artery, eg, there was insufficient macrophage recruitment to the arterial intima to metabolize modified LDL, or insufficient extracellular matrix to bind LDLs. CEE treatment significantly decreased atherosclerosis in a long-term portion of a study of similar design,[27] providing further evidence that

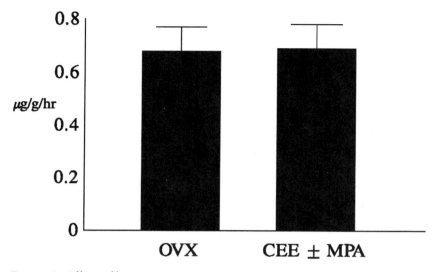

FIGURE 2. *Effect of hormone treatment on coronary artery LDL degradation (µg/g per hour) for ovariectomized control monkeys (OVX) and monkeys treated with either conjugated equine estrogens alone (CEE) or CEE and medroxyprogesterone acetate (MPA); P > 0.05.*

the lack of effect in the 12-week period was due to the brevity of atherogenic stimulus.

Study 3: Oral Esterified Estrogens With or Without Methyltestosterone

Estrogen/androgen combinations appear to be as effective as other modalities in ameliorating or preventing somatic complaints associated with estrogen deficiency and, in addition, have been shown to improve multiple psychological symptoms, libido, and sexual satisfaction,[28,29] yet may result in lowered plasma HDL-C concentrations.[7,8] The objective of the next study was to examine the effects of oral esterified estrogens alone or in combination with an androgen, methyltestosterone, on LDL metabolism and early atherogenesis after 16 weeks of atherogenic stimulus.[30] Three treatment groups were: no drug treatment (controls, n=11), esterified estrogens (EE, Estratab, Solvay Pharmaceuticals, Marietta, GA) (n=11), and EE plus methyltestosterone (MT, Estratest, Solvay Pharmaceuticals) (n=10). Drugs were given via a dosing solution calculated to be equivalent to a 60-kg woman receiving 2.5 mg EE and 5.0 mg of MT and resulted in estrone and equilin levels similar to women taking 1.25 mg EE.

Unlike the studies described above, in which there were no significant changes in plasma lipids, in this study TPC was decreased by 30% in the EE group and 35% in the EE + MT group compared with the control group. Although plasma HDL-C concentrations were not significantly different among treatment groups, triglyceride concentrations were increased in both EE and EE+MT groups compared with the control group. Also, as in both studies above, LDL particle size was reduced in both treatment groups ($P < 0.01$).

Arterial LDL metabolism again was assessed using dual labeled LDL. LDL isolated from pooled plasma from control animals were labeled and injected 24 hours before necropsy. All indices of arterial LDL metabolism were decreased with both treatments. As in the first study, the greatest effect induced by the hormone treatments was on the rate of arterial LDL degradation (Figure 3), which was reduced an average of 73% with EE and 75% with EE+MT. This is consistent with our previous study of the effects of combined estradiol and progesterone, in which treatment decreased LDL degradation rate by 78% compared with ovariectomized controls. Whereas hormone

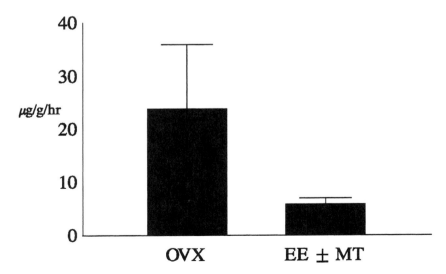

FIGURE 3. *Effect of hormone treatment on coronary artery LDL degradation (µg/g per hour) for ovariectomized control monkeys (OVX) and those treated with either esterified estrogens (EE) alone or with EE and methyltestosterone (MT); P < 0.05.*

treatment decreased arterial LDL metabolism, treatment with EE alone significantly increased the whole body FCR for LDL ($P < 0.05$), with a similar trend for treatment with EE+MT.

To investigate the role of estrogens as antioxidants, we assessed lipid peroxidation products by the thiobarbituric acid reaction (TBARS).[30] TBARS were decreased by >50% in the abdominal aorta of animals treated with EE compared with controls with a similar trend (23% reduction) with EE + MT. There were no apparent effects of treatment on TBARS in serum or liver. Aortic TBARS did not correlate significantly with the abdominal aortic cholesterol content ($r = -0.26$, $P > 0.05$) or aortic LDL degradation ($r = 0.24$, $P > 0.05$). The combination of decreased arterial lipid peroxidation and improved plasma lipoprotein metabolism may account for the decreased arterial LDL metabolism found in this study. Furthermore, the addition of an androgen, methyltestosterone, did not detract from the beneficial effects of estrogens.

Study 4: 17α-Dihydroequilenin in Rhesus Monkeys

CEE is the most commonly prescribed estrogen for replacement therapy in the United States. However, as this drug is a complex mixture of ~10 estrogens extracted from pregnant mares' urine,[31] it is unknown which of the components are most responsible for the cardioprotective effects. Earlier studies from our group suggested that one component, 17α-dihydroequilenin (DHEN), was more potent in reducing the plasma cholesterol concentrations of ovariectomized rats than the CEE mixture and had no effect on uterine weight, whereas the CEE mixture increased uterine weight considerably.[32] Thus, these data suggested that DHEN may not be feminizing for male monkeys.

Unlike the studies described above, this study used both male and female rhesus monkeys fed an atherogenic diet for 2–16 years. Monkeys were randomized into treatment groups by their total lifetime dietary cholesterol exposure (both time and amount of cholesterol in the diet) and their plasma TPC/HDL-C ratio. Treatment was for only 5 weeks to avoid any changes in plaque size that might confound the LDL metabolism studies. Males received 1.25 mg/kg per day of DHEN mixed into a moderately atherogenic diet (0.3 mg/Cal cholesterol) or this diet alone. The ovariectomized females received 25% of the male dose (0.3 mg/kg per day DHEN) or the diet alone.

No significant differences were found in plasma lipid or lipo-protein concentrations with treatment. However, plasma apoprotein A-I levels and insulin sensitivity were improved with DHEN in male monkeys. Plaque extent was similar between males with and without treatment and between females with and without treatment. When arterial LDL metabolism was assessed using dual-radiolabeled LDL, DHEN treatment significantly decreased coronary LDL degradation by 60% in males (Figure 4), but did not affect LDL degradation in females.[33]

Lipid peroxidation products (TBARS) also were assessed in se-rum, artery, and liver. Despite no treatment difference in the amount of serum or liver TBARS, DHEN significantly decreased arterial TBARS by 55% in females, with a similar trend in males (24% de-crease, $P > 0.05$). Thus, in females DHEN appeared to have signifi-cant arterial antioxidant activity, whereas in males, even though the dose was four times greater, this was not significant. However, in males, arterial degradation was decreased. This suggests that there is a complex interaction among antioxidant activity (as determined by TBARS), arterial LDL degradation, and activity of estrogens in males and females. However, nonfeminizing estrogens and related compounds may protect males as well as females against cardiovas-cular disease.

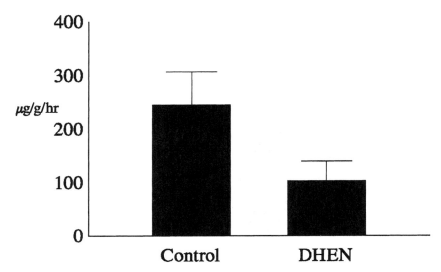

Figure 4. *Effect of hormone treatment on coronary artery LDL degradation (µg/g per hour) for male control monkeys and monkeys treated with 17α-dihydroequilenin (DHEN); P < 0.05.*

Study 5: Oral Contraceptive Agents

As with hormone replacement therapy, OC also attenuate the arterial accumulation of products of LDL degradation.[34] In a 16-week study, intact female monkeys were fed an atherogenic diet alone (controls, $n = 7$) or with one of two OCs; a monophasic formulation (Ovral, Wyeth-Ayerst, equivalent to a human dose of 50 μg ethinyl estradiol and 500 μg of norgestrel per day, $n = 8$), or a triphasic formulation (Triphasil, Wyeth-Ayerst, equivalent to a human dose of 30–40 μg ethinyl estradiol and 50–125 μg of levonorgestrel per day, $n = 8$). Despite causing a slightly more atherogenic lipoprotein profile (decreased HDL-C and increased TPC:HDL-C ratio) than diet alone, both OCs decreased arterial LDL degradation by >80% (Figure 5). As in the studies described previously, treatment also resulted in significantly lower LDL molecular weights. Again, these changes occurred prior to changes in arterial morphology.

Both OC treatments also resulted in a decrease in hepatic cholesterol content, which was independent of differences in LDL receptor and HMG-CoA reductase mRNA.[35] This occurred despite about a 30% increase in whole body LDL removal and a 50% increase in hepatic LDL uptake. The decreased hepatic cholesterol content in the face of increased plasma removal is consistent with

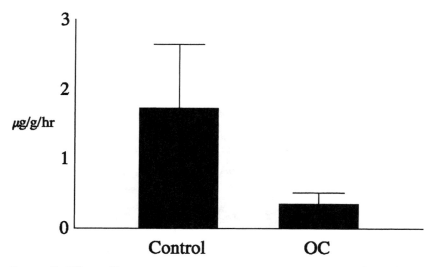

FIGURE 5. *Effect of hormone treatment on coronary artery LDL degradation (μg/g per hour) for intact control monkeys and monkeys treated with either a monophasic or triphasic oral contraceptive (OC); P < 0.05.*

an increased secretion of cholesterol into the bile acid biosynthetic pathway.

We observed, as expected, a strong positive correlation between plasma LDL cholesterol concentrations and hepatic LDL uptake (r = 0.88) and a strong negative correlation between plasma LDL and HMG-CoA reductase mRNA (-0.90) in control monkeys. However, there were no such correlations among OC-treated animals. Thus, in control animals, as plasma LDL cholesterol concentrations increased, hepatic LDL uptake and degradation increased significantly and HMG-CoA reductase mRNA decreased. As plasma cholesterol concentrations increased, a negative feedback relation was present in controls to decrease further hepatic cholesterol synthesis, but it appears this feedback relation is disrupted with OC treatment. The relation between HMG-CoA reductase mRNA and coronary artery LDL degradation was not significantly different between treatment groups, and when analyzed by multiple regression analysis, both HMG-CoA reductase mRNA and LDL molecular weight were significant predictors alone, and together they accounted for 48% of the variability in arterial LDL degradation.

Although the uncoupling of hepatic cholesterol metabolism with OC treatment was unexpected, it is consistent with studies of women,[36] where contraceptive steroids were found to increase cholesterol secretion in the bile. In these women, cholesterol synthesis (as measured in mononuclear cells) was correlated positively with biliary cholesterol secretion only during contraceptive steroid treatment. These results agree with the present study in monkeys, in which a decreased hepatic cholesterol content was observed with OC treatment and the expected strong positive correlation between HMG-CoA reductase mRNA concentrations and plasma LDL cholesterol concentrations was present in control monkeys but not present with OC treatment. Furthermore, it also appears that although there was a dietary down-regulation of cholesterol synthesis, newly synthesized cholesterol by HMG-CoA reductase may be an important regulatory cholesterol pool.

Studies in Other Animal Models

We believe that the decrease in arterial LDL degradation and accumulation is one mechanism by which hormone therapy may decrease arterial cholesterol accumulation and atherosclerosis in animal models and the incidence of coronary heart disease in women. In the studies described above, we found that in early atherogenesis ~60% to 70% of the LDL is present in the artery as degraded LDL and that hormone treatments decreased intracellular degradation rates more than concentrations of undegraded LDL. Our findings are consistent with the findings of Hough and Zilversmit,[37] who reported that estrogen treatment (estradiol-17β cypionate) in intact female rabbits decreased the arterial cholesteryl ester influx and hydrolysis. These findings occurred independently of plasma cholesterol concentrations and lipoprotein patterns.

Thus, in both our studies and those of Hough and Zilversmit,[37] estrogens (alone or with additional hormones) favorably decreased arterial LDL degradation and cholesteryl ester hydrolysis, which suggests that estrogens may be acting intracellularly. Furthermore, the findings of Haarbo et al.[38] suggest that intracellular mechanisms are more important in decreasing cholesterol accumulation, because in that study, estrogens had no effect on aortic permeability to LDL. However, whereas in monkeys, the greatest effect of estrogen treatment is decreased arterial LDL degradation, arterial content of undegraded LDL (which is primarily extracellular) also is decreased. The studies described here do not assess the intra-arterial retention of LDL, which could be an important factor in determining the subsequent LDL degradation because the longer LDL are retained in the intimal space, the greater the potential for oxidative modification of LDL.

Other studies in rabbits have found protective effects of estrogens independent of plasma cholesterol concentrations. Kushwaha and Hazzard[39] found that estradiol cypionate decreased both hypercholesterolemia and atherosclerosis. However, in some animals fed different amounts of cholesterol to induce similar levels of plasma cholesterol, estrogen-treated rabbits still had significantly less aortic cholesterol. A similar result was reported by Haarbo et al.,[40] who studied orally administered 17β-estradiol alone or with the progestins norethisterone and levonorgestrel. All hormone therapies reduced plasma cholesterol as well as aortic cholesterol accumulation. As with the study by Kushwaha and Hazzard,[39] the reduction in aortic cholesterol was again found to be independent of either total or very LDL (VLDL) cholesterol concentrations. However, a subsequent study by Haarbo et al.[41] found no effect of oral estradiol on plasma cholesterol concentrations, yet still found a 50% reduction in aortic cholesterol. A recent study by Sulistiyani et al.,[42] also in rabbits, reported the effects of two oral estrogens, ethinyl estradiol and 17α-dihydroequilin sulfate (a component of CEE). Neither estrogen affected plasma cholesterol concentrations, yet aortic cholesterol was reduced by up to 80%. Thus, studies in both monkeys and rabbits suggest that estrogens decrease atherogenesis independent of plasma lipoprotein concentrations.

Mechanistic Considerations

The mechanisms by which some estrogen treatments lower plasma LDL cholesterol concentrations are unclear. However, the oral route of administration[5,43] and the subsequent first-pass effect, along with dose and potency, appear to be important factors. Studies in animal models and in cell culture suggest that catabolism of LDL may be increased due to upregulation of the hepatic LDL receptor by estrogen.[44-48] However, because hepatic cholesterol content also is decreased with estrogen, the rise in LDL receptor activity may be a secondary response. Increased catabolism of LDL also has been shown in women treated orally with CEE but not in women given transdermal estradiol.[43] This is similar to our findings in monkeys: oral EE, CEE, and OCs all increased the LDL fractional catabolic rate by 30% to 40%, whereas with parenteral hormone therapy, no increase was found. However, the FCR measured in our studies and those in women do not differentiate among LDL receptor-mediated catabolism and other receptor or nonreceptor-mediated catabolism.

In addition to affecting plasma lipid and lipoprotein concentrations, sex steroids may affect lipoprotein composition and/or size heterogeneity. In our studies, the most consistent lipoprotein parameter to be affected by the various sex steroids is LDL size. Importantly, LDL particle size has been found to be associated with coronary artery disease in both human[49] and nonhuman primates.[21] In monkeys, LDL molecular weight is highly correlated with arterial LDL degradation[19,34] and is one of the strongest predictors of extent of coronary artery atherosclerosis, with animals having the largest LDL developing more extensive atherosclerosis.[21] Although increased LDL size appears to be more atherogenic in monkeys, smaller LDLs are associated with increased CHD risk in people.[49] However, in agreement with our studies in monkeys, a recent study in normolipidemic men by Campos et al.[50] found a predominance of larger LDL in those men at greater risk of coronary artery disease. This suggests that in dyslipidemic people small LDL may be a secondary response to other metabolic changes (eg, increased triglyceride concentrations associated with insulin resistance, etc.).

As in studies of women,[51-54] we have found that sex steroids decrease LDL size and alter composition in nonhuman primates. The decrease in LDL size may be secondary to estrogen-induced increases in plasma triglyceride concentrations and the enrichment of VLDL with triglyceride, which promotes the exchange with LDL cholesteryl esters.[49,55] The lipolysis of LDL triglycerides then results in smaller LDL particles.[56] This is consistent with the negative correlation seen with plasma triglycerides and LDL size in our studies and in humans.[30,49,55] Furthermore, if the increased atherogenicity of smaller particles is due to their greater oxidizability, this may be less important in the presence of an antioxidant, such as estrogen.

Alternatively, or in addition to this mechanism, larger lipoprotein particles may be removed selectively with estrogen treatment, leaving behind smaller particles. As was reported in monkeys, larger LDL particles are more apo E-enriched,[57] which may account for selective removal of large LDL particles via either the apo B/E receptor or the lipoprotein-related protein (LRP) receptor, for which apo E is the principal apoprotein ligand.[58] This also is consistent with a number of reports where estrogens resulted in a selective removal of either larger apo B particles or apo E-rich VLDL.[43,59–61] This decrease in larger, apo E-enriched particles may be responsible for the decreased plasma apo E concentrations reported in women[20] and baboons[62] and the similar trend in our monkeys[22] with estrogen treatment.

Although there tends to be an increase in the removal of apo B/E-containing particles with hormone treatment, an important feature in preventing subsequent downregulation of LDL receptor activity is the increase in biliary cholesterol secretion with estrogens.[24–26,36] Also, the decrease in hepatic cholesteryl ester content that we found with both OC[35] and CEE treatment,[23] may be responsible subsequently for smaller LDL particles, as suggested by studies of Parks et al.,[63] where a correlation among hepatic cholesteryl ester content, VLDL cholesterol secretion, and LDL size was found.

Thus, it seems clear that estrogens attenuate atherosclerosis progression, but the mechanisms of action remain unclear. In experimental studies in monkeys and rabbits and epidemiological studies in women, the "anti-atherogenic" effect of estrogens on plasma lipid and lipoprotein concentration explains little of their beneficial effects on cardiovascular disease. However, more subtle changes in plasma lipoproteins may be important. Because LDL size is highly correlated with coronary atherosclerosis[21] and because sex steroid use alters LDL size, this may be a way in which sex steroids affect atherosclerosis. LDL size has been found to affect binding to LDL receptors,[64,65] binding to proteoglycans,[66,67] the temperature of the liquid crystalline to liquid transition of the cholesteryl ester core,[56] and the oxidative potential of the particle,[68,69] all of which could affect atherogenesis.

Although there are differences in circulating LDL particles with estrogen treatments, estrogens also may affect modification of the particles in the artery. Oxidation of LDL occurs in vitro in the presence of endothelial cells, smooth muscle cells, and macrophages,[70] and evidence also exists that this process may occur in vivo.[71] An additional mechanism for estrogen cardioprotection may be related to its antioxidant activity. Estrogens inhibit LDL oxidation in vitro[72] and LDL isolated from estrogen-treated women[73] has increased resistance to lipid peroxidation. Estrogen treatment of LDL also inhibits LDL accumulation in macrophages.[74] Furthermore, we have found in two studies that estrogens decrease TBARs levels in the artery wall. The lack of treatment effect on serum TBARS in our studies is not surprising, because there are a number of antioxidants present in the serum.[75] However, the significant decrease in lipid peroxidation in the artery suggests that estrogens may attenuate the oxidative modification of LDL or other lipids in the artery and may decrease the subsequent unregulated uptake and accumulation in macrophages.

The lack of effect of CEE treatment in our 12-week study may be explained by the fact that there was not enough atherogenic stimulus to recruit sufficient macrophage numbers to detect any difference in arterial LDL degradation.[23] This is consistent with studies in rabbits where an antioxidant, probucol, inhibited lesion progression and also decreased rates of LDL degradation but only in lesioned areas rich in macrophage-derived foam cells.[76] No differences in rates of LDL degradation were found in nonlesioned areas, where degradation was predominantly in smooth muscle cells.

Conclusions

Estrogens may decrease the risk of coronary atherosclerosis and heart disease through a number of mechanisms. The decrease in arterial LDL degradation and accumulation seems to be a key event in preventing atherosclerosis progression. Furthermore, we have seen a similar decrease in LDL degradation in three short-term studies of parenteral estrogen and progesterone, in which there were no changes in plasma lipids and lipoproteins, oral esterified estrogens with or without methyltestosterone, in which there was a decrease in apo B-containing lipoproteins, and oral contraceptive agents, in which there was an increase in the TPC/HDLC ratio. These studies strongly suggest that estrogens decrease arterial LDL accumulation independently of plasma lipids and lipoproteins. A consistent change in all the short-term studies was a decrease in LDL size. This was not found in the 5-week DHEN study, most likely due to the very short period of study. Whether the decrease in LDL size is responsible for the decrease in arterial LDL degradation or just a marker for changes in lipoprotein metabolism (ie, changes in hepatic lipo-protein metabolism) that indirectly affect arterial metabolism is un-known. Also, estrogen's role as an antioxidant in affecting athero-sclerosis and LDL metabolism may be primary to estrogen's cardioprotection. Further studies are now underway in an attempt to determine if the decrease in arterial LDL metabolism is due to a direct effect on the artery or due to changes in LDL metabolism resulting from changes in composition or oxidation.

References

1. Godsland IF, Wynn V, Crook D, et al. Sex, plasma lipoproteins, and atherosclerosis: Prevailing assumptions and outstanding questions. *Am Heart J* 1987;114:1467–1503.
2. Stampfer MJ, Colditz GA. Estrogen replacement therapy and coronary heart disease: A quantitative assessment of the epidemiologic evidence. *Prevent Med* 1991;20:47–63.
3. Barrett-Connor E, Bush TL. Estrogen and coronary heart disease in women. *JAMA* 1991;265:1861–1867.
4. Kannel WB. Metabolic risk factors for coronary heart disease in women: Perspective from the Framingham Study. *Am Heart J* 1987;114: 413-419.
5. Crook D, Seed M. Endocrine control of plasma lipoprotein metabolism: Effects of gonadal steroids. *Bailliere's Clin Endocrinol Metab* 1990;4: 851-875.
6. Knopp RH, Walden CE, Wahl PW, et al. Oral contraceptive and post-menopausal estrogen effects on lipoprotein triglyceride and cholesterol in an adult female population. Relationships to estrogen and progestin potency. *J Clin Endocrinol Metab* 1981;53:1123-1132.
7. Hickock LR, Toomey C, Speroff L. A comparison of esterified estrogens with and without methyltestosterone: Effects on endometrial histology and serum lipoproteins in postmenopausal women. *Obstet Gynecol* 1993;82:919-924.
8. Watts NB, Notelovitz M, Timmons MC, et al. Comparison of oral estrogens and estrogens plus androgen on bone mineral density, menopausal symptoms, and lipid-lipoprotein profiles in surgical menopause. *Obstet Gynecol* 1995;85:529-537.
9. Washburn SA, Wagner JD, Adams MR, et al. Effects of contraceptive steroids on plasma lipoprotein levels and coronary artery atheroscle-rosis. In: Goldzieher JW, Fotherby K, eds. *Pharmacology of Contracep-tive Steroids.* New York: Raven Press; 1994:335-343.
10. Stampfer MJ, Willett WC, Colditz GA, et al. A prospective study of past use of oral contraceptive agents and risk of cardiovascular diseases. *N Engl J Med* 1988;319:1313-1317.
11. Clarkson TB, Adams MR, Williams JK, et al. Clinical implications of animal models of gender difference in heart disease. In: Douglas PS, ed. *Cardiovascular Health and Disease in Women.* Philadelphia: W.B. Saun-ders; 1993:283-302.

12. Adams MR, Kaplan JR, Manuck SB, et al. Inhibition of coronary artery atherosclerosis by 17-beta estradiol in ovariectomized monkeys. Lack of an effect of adding progesterone. *Arteriosclerosis* 1990;10:1051–1057.

13. Pittman RC, Carew TE, Glass CK, et al. A radioiodinated, intracellularly trapped ligand for determining the sites of plasma protein degradation *in vivo*. *Biochem J* 1983;212:791–800.

14. Carew TC, Pittman RC, Marchand ER, et al. Measurement *in vivo* of irreversible degradation of low density lipoprotein in the rabbit aorta. *Arteriosclerosis* 1984;4:214–224.

15. Schwenke DC, Carew TE. Quantification *in vivo* of increased LDL content and rate of LDL degradation in the normal rabbit aorta occurring at sites susceptible to early atherosclerotic lesions. *Circ Res* 1988; 62:699–710.

16. Newman HA, Zilversmit DB. Quantitative aspects of cholesterol flux in rabbit atheromatous lesions. *J Biol Chem* 1962;237:2078–2084.

17. Dayton S, Hashimoto S. Recent advances in molecular pathology: A review. Cholesterol flux and metabolism in arterial tissue in atheroma. *Exp Mol Pathol* 1970;13:253–268.

18. Wagner JD, Clarkson TB, St. Clair RW, et al. Estrogen and progesterone replacement therapy reduces LDL accumulation in the coronary arteries of surgically postmenopausal cynomolgus monkeys. *J Clin Invest* 1991;88:1995–2002.

19. Wagner JD, St. Clair RW, Schwenke DC, et al. Regional differences in arterial low density lipoprotein metabolism in surgically postmenopausal cynomolgus monkeys: Effects of estrogen and progesterone therapy. *Arterioscler Thromb* 1992;12:717–726.

20. Applebaum DM, Goldberg AP, Pykalisto OJ, et al. Effect of estrogen on post–heparin lipolytic activity: Selective decline in hepatic triglyceride lipase. *J Clin Invest* 1977;59:601–608.

21. Rudel LL, Bond MG, Bullock BC. LDL heterogeneity and atherosclerosis in nonhuman primates. *Ann NY Acad Sci* 1985;454:248–253.

22. Wagner JD, Schwenke DC, Zhang L, et al. Effects of short-term hormone replacement therapies on low-density lipoprotein metabolism in cynanolgus monkeys. *Arterioscler Thromb Vasc Biol*, In press.

23. Manning JM, Campos G, Edwards IJ, et al. Effects of hormone replacement modalities on low density lipoprotein composition and distribution in ovariectomized cynomolgus monkeys. *Atherosclerosis* In press.

24. Colvin PL Jr, Wagner JD, Adams MR, et al. Sex steroid replacement increases hepatic 7 alpha–hydroxylase mRNA. Abstract. *Circulation* 1994;90(suppl I):I–351.

25. Kushwaha RS, Born KM. Effect of estrogen and progesterone on the hepatic cholesterol 7α-hydroxylase activity in ovariectomized baboons. *Biochim Biophys Acta* 1991;1084:300–302.

26. Everson GT, McKinley C, Kern F Jr. Mechanisms of gallstone formation in women. Effects of exogenous estrogen (Premarin) and dietary cholesterol on hepatic lipid metabolism. *J Clin Invest* 1991;87:237–246.

27. Adams MR, Register TC, Golden DL, et al. Medroxyprogesterone acetate antagonizes inhibitory effects of conjugated equine estrogens on coronary artery atherosclerosis. *Arterioscler Thromb Vasc Biol.* 1997;17:217–221.

28. Burger HG, Hailes J, Menelaus M, et al. The management of persistent menopausal symptoms with oestradiol-testosterone implants: Clinical, lipid and hormonal results. *Maturitas* 1984;6:351–358.

29. Sherwin BB, Gelfand MM. Transaction of the 40th annual meeting of the Society of Obstetricians and Gynaecologists of Canada: Differential symptom response to parenteral estrogen and/or androgen administration in the surgical menopause. *Am J Obstet Gynecol* 1985;151:153–160.
30. Wagner JD, Zhang L, Williams JK, et al. Esterified estrogens with and without methyltestosterone decrease arterial LDL metabolism in cynomolgus monkeys. *Arterioscler Thromb Vasc Biol* 1996;16:1473–1480.
31. Stern MD. Pharmacology of conjugated oestrogens. *Maturitas* 1982; 4:333–339.
32. Washburn SA, Adams MR, Clarkson TB, et al. A conjugated equine estrogen with differential effects on uterine weight and plasma cholesterol in the rat. *Am J Obstet Gynecol* 1993;169:251–256.
33. Wagner JD, Washburn SA, Zhang L, et al. A non-feminizing conjugated equine estrogen decreases arterial LDL degradation and improves vascular reactivity in male rhesus monkeys. Abstract. *Circulation* In press.
34. Wagner JD, Adams MR, Schwenke DC, et al. Oral contraceptive treatment decreases arterial LDL degradation in female cynomolgus monkeys. *Circ Res* 1993;72:1300–1307.
35. Colvin PL Jr, Wagner JD, Heuser MD, et al. Oral contraceptives decrease hepatic cholesterol independent of the low density lipoprotein receptor in nonhuman primates. *Arterioscler Thromb* 1993;13:1645–1649.
36. Kern F Jr, Everson GT. Contraceptive steroids increase cholesterol in bile: Mechanisms of action. *J Lipid Res* 1987;28:828–839.
37. Hough JL, Zilversmit DB. Effect of 17-β estradiol on cholesterol content and metabolism in cholesterol-fed rabbits. *Arteriosclerosis* 1986; 6:57–63.
38. Haarbo J, Nielsen LB, Stender S, et al. Aortic permeability to LDL during estrogen therapy. A study in normocholesterolemic rabbits. *Arterioscler Thromb* 1994;14:243–247.
39. Kushwaha RS, Hazzard WR. Exogenous estrogens attenuate dietary hypercholesterolemia and atherosclerosis in the rabbits. *Metabolism* 1981; 30:359–366.
40. Haarbo J, Leth-Espensen P, Stender S, et al. Estrogen monotherapy and combined estrogen-progestogen replacement therapy attenuate aortic accumulation of cholesterol in ovariectomized cholesterol-fed rabbits. *J Clin Invest* 1991;87:1274–1279.
41. Haarbo J, Svendsen OL, Christiansen C. Progestogens do not affect aortic accumulation of cholesterol in ovariectomized cholesterol-fed rabbits. *Circ Res* 1992;70:1198–1202.
42. Sulistiyani, Adelman SJ, Chandrasekaran A, et al. Effect of 17α-dihydroequilin sulfate, a conjugated equine estrogen, and ethynylestradiol on atherosclerosis in cholesterol-fed rabbits. *Arterioscler Thromb Vasc Biol* 1995;15:837–846.
43. Walsh BW, Schiff I, Rosner B, et al. Effects of postmenopausal estrogen replacement on the concentrations and metabolism of plasma lipoproteins. *N Engl J Med* 1991;325:1196–1204.
44. Windler EET, Kovanen PT, Chao YS, et al. The estradiol-stimulated lipoprotein receptor of rat liver. A binding site that mediates the uptake of rat lipoproteins containing apoproteins B and E. *J Biol Chem* 1980;225:10464–10471.
45. Veldhuis JD, Gwynne JT. Estrogen regulates low density lipoprotein metabolism by cultured swine granulosa cells. *Endocrinology* 1985; 117:1321–1327.

46. Chao Y-S, Windler EE, Chen GC, et al. Hepatic catabolism of rat and human lipoproteins in rats treated with 17α-ethinyl estradiol. *J Biol Chem* 1979;254:11360–11366.
47. Kovanen PT, Brown MS, Goldstein JL. Increased binding of low density lipoprotein to liver membranes from rats treated with 17α-ethinyl estradiol. *J Biol Chem* 1979;254:11367–11373.
48. Ma PT, Yamamoto T, Goldstein JL, et al. Increased mRNA for low density lipoprotein receptors in livers of rabbits treated with 17α-ethinyl estradiol. *Proc Natl Acad Sci USA* 1986;83:792–796.
49. Crouse JR, Parks JS, Schey HM, et al. Studies of low density lipoprotein molecular weight in human beings with coronary artery disease. *J Lipid Res* 1985;26:566–573.
50. Campos H, Roederer GO, Lussier-Cacan S, et al. Predominance of large LDL and reduced HDL₂ cholesterol in normolipidemic men with coronary artery disease. *Arterioscler Thromb Vasc Biol* 1995;15:1043–1048.
51. van der Mooren MJ, de Graaf J, Demacker PN, et al. Changes in the low-density lipoprotein profile during 17β-estradiol-dydrogesterone therapy in postmenopausal women. *Metab Clin Exp* 1994;43:799–802.
52. Campos H, Sacks FM, Walsh BW, et al. Differential effects of estrogen on low-density lipoprotein subclasses in healthy postmenopausal women. *Metabolism* 1993;42:1153–1158.
53. Campos H, McNamara JR, Wilson PWF, et al. Differences in low density lipoprotein subfractions and apolipoproteins in premenopausal and postmenopausal women. *J Clin Endocrinol Metab* 1988;67:30–35.
54. Granfone A, Campos H, McNamara JR, et al. Effects of estrogen replacement on plasma lipoproteins and apolipoproteins in postmenopausal, dyslipidemic women. *Metabolism* 1992;41:1193–1198.
55. McNamara JR, Jenner JL, Zhengling L, et al. Change in LDL particle size is associated with change in plasma triglyceride concentration. *Arterioscler Thromb* 1992;12:1284–1290.
56. Rudel LL, Parks JS, Johnson FL, et al. Low density lipoproteins in atherosclerosis. *J Lipid Res* 1986;27:465–474.
57. Stevenson SC, Sawyer JK, Rudel LL. Role of apolipoprotein E on cholesteryl ester-enriched low density lipoprotein particles in coronary artery atherosclerosis of hypercholesterolemic nonhuman primates. *Arterioscler Thromb* 1992;12:28–40.
58. Hazzard WR, Applebaum-Bowden D, Terry JG. Apolipoprotein E: Paradoxes abound. In: LL Gallo, ed. *Cardiovascular Disease 2* New York: Plenum Press; 1995:57–66.
59. Floren C-H, Kushwaha RS, Hazzard WR, et al. Estrogen-induced increase in uptake of cholesterol-rich very low density lipoproteins in perfused rabbit liver. *Metabolism* 1981;30:367–375.
60. Demacher PNM, Mol MJTM, Stalenhoef AFH. Increased hepatic lipase activity and increased direct removal of very low density lipoprotein remnants in Watanabe heritable hyperlipidemic (WHHL) rabbits treated with ethinyl estradiol. *Biochem J* 1990;272:647–651.
61. Westerveld HT, Kock LAW, van Rijn JM, et al. 17β-estradiol improves postprandial lipid metabolism in postmenopausal women. *J Clin Endocrinol Metab* 1995;80:249–253.
62. Kushwaha RS, Foster DM, Barrett PHR, et al. Metabolic regulation of plasma apolipoprotein E by estrogen and progesterone in the baboon (*Papio* sp). *Metabolism* 1991;40:93–100.

63. Parks JS, Wilson MD, Johnson FL, et al. Fish oil decreases hepatic cholesteryl ester secretion but not apoB secretion in African green monkeys. *J Lipid Res* 1989;30:1535–1544.
64. St Clair RW, Mitschelen JJ, Leight MA. Metabolism by cells in culture of low-density lipoproteins of abnormal composition from non-human primates with diet-induced hypercholesterolemia. *Biochim Biophys Acta* 1980;618:63–79.
65. St. Clair RW, Greenspan P, Leight MA. Enhanced cholesterol delivery to cells in culture by low density lipoproteins from hypercholesterolemic monkeys. Correlation of cellular cholesterol accumulation with low density lipoprotein molecular weight. *Arteriosclerosis* 1983;3:77–86.
66. Bondjers G, Wiklund O, Fage G, et al. Transfer of lipoproteins from plasma to the cell populations of the normal and atherosclerotic arterial tissue. *Eur Heart J* 1990;11(suppl E):158–163.
67. Camejo G, Mateu L, Lalaguna F, et al. Structural individuality of human serum LDL associated with a differential affinity for a macromolecular component of the arterial wall. *Artery* 1976;2:79–97.
68. de Graaf J, Hak-Lemmers HLM, Hectors MPC, et al. Enhanced susceptibility to in vitro oxidation of the dense low density lipoprotein subfraction in healthy subjects. *Arterioscler Thromb* 1991;11:298–306.
69. Tribble DL, Holl LG, Wood PD, et al. Variations in oxidative susceptibility among six low-density lipoprotein subfractions of differing density and particle size. *Atherosclerosis* 1992;93:189–199.
70. Steinberg D, Parthasarathy S, Carew TE, et al. Beyond cholesterol. Modifications of low density lipoprotein that increase its atherogenicity. *N Engl J Med* 1989;320:915–924.
71. Palinski W, Rosenfeld ME, Yla-Herttuala S, et al. Low density lipoprotein undergoes oxidative modification *in vivo*. *Proc Natl Acad Sci USA* 1989;86:1372–1376.
72. Subbiah MTR, Kessel B, Agrawal M, et al. Antioxidant potential of specific estrogens on lipid peroxidation. *J Clin Endocrinol Metab* 1993;77:1095–1097.
73. Sack MN, Rader DJ, Cannon RO III. Oestrogen and inhibition of oxidation of low–density lipoproteins in postmenopausal women. *Lancet* 1994;343:269–270.
74. Huber LA, Scheffler E, Poll T, et al. 17 Beta-estradiol inhibits LDL oxidation and cholesteryl ester formation in cultured macrophages. *Free Rad Res Commun* 1990;8:167–173.
75. Witztum JL, Steinberg D. Role of oxidized low density lipoprotein in atherogenesis. *J Clin Invest* 1991;88:1785–1792.
76. Carew TE, Schwenke DC, Steinberg D. Antiatherogenic effect of probucol unrelated to its hypocholesterolemic effect: Evidence that antioxidants in vivo can selectively inhibit low density lipoprotein degradation in macrophage-rich fatty streaks and slow the progression of atherosclerosis. *Proc Natl Acad Sci USA* 1987;84:7725–7729.

Chapter 11

Effects of Estrogen on the Anatomic and Functional Sequelae of Coronary Atherosclerosis

David M. Herrington, MD, MHS

Meta-analyses of numerous observational studies have shown that postmenopausal estrogen replacement therapy is associated with lower risk of clinical cardiovascular events.[1-3] These clinical events are the result of both anatomic and functional abnormalities of the coronary and other arteries that occur as a result of the atherosclerotic process. The purpose of this chapter is to review the currently available data on the effects of estrogen on these anatomic and functional abnormalities, which are the final steps in the pathogenesis of clinically evident coronary artery disease. Others in this book will review the effects of estrogen on the molecular, cellular, and metabolic processes that lead to these abnormalities and provide a mechanistic framework to understand how estrogen may be beneficial in attenuating the atherosclerotic process and its attendant clinical events.

Anatomic and Functional Sequelae of Atherosclerosis

Medicine's foundation in pathological studies has left us with largely anatomic paradigms for describing chronic diseases such as atherosclerosis. Medical textbooks and practicing clinicians typically define and quantify atherosclerosis in anatomic terms related to thickening of the arterial wall and encroachment on the arterial lumen. This approach has proven very useful both in clinical inves-

From: Forte TM, (ed). *Hormonal, Metabolic, and Cellular Influences on Cardiovascular Disease in Women.* Armonk, NY: Futura Publishing Company, Inc.; © 1997.

tigation and clinical management of patients with atherosclerosis. For example, the extent and severity of coronary stenoses by angiography has been used to study the natural history of risk factors for, and the effects of, interventions on coronary artery disease. However, current understanding of the pathogenesis of coronary artery disease suggests that we should define atherosclerosis more broadly to include the associated functional derangements that also occur as a result of atherosclerosis and that share in the responsibility for the resulting clinical events. Therefore, this chapter will focus on studies that relate to three different sequelae of atherosclerosis in the coronary arteries: abnormal wall thickening and lumenal encroachment, abnormal endothelial-dependent vasodilator capacity, and abnormal thrombogenic potential. The abnormal wall thickening, which can be quite extensive before actual lumenal encroachment occurs,[4] is the result of intimal and medial cellular proliferation and intimal accumulation of intra- and extracellular lipid, extracellular matrix elements such as collagen, fibrin, fibronectin, and calcium as well as necrotic cellular debris.[5,6] However, atherosclerosis is also accompanied by significant abnormalities in endothelial-dependent vasomotor regulation. One abnormality is the impairment of nitric oxide (NO)-mediated vasodilator response to endothelial vasodilator stimuli such as acetylcholine or serotonin.[7,8] In the face of this atherosclerosis-associated endothelial dysfunction, some endothelial targeted stimuli can paradoxically result in a vasoconstrictor response because of a concomitant weak vasoconstrictor effect of these stimuli on the vascular smooth muscle.[9,10] This shift in the balance of vasodilators and vasoconstrictors may exacerbate the development of exertional angina and may also cause or complicate acute coronary syndromes by promoting plaque rupture and/or producing a more vigorous vasoconstrictor response to the ensuing aggregate of degranulating platelets.[11]

The third sequela of atherosclerosis considered here is an impairment of the antithrombotic function of the endothelium. This capacity of the endothelium to prevent thrombosis stems from the physical barrier function that protects the blood elements from the highly thrombogenic material in the intimal and subintimal space and the functional effect of intact endothelium to attenuate platelet aggregation[8] through the secretion of NO and other compounds.[12-15] A breach in the physical and functional integrity of the endothelium that occurs during rupture of an atherosclerotic plaque results in thrombus formation, which, if left unchecked, can propagate into and occlude the adjacent coronary lumen. Although there are no data on estrogen's ability to modulate risk for plaque rupture, there are considerable data concerning the effects of estrogen on the coagulation and fibrinolytic cascades and on platelet function that may determine the extensiveness of a thrombotic response.

Does Estrogen Alter the Development of Wall Thickness/Lumenal Encroachment?

There are three classes of data to draw on to examine this question: cross-sectional studies of coronary angiograms and carotid ultrasounds in women, nonrandomized prospective studies of coronary angiographic and carotid ultrasound studies in women, and clinical trials in nonhuman primates using pathological measures of coronary disease at necropsy. There are three angiographic cross-sectional studies published to date examining the extent of angiographically defined coronary artery disease in postmenopausal women with and without estrogen replacement therapy (Figure 1).[16–18] Sullivan et al. compared 1,444 postmenopausal women with at least one ≥70% coronary stenosis by angiography with 744 women who had no angiographic evidence of disease. Only 2.7% of the women with significant coronary disease were current users of

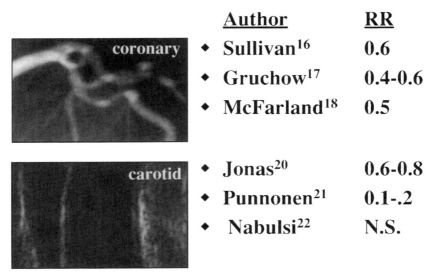

	Author	RR
coronary	◆ Sullivan[16]	0.6
	◆ Gruchow[17]	0.4-0.6
	◆ McFarland[18]	0.5
carotid	◆ Jonas[20]	0.6-0.8
	◆ Punnonen[21]	0.1-.2
	◆ Nabulsi[22]	N.S.

FIGURE 1. *Cross sectional studies of estrogen use and risk of coronary or carotid atherosclerotic lesions. RR, relative risk of disease among users versus nonusers. All RRs are significantly <1.0 (P < 0.05) except for Nabulsi et al.[22]*

postmenopausal estrogen compared with 7.7% of the women with normal angiograms. After adjustment for age and other risk factors, the odds ratio for significant coronary disease among users of postmenopausal estrogen relative to nonusers was 0.44 ($P = 0.04$). Gruchow et al.[17] reported age-adjusted odds ratios of 0.59 and 0.37 for use of postmenopausal estrogen in 933 women with moderate and severe coronary occlusion scores respectively ($P < 0.05$). This association was independent of type of menopause and conventional cardiovascular disease risk factors except high-density lipoprotein (HDL) cholesterol levels. The authors concluded that modulation of HDL levels was one of the mechanisms that could account for an association between estrogen use and stenotic coronary disease. McFarland et al.[18] also reported on a group of 345 women aged 35–59 years who had undergone coronary angiography. Women with a ≥70% coronary stenosis (n=137) were compared with women with angiographically normal coronaries (n=208). The odds ratio for estrogen use for greater than 6 months duration was 0.50 ($P < 0.01$).

Angiographic studies have the advantage of using direct measures of an anatomic manifestation of coronary atherosclerosis ie, lumenal encroachment. However, they are subject to the potential for misclassification of cases because early atherosclerosis may be present without any angiographically detectable changes. Furthermore, these cross-sectional angiographic cohorts may be subject to diagnosis or detection biases because only symptomatic subjects undergo coronary angiography in the first place. Carotid ultrasound provides a mechanism to directly measure extent of arterial intimal thickening even at early stages of the disease process. In addition, large cohort studies using noninvasive techniques such as carotid ultrasound are less subject to selection biases that could bias results from studies of catheterization laboratory cohorts.

In a large cross-sectional study of estrogen use and carotid wall thickness in 2,962 women >65 years, CHS investigators[19,20] reported significantly lower internal and common carotid artery wall thickness among current users of estrogen replacement when compared to nonusers ($P < 0.01$). The risk of any wall thickening (≥1% stenosis) was also significantly lower among estrogen users ($P < 0.05$; Figure 1). Similar results were observed in a much smaller vascular ultrasound study of women on estradiol valerate alone or in combination with levonorgestrel when compared with women who had never used hormone replacement therapy.[21] In that study, the total number of fibrous and calcific plaques in the abdominal aorta and the carotid and femoral arteries was significantly less in the women who were current users of estradiol valerate with or without levonorgestrel when compared with similar aged women who were not hormone users ($P = 0.001$ and 0.01, respectively). In contrast, Na-bulsi et al.[22] found no difference in wall thickness between users and nonusers of hormone replacement therapy among postmenopausal women enrolled in the Atherosclerosis Risk in Communities (ARIC) Study. Interestingly, in the studies by Jonas et al.[20] and Punnonen et al.,[21] the addition of progestins did not attenuate the apparent favorable effect of estrogen on extent of measurable carotid atherosclerosis.

There are very few prospective data concerning estrogen use and prospectively measured progression of coronary artery disease. Recently, O'Brien et al.[23] reported a secondary analysis of 197 post-menopausal women from the Coronary Angioplasty versus Exci-sional Atherectomy Trial (CAVEAT I). At 6 months after either per-cutaneous transluminal coronary angioplasty (PTCA) or directional atherectomy, the 39 postmenopausal women who were taking estro-gen replacement therapy had significantly less restenosis than the women who were not on estrogen therapy ($P < 0.01$). Furthermore, the effect of estrogen was most pronounced in the subset of women who underwent atherectomy, the technique postulated to result in a more vigorous inflammatory response following the procedure. This suggests that estrogen may play an important role in modulat-ing the inflammatory component of the pathogenesis of restenosis and possibly atherosclerosis.

Similar differences between users and nonusers of estrogen were observed in a secondary analysis of the Asymptomatic Carotid Atherosclerosis Progression Study (ACAPS)—a clinical trial testing the effects of lovastatin or placebo on progression of carotid intimal-medial wall thickness (IMT).[24] Among the 186 postmenopausal women enrolled, those who were on estrogen replacement (n=63) had regression of their IMT regardless of their assignment to lovas-tatin or placebo. In contrast, nonusers of estrogen in the placebo group had significant progression of their carotid disease during 3 years. The differences between users and nonusers was significant at the 0.05 level.

The only clinical trial evidence to date suggesting that post-menopausal hormone replacement therapy can alter the progression of coronary atherosclerosis in women comes from clinical trials con-ducted in nonhuman primates. Adams et al.[25] demonstrated in two separate studies that ovariectomized cynomolgus macaques on ath-erogenic diet had less coronary atherosclerotic plaque when treated concurrently with either estradiol or conjugated equine estrogen compared to placebo-treated animals[26] (Figure 2). These studies were supported by earlier work demonstrating increased extent of coronary atherosclerosis in ovariectomized monkeys and in mon-

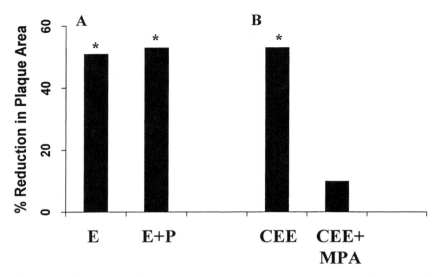

FIGURE 2. *Percent reduction in coronary artery plaque area (compared with control) in ovariectomized atherosclerotic monkeys treated with various hormone replacement regimens. E, subcutaneous estradiol; P, cyclic subcutaneous progesterone; CEE, conjugated equine estrogen; MPA, continuous medroxyprogesterone acetate; *P < 0.05. Adapted with permission from Reference 25 and Reference 26.*

keys with relative estrogen deficiency due to low-social status[27] and almost complete protection from atherosclerosis in monkeys with elevated endogenous estradiol due to pregnancy.[28] In the clinical trials, the addition of cyclicly administered subcutaneous progesterone had no adverse impact on the protective effect of estrogen,[25] whereas continuous low-dose medroxyprogesterone acetate was associated with blunted or abolished estrogenic protection against plaque formation.[26] This observation raises important questions about the types of progestational agents and their method of delivery with respect to use of hormone replacement for protection against heart disease.

Definitive proof of the benefit of estrogen, with or without progestins, on progression of coronary atherosclerosis in women will await completion of the various angiographic endpoint trials, which are in the planning stages or currently underway. The Estrogen Replacement and Atherosclerosis (ERA) Trial is the largest of the active trials with an anticipated enrollment of 375. This is a three-arm trial comparing the effects of conjugated oral estrogen (0.625 mg q.d.) with or without low-continuous dose medroxyprogesterone acetate

(MPA) (2.5 mg q.d.) and placebo on progression of coronary stenoses in women with established coronary artery disease. Intracoronary ultrasound and measures of potential mechanisms through which hormone replacement might exert its effects will supplement the angiographic outcomes (Table 1). The Women's Estrogen-Progestin Lipid Lowering Hormone Atherosclerosis Regression Trial (WELL-HART) will test the efficacy of oral estradiol (1 mg q.d.) with or without cyclic MPA (cMPA) (5 mg days 1–10) in slowing the progression of established coronary stenoses (H. Hodis MD, personal communication). A third trial called the Angiographic Trials in Women, currently in the planning phase, is a 2 × 2 factorial design comparing the effects of hormone replacement therapy and/or an antioxidant intervention on progression of coronary stenoses. The actual interventions for this trial are not yet known.

In summary, cross-sectional angiographic and carotid ultrasound studies and nonrandomized prospective angiographic and carotid ultrasound data all suggest that estrogen replacement therapy can slow the development or progression of arterial atherosclerosis or restenosis. These observations are supported by observational studies and clinical trials in nonhuman primates. The human angiographic trials will ultimately confirm or refute the hypothesis that estrogen replacement therapy can slow, or possibly reverse, the cor-

---

TABLE 1

Plasma Factors to be Measured in the ERA Trial

Lipids
  Lipid profile
  LDL/VLDL beta quant
  HDL subfractions
  Apo-A-I, B, E, Lp(a)
  Apo E isoforms
Carbohydrate metabolism
  Insulin/glucose during 2-hr OGTT
Estrogens
  Estradiol, estrone, SHBG
Blood pressure
  Renin
  Angiotensin II,(I-7)
Hemostasis
  Fibrinogen
  Factor VII
  PAI-1
Antioxidants
  Plasma antioxidant activity

onary lumenal encroachment in women that constitutes one of the anatomic sequelae of atherosclerosis. The intracoronary ultrasound data from the ERA trial may also address the issue of progression of wall thickening, which can occur in the absence of lumenal encroachment.

Does Estrogen Influence Endothelial-Dependent Vasomotor Function in Women?

In vitro studies demonstrate that estrogen can enhance the vasodilator response to acetylcholine in rabbit femoral arteries[29] and pig coronary arteries.[30] In vivo angiographic studies in both non-human primates and postmenopausal women have confirmed that chronic[31,32] and acute[33-37] estrogen administration can attenuate or even reverse the abnormal coronary vasomotor response to acetylcholine that occurs as a consequence of atherosclerosis (Figure 3). This effect of estrogen has also been demonstrated in the brachial artery in response to either acetylcholine[38-40] or increase in flow,[41,42] and the effects can be documented both in the macrovasculature[32,35-37] and in the resistance arterioles.[35-39] The effects of estrogen on endothelial-dependent vasomotor tone are likely mediated

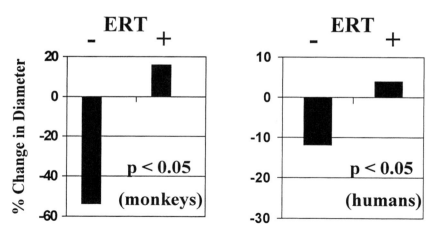

FIGURE 3. *Percent change in coronary artery diameter in response to 10^{-6} M acetylcholine in ovariectomized monkeys (left) and postmenopausal women (right) according to estrogen replacement status. +, chronic estrogen replacement therapy; −, no estrogen replacement. Adapted with permission from References 31 and 32.*

through an effect on synthesis, release, or delivery of NO from the endothelium to the encircling vascular smooth muscle cells. In the central nervous system, estrogen upregulates muscarinic receptors.[43] Whether or not some of the effects of estrogen on the vascular responses to acetylcholine can be attributed to a similar effect on vascular endothelial cells is unknown. Hishikawa et al.[44] reported that estrogen upregulates NO synthase in human aortic endothelial cells. Estrogen treatment of hypertensive rats results in greater dependency on NO for maintenance of resting blood pressure,[45] further supporting an effect of estrogen on the NO axis. In addition to the effects of estrogen on endothelial-dependent vasomotor function, high doses of estrogen also appear to have a direct vasodilating effect on rabbit,[46] canine,[47] and human[48] coronary arteries in vitro mediated through a calcium channel antagonist effect[37,49] or by rendering coronaries less responsive to vasoconstrictor stimuli.[50]

Ultimately, the question remains whether estrogen has an effect on vasomotor function that is of clinical relevance. The best evidence currently available comes from a study of exercise treadmill performance in postmenopausal women.[51] A single dose of sublingual estradiol resulted in a 27% increase in time to 1 mm ST segment depression and a 25% reduction in maximum ST segment depression ($P < 0.05$ for both). It is unknown whether this reflects a direct vasodilating effect of estrogen or an estrogen effect on endothelially regulated vasomotor tone; however, the clinical implications for chronic ischemic syndromes including stable exertional angina are clear. Whether or not an estrogen-mediated shift away from vasoconstriction toward vasodilation will minimize the initiation of plaque rupture and the ensuing acute ischemic syndromes is unknown.

Does Estrogen Influence Thrombogenic Potential?

The third sequela of atherosclerosis that is responsible for acute ischemic syndromes is enhanced thrombogenic potential. This is due to a combination of plaque ulceration that exposes highly thrombogenic material in the intimal space to the lumen and the thrombotic response to this stimulus, which may be enhanced as a result of endothelial dysfunction.[8] Clearly a plaque cannot ulcerate if it does not exist. As discussed above, estrogen may reduce thrombotic potential by decreasing the substrate of coronary lesions available to ulcerate. However, once a lesion has formed, there is no direct evidence to suggest that estrogen helps stabilize plaques, rendering them less prone to ulcerate. Whether or not estrogen's ability to blunt vasoconstrictor or enhance vasodilator responses helps minimize the likelihood of ulceration is unknown. On the other hand, there are ample data to suggest that estrogen may attenuate the thrombotic response that occurs in the face of plaque ulceration through effects on coagulation, fibrinolysis, and platelet aggregation. The effects of estrogen on the coagulation cascade are complex and depend on dose and route of administration.[52,53] The effects of oral replacement therapy doses of estrogen are summarized in Figure 4. Many studies have shown that replacement therapy doses of oral estrogen are associated with small increases in the procoagulant factor VII[19,54–56] and transient increases in factors IX and X.[57] The increases in factor VII may be related to estrogen-associated increases in triglycerides, which are known to increase levels and activation of factor VII.[58,59] The increases in factor VII are not seen with hormone replacement regimens that include low-dose progestins[54,56,60,61] or nonoral estrogen regimens that avoid the first-pass effects on hepatic protein synthesis.[62]

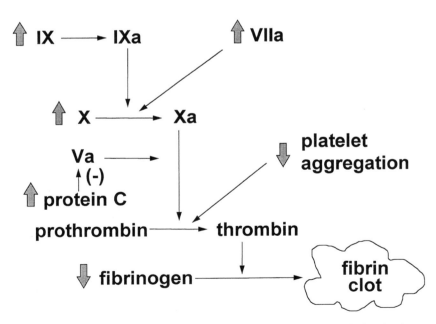

FIGURE 4. *Effects of estrogen on the coagulation cascade and platelet function. Changes reported to be associated with hormone replacement therapy are indicated by gray arrows.*

Any procoagulant effect of estrogen through elevations in factor VII is likely offset by concomitant increases in protein C, the enzyme substrate that degrades factor V^{54} and lowers levels of fibrinogen,[19,54,61,63] which, when cleaved by thrombin, leads to fibrin clot formation. The importance of the estrogen-associated reductions in fibrinogen are emphasized by the numerous epidemiological studies showing that elevated fibrinogen is an independent risk factor for cardiovascular disease.[64–67] The effects of estrogen on the anticoagulant antithrombin III (AT-III) are unclear, with some studies reporting a decrease in AT-III levels[54,56] and others reporting no effect.[68,69]

The effects of estrogen on the fibrinolytic pathway include reductions in plasma levels of plasminogen activator inhibitor-1 (PAI-1) antigen[69–72] and lower levels of lipoprotein(a) [Lp(a)] (Figure 5).[54,73,74] Because both PAI-1 and Lp(a) are inhibitors of fibrinolysis, these effects should enhance fibrinolysis. In addition, physiological increases in endogenous estradiol are accompanied by higher levels of plasminogen[75,76] and combination conjugated oral estrogen and medroxyprogesterone acetate results in enhanced plasminogen ac-

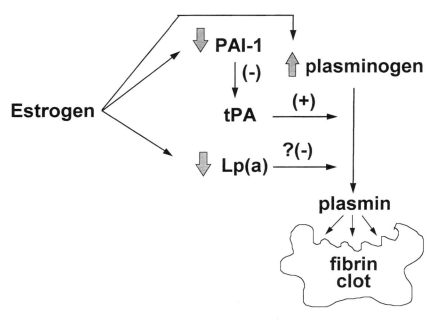

FIGURE 5. *Effects of estrogen replacement therapy on the fibrinolytic cascade. Changes reported to be associated with estrogen replacement therapy are indicated by the gray arrows.*

tivity.[56,62,68,69] The net effect of these changes is consistent with enhanced fibrinolytic activity.

Finally, there are numerous studies suggesting that estrogen attenuates platelet aggregation. In vivo studies of platelets that were incubated with estrogen or obtained from women on hormone replacement show reductions in vasopressin-induced calcium uptake,[77] impaired adherence to endothelial cell matrix,[78] and attenuated aggregation and adenosine triphosphate (ATP) release in response to adrenalin.[79] Similar effects of estrogen have been reported in platelets from rats.[80] These effects of estrogen are not changed by the addition of low-dose progestin.[60,79] The mechanism for the effects of estrogen on platelet function is unknown. However, in view of the central role of NO in attenuating platelet aggregation[12-15] and the mounting evidence that estrogen enhances the NO pathways related to vasomotor function, it is an attractive hypothesis that estrogen may blunt platelet aggregation through an increase in endothelial synthesis and/or release of NO.

In the aggregate, the data suggest that estrogen may blunt the enhanced thrombogenic potential created by atherosclerosis by inhibiting coagulation and platelet aggregation and enhancing the fibrinolytic system. Thus, estrogen may offset the threat of thrombotic occlusions from ulcerated plaques by minimizing the response to the thrombotic stimulus. Whether estrogen also prevents plaques from becoming unstable and ulcerating remains unknown.

Summary

In summary, the three anatomic and functional sequelae of atherosclerosis that are directly responsible for the majority of both acute and chronic cardiovascular clinical events are wall thickening and lumenal encroachment, abnormal vasomotor function, and enhanced thrombogenic potential. In each instance, the currently available data suggest that estrogen should have a favorable effect, thereby reducing clinical cardiovascular events (Figure 6). Despite the abundance of epidemiological data supporting this contention, actual proof will await the results of the primary and secondary prevention trials that are currently underway. These trials include the Women's Health Initiative (WHI), the Heart Estrogen/Progestin Replacement Study (HERS), and the Women's Estrogen for Stroke Trial (WEST). WHI has, as a component, a trial of hormone replacement therapy for primary prevention of cardiovascular disease. The intervention is 0.625 mg/day of oral conjugated estrogen with or

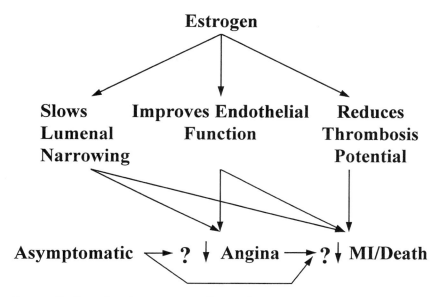

FIGURE 6. *Postulated or proven effects of estrogen on the anatomic and functional sequelae of atherosclerosis. Whether or not estrogen replacement therapy actually reduces the clinical manifestations of atherosclerosis will be determined by the outcome of the various primary and secondary prevention trials that are currently underway.*

without low-dose progestin depending on the hysterectomy status of the woman. Overall, the women in the WHI will be followed for 9 years. However, there may be interim analyses for the cardiovascular endpoints that will provide answers to the question of primary prevention of cardiovascular disease before the scheduled end of the trial in 2005. The two trials of hormone replacement for secondary prevention are HERS and WEST. The HERS trial has enrolled 2,762 women with established coronary artery disease into a two-arm trial of continuous combined oral conjugated estrogen (0.625 mg) and low-dose medroxyprogesterone acetate (2.5 mg) versus placebo. The women will be followed for fatal and nonfatal myocardial infarctions for an average of 4.75 years. In the HERS trial, women with a prior hysterectomy were ineligible. The WEST trial currently is seeking to complete enrollment of 652 women with documented transient ischemic attack or stroke for a 3-year trial of daily estradiol-17β (1.0 mg) versus placebo. The primary outcome is a combined outcome of stroke or death. These trials will provide important data concerning the actual efficacy of estrogen replacement therapy for prevention of cardiovascular disease.

Even after these trials are completed there will remain numerous additional questions to be answered concerning the mechanisms through which estrogen exerts its vascular effects, the efficacy of other estrogenic agonists in both women and men, the effects of concurrent progestins on the atherosclerotic process, and strategies to enhance compliance in order that the fullest benefits of estrogen and related therapies can be realized by the greatest number of individuals.

References

1. Stampfer MJ, Colditz GA. Estrogen replacement therapy and coronary heart disease: A quantitative assessment of the epidemiological evidence. *Prev Med* 1991;20:47–63.
2. Grady D, Rubin SM, Petitti DB, et al. Hormone therapy to prevent disease and prolong life in postmenopausal women. *Ann Intern Med* 1992;117:1016–1037.
3. Bush TL. Noncontraceptive estrogen use and risk of cardiovascular disease: An overview and critique of the literature. In: Korenman SG, ed. *The Menopause. Biological and Clinical Consequences of Ovarian Failure: Evaluation and Management.* Norwell, MA; Serono Symposia; 1990:211–223.
4. Glagov S, Weisenberg E, Zarins CK, et al. Compensatory enlargement of human arthrosclerotic coronary arteries. *N Engl J Med* 1987;316:1371–1375.
5. Stary HC, Chandler AB, Dinsmore RE, et al. A definition of advanced types of atherosclerotic lesions and a histological classification of atherosclerosis. A report from the Committee on Vascular Lesions of the Council on Arteriosclerosis, American Heart Association. *Arterioscler Thromb Vasc Biol* 1995;15:1512–1531.
6. Ross R. The pathogenesis of atherosclerosis—an update. *N Engl J Med* 1986;314:488–500.
7. Shimokawa H, Flavahan NA, Shepherd JT, et al. Endothelium-dependent inhibition of ergonovine-induced contraction is impaired in porcine coronary arteries with regenerated endothelium. *Circulation* 1989;80:643–650.
8. Badimon L, Badimon JJ, Penny W, et al. Endothelium and atherosclerosis. *J Hypertens* 1992;10(suppl):S43–50.
9. Vanhoutte PM. Endothelium and control of vascular function. State of the Art lecture. *Hypertension* 1989;13:658–667.
10. Luscher TF, Richard V, Tschudi M, et al. Serotonin and the endothelium. *Clin Physiol Biochem* 1990;8(suppl 3):108–119.
11. Feldman RL. Coronary thrombosis, coronary spasm and coronary atherosclerosis and speculation on the link between unstable angina and acute myocardial infarction. *Am J Cardiol* 1987;59:1187–1190.
12. Pearson JD. Endothelial cell function and thrombosis. *Baillieres Clin Haematol* 1994;7:441–452.

13. Vanhoutte PM, Scott-Burden T. The endothelium in health and disease. *Texas Heart Inst J* 1994;21:62–67.
14. Radomski MW, Moncada S. The biological and pharmacological role of nitric oxide in platelet function. *Adv Exp Med Biol* 1993; 344:251–264.
15. Loscalzo J. Antiplatelet and antithrombotic effects of organic nitrates. *Am J Cardiol* 1992;70:18B-22B.
16. Sullivan JM, Vander Zwaag R, Lemp GF, et al. Postmenopausal estrogen use and coronary atherosclerosis. *Ann Intern Med* 1988;108:358–363.
17. Gruchow HW, Anderson AJ, Barboriak JJ, et al. Postmenopausal use of estrogen and occlusion of coronary arteries. *Am Heart J* 1988;115:954–963.
18. McFarland KF, Boniface ME, Hornung CA, et al. Risk factors and non-contraceptive estrogen use in women with and without coronary disease. *Am Heart J* 1989;117:1209–1214.
19. Manolio TA, Furberg CD, Shemanski L, et al. Associations of post-menopausal estrogen use with cardiovascular disease and its risk factors in older women. The CHS Collaborative Research Group. *Circulation* 1993;88:2163–2171.
20. Jonas HA, Kronmal RA, Psaty BM, et al. Current estrogen-progestin and estrogen replacement therapy in elderly women: Association with ca-rotid atherosclerosis. Abstract. *Am J Epidemiol* 1995;41:S56.
21. Punnonen RH, Jokela HA, Dastidar PS, et al. Combined oestrogen-pro-gestin replacement therapy prevents atherosclerosis in postmenopausal women. *Maturitas* 1995;21:179–187.
22. Nabulsi A, Folsom A. Is menopause status or hormone replacement therapy associated with carotid intimal-medial wall thickness? Abstract. *Am J Epidemiol* 1992;136:1003–1004.
23. O'Brien JE, Peterson ED, Keeler GP, et al. Impact of estrogen replace-ment therapy on restenosis following percutaneous coronary interven-tions. Abstract. *Circulation* 1995;92:I-345.
24. Espeland MA, Applegate W, Furberg C, et al. Estrogen replacement therapy and progression of intimal-medial thickness in the carotid ar-teries of postmenopausal women. *Am J Epidemiol* 1995;142:1–9.
25. Adams MR, Kaplan JR, Manuck SB, et al. Inhibition of coronary artery atherosclerosis by 17-beta estradiol in ovariectomized monkeys. Lack of an effect of added progesterone. *Arteriosclerosis* 1990;10:1051–1057.
26. Adams MR, Register TC, Golden DL, et al. Medroxyprogesterone acetate antagonizes inhibitory effects of conjugated equine estrogens on coro-nary artery atherosclerosis. *Arterioscler Thromb Vasc Biol.* 1997;17:217–221.
27. Adams MR, Kaplan JR, Clarkson TB, et al. Ovariectomy, social status, and atherosclerosis in cynomolgus monkeys. *Arteriosclerosis* 1985;5:192–200.
28. Adams MR, Kaplan JR, Koritnik DR, et al. Pregnancy-associated inhi-bition of coronary artery atherosclerosis in monkeys: Evidence of a re-lationship with endogenous estrogen. *Arteriosclerosis* 1987;7:378–384.
29. Gisclard V, Miller VM, Vanhoutte PM. Effect of 17 beta-estradiol on endothelium-dependent responses in the rabbit. *J Pharmacol Exp Ther* 1988;244:19–22.
30. Bell DR, Rensberger HJ, Koritnik DR, et al. Estrogen pretreatment di-rectly potentiates endothelium-dependent vasorelaxation of porcine coronary arteries. *Am J Physiol* 1995;268:H377–H383.

31. Williams JK, Adams MR, Klopfenstein HS. Estrogen modulates responses of atherosclerotic coronary arteries. *Circulation* 1990;81: 1680–1687.
32. Herrington DM, Braden GA, Williams JK, et al. Endothelial-dependent coronary vasomotor responsiveness in postmenopausal women with and without estrogen replacement therapy. *Am J Cardiol* 1994;73:951–952.
33. Williams JK, Adams MR, Herrington DM, et al. Short-term administration of estrogen and vascular responses of atherosclerotic coronary arteries. *J Am Coll Cardiol* 1992;20:452–457.
34. Williams JK, Honore EK, Washburn SA, et al. Effects of hormone replacement therapy on reactivity of atherosclerotic coronary arteries in cynomolgus monkeys. *J Am Coll Cardiol* 1994;24:1757–1761.
35. Reis SE. Oestrogens attenuate abnormal coronary vasoreactivity in postmenopausal women. *Ann Med* 1994;26:387–388.
36. Gilligan DM, Quyyumi AA, Cannon RO III. Effects of physiological levels of estrogen on coronary vasomotor function in postmenopausal women. *Circulation* 1994;89:2545–2551.
37. Collins P, Rosano GM, Sarrel PM, et al. 17 beta-Estradiol attenuates acetylcholine-induced coronary arterial constriction in women but not men with coronary heart disease. *Circulation* 1995; 92:24–30.
38. Gilligan DM, Badar DM, Panza JA, et al. Acute vascular effects of estrogen in postmenopausal women. *Circulation* 1994;90:786–791.
39. Gilligan DM, Badar DM, Panza JA, et al. Effects of estrogen replacement therapy on peripheral vasomotor function in postmenopausal women. *Am J Cardiol* 1995;75:264–268.
40. Lieberman EH, Gerhard MD, Uehata A, et al. Estrogen improves endothelium-dependent, flow-mediated vasodilation in postmenopausal women. *Ann Intern Med* 1994;121:936–941.
41. Gerhard MD, Roddy M, Knab ST, et al. Acute estrogen administration improves endothelium-dependent vasodilation in postmenopausal women. Abstract. *Circulation* 1994;90:I-86.
42. Bush DE, Bruza JM, Bass KM, et al. Estrogen replacement increases flow mediated vasodilation in postmenopausal women. Abstract. *Circulation* 1994;90:I-86.
43. Dohanich GP, Fader AJ, Javorsky DJ. Estrogen and estrogen-progesterone treatments counteract the effect of scopolamine on reinforced T-maze alternation in female rats. *Behav Neurosci* 1994;108:988–992.
44. Hishikawa K, Nakaki T, Marumo T, et al. Up-regulation of nitric oxide synthase by estradiol in human aortic endothelial cells. *FEBS Lett* 1995;360:291–293.
45. Brosnihan KB, Ping L, Ferrario CM. Angiotensin-(1–7) elicits nitric oxide-dependent vasodilation in canine coronary arteries. Abstract. *Hypertension* 1995;26:544.
46. Jiang CW, Sarrel PM, Lindsay DC, et al. Progesterone induces endothelium-independent relaxation of rabbit coronary artery in vitro. *Eur J Pharmacol* 1992;211:163–167.
47. Sudhir K, Chou TM, Mullen WL, et al. Mechanisms of estrogen-induced vasodilation: In vivo studies in canine coronary conductance and resistance arteries. *J Am Coll Cardiol* 1995;26:807–814.
48. Chester AH, Jiang C, Borland JA, et al. Oestrogen relaxes human epicardial coronary arteries through non-endothelium-dependent mechanisms. *Coron Artery Dis* 1995;6:417–422.

49. Collins P, Rosano GM, Jiang C, et al. Cardiovascular protection by oestrogen—a calcium antagonist effect?. *Lancet* 1993;341:1264–1265.
50. Harder DR, Coulson PB. Estrogen receptors and effects of estrogen on membrane electrical properties of coronary vascular smooth muscle. *J Cell Physiol* 1979;100:375–382.
51. Rosano GM, Sarrel PM, Poole-Wilson PA, et al. Beneficial effect of oestrogen on exercise-induced myocardial ischaemia in women with coronary artery disease. *Lancet* 1993;342:133–136.
52. Weksler BB. Hemostasis and thrombosis. In: Douglas PS, ed. *Cardiovascular Health and Disease in Women*. Philadelphia: W.B. Saunders; 1993:231–251.
53. Herrington DM. Sex hormones and normal cardiovascular physiology in women. In: Burgess A, ed. *Women and Heart Disease*. London: Martin Dunitz; 1991;243–264.
54. Nabulsi AA, Folsom AR, White A, et al. Association of hormone-replacement therapy with various cardiovascular risk factors in postmenopausal women. The Atherosclerosis Risk in Communities Study Investigators. *N Engl J Med* 1993;328:1069–1075.
55. Meade TW. Clotting factors and ischaemic heart disease: The epidemiologic evidence. In: Meade TW, ed. *Anticoagulants and Myocardial Infarction: A Reappraisal*. New York: John Wiley; 1984:91–111.
56. Lobo RA, Pickar JH, Wild RA, et al. Metabolic impact of adding medroxyprogesterone acetate to conjugated estrogen therapy in postmenopausal women. The Menopause Study Group. *Obstet Gynecol* 1994;84:987–995.
57. Bonnar J, Haddon M, Hunter DH, et al. Coagulation system changes in post-menopausal women receiving oestrogen preparations. *Postgrad Med J* 1976;52(suppl 6):30–36.
58. Skartlien AH, Lyberg-Beckmann S, Holme I, et al. Effect of alteration in triglyceride levels on factor VII-phospholipid complexes in plasma [see Comments]. *Arteriosclerosis* 1989;9:798–801.
59. Dahlback B, Carlsson M, Svensson PJ. Familial thrombophilia due to a previously unrecognized mechanism characterized by poor anticoagulant response to activated protein C: Prediction of a cofactor to activated protein C. *Proc Natl Acad Sci USA* 1993;90:1004–1008.
60. Aylward M. Coagulation factors in opposed and unopposed oestrogen treatment at the climacteric. *Postgrad Med J* 1978;54(suppl 2):31–37.
61. Scarabin PY, Plu-Bureau G, Bara L, et al. Haemostatic variables and menopausal status. Influence of hormone replacement therapy. *Thromb Haemost* 1993;70:584–587.
62. Alkjaersig N, Fletcher AP, de Ziegler D, et al. Blood coagulation in postmenopausal women given estrogen treatment: Comparison of transdermal and oral administration. *J Lab Clin Med* 1988;111:224–228.
63. The Writing Group for the PEPI Trial. Effects of estrogen or estrogen/progestin regimens on heart disease risk factors in postmenopausal women. The Postmenopausal Estrogen/Progestin Interventions (PEPI) Trial. *JAMA* 1995;273:199–208.
64. Meade TW. Orchidectomy versus oestrogen for prostatic cancer: Cardiovascular effects. Letter. *Br Med J* 1986;293(Clin Res Ed):953–954.
65. Kannel WB, Wolf PA, Castelli WP, et al. Fibrinogen and risk of cardiovascular disease. The Framingham Study. *JAMA* 1987;258:1183–1186.
66. Yarnell JW, Baker IA, Sweetnam PM, et al. Fibrinogen, viscosity, and white blood cell count are major risk factors for ischemic heart disease.

The Caerphilly and Speedwell collaborative heart disease studies. *Circulation* 1991;83:836–844.
67. Balleisen L, Schulte H, Assmann G, et al. Coagulation factors and the progress of coronary heart disease. Letter. *Lancet* 1987;2:461.
68. Notelovitz M, Kitchens C, Ware M, et al. Combination estrogen and progestogen replacement therapy does not adversely affect coagulation. *Obstet Gynecol* 1983;62:596–600.
69. Notelovitz M, Kitchens CS, Ware MD. Coagulation and fibrinolysis in estrogen-treated surgically menopausal women. *Obstet Gynecol* 1984; 63:621–625.
70. Gebara OC, Mittleman MA, Sutherland P, et al. Association between increased estrogen status and increased fibrinolytic potential in the Framingham Offspring Study. *Circulation* 1995;91:1952–1958.
71. Jespersen J, Petersen KR, Skouby SO. Effects of newer oral contraceptives on the inhibition of coagulation and fibrinolysis in relation to dosage and type of steroid. *Am J Obstet Gynecol* 1990;163:396–403.
72. Meilahn EN, Kuller LH, Matthews KA, et al. Hemostatic factors according to menopausal status and use of hormone replacement therapy. *Ann Epidemiol* 1992;2:445–455.
73. Soma M, Fumagalli R, Paoletti R, et al. Plasma Lp(a) concentration after oestrogen and progestagen in postmenopausal women. Letter. *Lancet* 1991;337:612
74. van der Mooren MJ, Demacker PN, Thomas CM, et al. Beneficial effects on serum lipoproteins by 17 beta-oestradiol-dydrogesterone therapy in postmenopausal women; a prospective study. *Eur J Obstet Gynecol Reprod Biol* 1992;47:153–160.
75. Bonnar J, Davidson JF, Pidgeon CF, et al. Fibrin degradation products in normal and abnormal pregnancy and parturition. *Br Med J* 1969; 3:137–140.
76. Shaper AG, Evans CM, Macintosh DM, et al. Fibrinolysis and plasminogen levels in pregnancy and the puerperium. *Lancet* 1965;2:706–708.
77. Raman BB, Standley PR, Rajkumar V, et al. Effects of estradiol and progesterone on platelet calcium responses. *Am J Hypertens* 1995;8: 197–200.
78. Miller ME, Dores GM, Thorpe SL, et al. Paradoxical influence of estrogenic hormones on platelet-endothelial cell interactions. *Thromb Res* 1994;74:577–594.
79. Bar J, Tepper R, Fuchs J, et al. The effect of estrogen replacement therapy on platelet aggregation and adenosine triphosphate release in postmenopausal women. *Obstet Gynecol* 1993;81:261–264.
80. Johnson M, Ramey E, Ramwell PW. Androgen-mediated sensitivity in platelet aggregation. *Am J Physiol* 1977;232:H381–H385.

Chapter 12

Antioxidant Properties of Estrogen
Selective Protection of High-Density Lipoprotein

Carole L. Banka, PhD

Antioxidants and Atherosclerosis

The "oxidation hypothesis" of atherogenesis emphasizes the role of oxidative modification of low-density lipoprotein (LDL) and/or other lipoproteins as a major contributing factor to the onset and progression of atherosclerosis. Evidence from studies conducted in vitro and in vivo has revealed biological properties of oxidized LDL that confer atherogenicity to the particle and that vary with the degree of modification.[1-3] A recent investigation has linked the oxidation hypothesis with the theory that high plasma cholesterol levels are a significant risk factor by demonstrating that older lipoproteins are more susceptible to oxidative modification.[4] The oxidation hypothesis predicts that any antioxidant that prevents lipoprotein oxidation should inhibit the onset or slow the progression of atherogenesis. Persuasive dietary studies in animal models document cardioprotective effects of natural and synthetic antioxidants (reviewed by Hoffman and Garewal[5]). In most cases, the antioxidant-mediated decrease in atherosclerotic lesion formation correlates with the inhibition of LDL oxidation.[6,7] However, in several studies, a reduction in LDL susceptibility to oxidation in vitro was not accompanied by a reduction in atherosclerotic lesion formation.[8,9] One explanation for this discrepancy may be that the doses of antioxidants sufficient to protect LDL from oxidation in vitro are not sufficient to protect LDL from oxidation in vivo. Furthermore, differ-

Grant support was provided by the National Institutes of Health Grant HL-50060.

From: Forte TM, (ed). *Hormonal, Metabolic, and Cellular Influences on Cardiovascular Disease in Women.* Armonk, NY: Futura Publishing Company, Inc.; © 1997.

ences in experimental protocols may confound comparisons. For example, vitamin E at 10 g/kg did not significantly reduce aortic lesion formation in cholesterol-fed New Zealand White rabbits,[9] whereas a lower dose (5 g/kg) significantly reduced restenosis in femoral arteries of the same species after angioplasty and a high-fat diet.[10] Although these observations indicate that caution must be used when interpreting the results of antioxidant treatments, the cumulative data from experimental animals suggest that natural antioxidants such as vitamin E and pharmacological antioxidants such as probucol are protective against cardiovascular disease.

The clinical data relevant to antioxidants and coronary heart disease have been reviewed recently by Steinberg.[11] Although there is not sufficient clinical information to draw conclusions, there is a trend suggesting the efficacy of several natural antioxidants in reducing cardiovascular risk and this has prompted the undertaking of large scale clinical trials. Most pertinent to the discussion here are the recently reported studies demonstrating a correlation between consumption of vitamin E and reduced risk of coronary heart disease.[12,13]

If one accepts with cautious optimism that antioxidants reduce the risk of heart disease by inhibiting lipoprotein oxidation, then a role for estrogens as antioxidants can be added to the growing list of multifactorial mechanisms of cardiovascular protection these hormones confer on women.

Estrogens as Antioxidants

The term "estrogen" refers to any member of a class of steroid hormones with eighteen carbons and a phenolic A ring (see Figure 1). This classification includes both physiological steroids and synthetic compounds used in clinical treatments. Estradiol-17β is the most potent natural estrogen in humans due to its high receptor affinity and will be the primary focus of this chapter. It is important to note, however, that the direct action of estrogens as antioxidants is not receptor mediated. Therefore, estrogens with little or no receptor activity may be important as antioxidants.

The generic term "oxidation" is used here and by others to include the process of lipid peroxidation and the protein modifications that accompany or result from lipid peroxidation. The majority of antioxidants that are thought to reduce the risk of atherosclerosis are "chain-breaking" antioxidants, which scavenge lipid peroxyl radicals and, therefore, inhibit the propagation of lipid peroxidation.

$$L^{\bullet} + O_2 \rightarrow LOO^{\bullet}$$

$$LOO^{\bullet} + LH \rightarrow LOOH + L^{\bullet}$$

$$LOO^{\bullet} + E2OH \rightarrow LOOH + E2O^{\bullet}$$

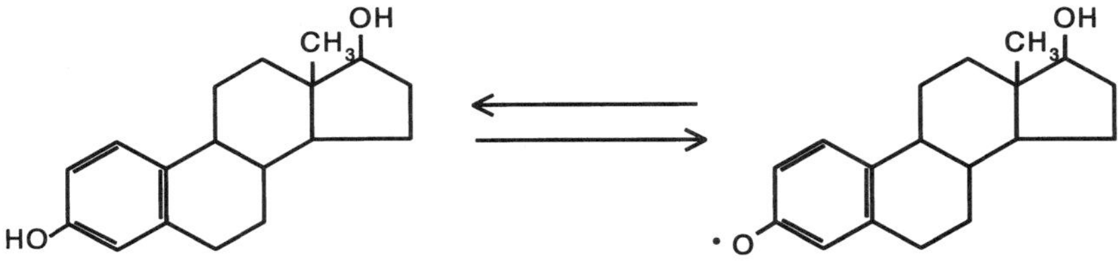

17β-Estradiol   Estradiol Radical

FIGURE 1. *Estradiol is a phenolic, chain-breaking, antioxidant. One cycle of the lipid peroxidation pathway is shown. A lipid radical (L•) interacts with molecular oxygen to form a lipid peroxyl radical (LOO•) that, in turn, attacks a fatty acyl chain (LH) to form a lipid peroxide (LOOH) and another lipid radical (L•). By giving up a hydrogen from the C-3 position hydroxyl group on the phenolic ring, estradiol (E2OH) forms an estradiol radical (E2O•) and interrupts the lipid peroxidation chain reaction.*

Figure 1 illustrates the lipid peroxidation pathway and the mechanism by which estrogens may act as chain-breaking antioxidants. The carbon-hydrogen bonds adjacent to double bonds in polyunsaturated fatty acids are susceptible to abstraction of the hydrogen through a variety of mechanisms. The lipid radical (L•) resulting from the removal of a hydrogen combines with molecular oxygen forming a lipid peroxyl radical (LOO•). The peroxyl radical is highly reactive and will subsequently abstract another hydrogen from the acyl chain creating another lipid radical (L•) and a lipid peroxide (LOOH), which is nonreactive, but unstable, and subject to fragmentation and the generation of aldehyde species. The lipid radical initiates yet another cycle of lipid peroxidation. This "chain reaction" continues until the lipid peroxyl radicals reach concentrations high enough to favor interaction between two radicals, resulting in a nonreactive species.

Alternatively, the chain reaction can be interrupted by a radical scavenging antioxidant. α-Tocopherol, butylated hydroxytoluene (BHT), and probucol are all phenolic antioxidants and, as such, are good radical scavengers. Estrogens, represented in Figure 1 by estradiol-17β, share a phenolic ring with these antioxidants. The estradiol-17β molecule (E2OH) is subject to hydrogen extraction by a lipid peroxyl radical resulting in formation of an estradiol radical (E2O•). Because the energy of the radical on the estradiol molecule can be distributed throughout the phenolic ring, the estradiol radical has a lower energy level and is significantly less reactive than the lipid peroxyl radical. Therefore, formation of the lower energy estradiol radical interrupts the lipid peroxidation cascade.

Several laboratories have demonstrated the inhibition of lipid peroxidation in membrane phospholipids by estrogens and related compounds.[14–17] All polyunsaturated fatty acids are subject to lipid peroxidation including those in phospholipids, triglycerides, and cholesteryl esters. Therefore, lipoproteins are particularly susceptible to lipid peroxidation and the resultant protein modifications should be protected by estrogen antioxidants. Much attention has been focused on the mechanisms and consequences of lipid peroxidation in LDL. It is presumed that lipid peroxidation in LDL begins in the acyl chains of the phospholipids and propagates to the neutral lipids in the core of the particle. In the process, polyunsaturated fatty acids and cholesterol are altered chemically, and the major protein component of LDL, apoprotein B, is modified chemically and fragmented (for review, see Steinberg et al.[1]). Antioxidant protection of LDL by estradiol-17β[18–20] and the related estrogenic phenolic compounds tamoxifen[21] and RU-486[22] has been demonstrated in vitro. Treatment of postmenopausal women with estrogens results in a decreased susceptibility of LDL to oxidation ex vivo[23,24,] and similar results have been documented in hypercholesterolemic swine.[25] The impact of estrogens as antioxidants for LDL is discussed more extensively in Chapter 13.

Although it is likely that the same progression of oxidative modification described above for LDL also occurs in high-density lipoproteins (HDL), the topic has not been widely discussed, nor has the impact of estrogens as antioxidants for HDL. The purpose of the remainder of this chapter is to focus on the role of estrogens (particularly estradiol-17β) in protecting HDL from oxidation. This is particularly relevant in a discussion of cardiovascular disease in women because a major factor in the protection of premenopausal women and postmenopausal women on hormone replacement therapy (HRT) is an increased level of circulating HDL.[26]

HDL Oxidation

Evidence for the atheroprotective role of HDL, due in part to its role in reverse cholesterol transport, is now quite compelling (for review, see Pieters et al.[27]). HDL mediates efflux of excess free cholesterol from peripheral cells.[28] The majority of cholesterol esterification in plasma occurs on HDL particles because of the action of lecithin:cholesterol acyltransferase (LCAT).[29] Thus, free cholesterol removed from peripheral tissues is esterified on HDL. The net result of these processes is the movement of cholesterol from the periphery to the liver for catabolism. HDL also delivers cholesterol to steroidogenic cells where it is used as substrate for steroid hormone synthesis.[30] If the apoproteins of HDL are modified during oxidation, then any of these protective processes that depend upon apoprotein interactions are expected to be impacted. Lipid peroxidation itself is also predicted to adversely effect HDL function and metabolism.

There is mounting evidence that HDL is more susceptible to oxidation than LDL.[31,32] Although numerous laboratories have reported that HDL protects LDL from oxidation,[33–37] none have addressed the possibility that components of the HDL particle may become oxidized in the process of inhibiting LDL oxidation. HDL acts as an acceptor for lipid peroxides from oxidized LDL.[38] Furthermore, cholesteryl ester transfer protein mediates transfer of oxidized cholesteryl ester molecules from LDL to HDL.[39] Thus, HDL carries a significant oxidative burden. Oxidative modification of HDL in vitro impacts adversely on HDL promotion of cholesterol efflux from peripheral cells.[40–42] Modifications of HDL apoproteins similar to those that accompany oxidation lead to increased clearance of HDL from the circulation.[43,44] Because of its protective properties, decreases in plasma HDL due to oxidation would be proatherogenic. Therefore, the oxidation of both LDL and HDL may contribute to atherogenesis.

The initial steps in the oxidation of HDL in vitro appear to involve lipid peroxidation as described above for LDL. Phenolic antioxidants that scavenge free radicals should be effective in protecting HDL from oxidation as has been reported for LDL. Therefore, experiments were conducted to examine the effectiveness of estradiol-17β as an inhibitor of lipid peroxidation in HDL.

Estrogens as HDL Antioxidants

The first experiment was designed to determine if HDL was susceptible to lipid peroxidation in vitro under circumstances known to lead to LDL oxidation and to ascertain whether estrogen influenced the oxidation. HDL (200 μg protein/ml) was dialyzed against saline to remove the aqueous antioxidants used during storage and then oxidized by exposure to 5 μmol/L copper acetate, a conventional method for oxidizing LDL in vitro. The degree of lipid peroxidation was measured using the thiobarbituric acid reactive substances (TBARS) assay. This assay detects aldehyde products of lipid peroxidation and has proven to be a reliable method for assessing lipid peroxidation in isolated lipoproteins.[45] The kinetics of TBARS generation in HDL alone and in the presence of increasing concentrations of estradiol-17β are shown in Figure 2. HDL was oxidized readily under these conditions and near maximal TBARS concentrations were reached at 6 hours with little increase in the subsequent 8 hours. At 2.5 and 6 hours, all concentrations of estradiol blocked oxidation. By 14 hours, estradiol was partially inhibitory at a concentration of 1.0 μmol/L and completely inhibitory at 3.0 μmol/L. Inhibition of oxidation by the lower concentrations of estradiol at 6 hours suggested that the steroid might be more effective in protecting HDL than LDL because higher concentrations had been required for the protection of LDL in vitro.[18–20]

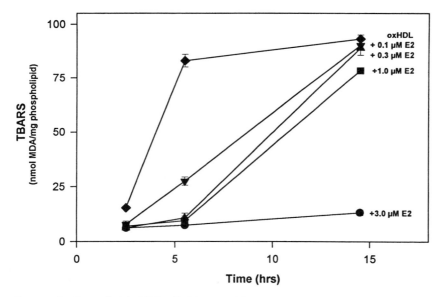

FIGURE 2. *Estradiol inhibits lipid peroxidation in HDL. HDL (200 μg protein/ml) was oxidized by incubation with copper acetate (5 μmol/L) in the absence (oxHDL) or presence (+ E2) of increasing concentrations of estradiol-17β (E2). Lipid peroxidation was quantified by measuring thiobarbituric acid reactive substances (TBARS), the aldehydes resulting from lipid peroxidation.*

To determine the relative efficacy of estrogen as an antioxidant for HDL and LDL, oxidation in the two lipoproteins from the same donor was examined in the presence of estradiol by monitoring the formation of conjugated dienes (transient rearrangements of bonds in polyunsaturated acyl chains).[46] HDL was protected longer than LDL at each concentration of estradiol tested. In this experiment, the HDL and LDL were oxidized at a lipoprotein concentration of 200 μg protein/ml. Under these conditions, significantly more conjugated dienes were generated in the LDL.[47] We subsequently determined empirically that normalizing the HDL and LDL to phospholipid concentrations led to near-identical lipid peroxidation in the two lipoproteins during a 4-hour period. Therefore, all further comparisons of antioxidant protection of the two lipoproteins were performed using the protocol outlined in Figure 3. HDL from a fasting, male, nonsmoking donor was oxidized at 200 μg protein/ml, which generally converted to phospholipid concentrations between 90 and 150 μg/ml, depending upon the donor. LDL from the same donor

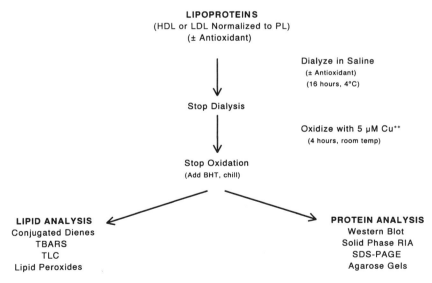

FIGURE 3. *Procedures for lipoprotein oxidation and analysis. Lipoproteins (HDL and/or LDL) were dialyzed for 16 hours, oxidized by exposure to copper acetate (Cu^{2+}) for 4 hours and analyzed for lipid and/or protein modifications. PL, phospholipid; BHT, butylated hydroxytoluene; TBARS, thiobarbituric reactive substances; TLC, thin layer chromatography; RIA, radioimmunoassay; and SDS-PAGE, sodium dodecyl sulfate polyacrylamide electrophoresis.*

was oxidized at the same phospholipid concentration. The lipoproteins were dialyzed against saline for 16 hours. Test antioxidants were introduced during the dialysis treatment. After dialysis, oxidation was initiated by the addition of copper acetate (5 μmol/L) and the reaction was allowed to proceed for 4 hours at room temperature. Oxidation was terminated by chilling the reaction mixtures and adding butylated hydroxytoluene (BHT, 40 μmol/L), a potent antioxidant for lipoproteins. Quantitative changes in lipids were assessed by measuring TBARS, conjugated dienes, or lipid peroxides. Qualitative lipid changes can be detected by thin layer chromatography (TLC). Protein modification was assessed by SDS-PAGE, Western blot, immunochemistry (solid phase radioimmunoassay), or agarose gel electrophoresis.

When estradiol-17β was introduced as an antioxidant to lipoproteins normalized on the basis of phospholipid concentration, partial inhibition of TBARS formation in LDL was accomplished at an estradiol concentration of 2.25 μmol/L, whereas 0.25 μmol/L estradiol completely blocked TBARS formation in HDL.[47] This prompted us to compare estradiol with other phenolic antioxidants to determine whether the selective protection of HDL was a characteristic of estradiol or a reflection of the different lipid and protein compositions of HDL and LDL. The results of a representative experiment are illustrated in Figure 4. The dialyzed lipoproteins (control, open bars) had very low levels of TBARS activity. After 4 hours of oxidation, the oxidized HDL and LDL (oxHDL and oxLDL, respectively, shaded bars) contained comparable levels of TBARS activity. The antioxidants were tested at a concentration of 2 μmol/L (hatched bars). Probucol inhibited both HDL and LDL oxidation by <50%. Trolox, a water-soluble analogue of α-tocopherol, was completely inhibitory for both lipoproteins as was BHT. In contrast, 2 μmol/L estradiol-17β (E2) (solid bars) inhibited TBARS formation in HDL completely but inhibited lipid peroxidation in LDL by <50%. A series of experiments including dose titrations of the phenolic antioxidants as well as ascorbic acid (an aqueous antioxidant) and lipoproteins from several donors revealed that only estradiol bestowed this differential antioxidant protection on the two lipoproteins.[47] Because the selective protection was not a characteristic shared by other phenolic antioxidants or by the aqueous antioxidant, ascorbic acid, we concluded that the selective protection of HDL by estradiol was not a reflection of differences in lipoprotein composition.

The next experiments were designed to determine if hormones representative of the other classes of sex steroids had antioxidant characteristics. The results of these experiments are summarized in

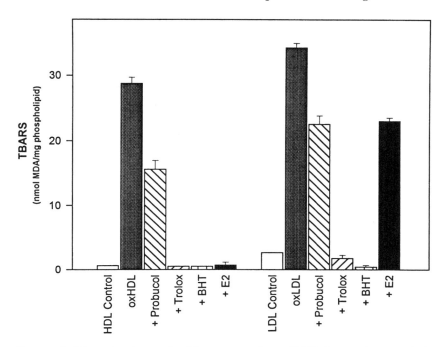

FIGURE 4. *The selective antioxidant protection of HDL is not characteristic of other phenolic antioxidants. HDL and LDL from the same male donor were oxidized as described in Figure 3 and analyzed by measuring TBARS. Lipid peroxidation in the absence of antioxidants (oxHDL and oxLDL; shaded bars) was comparable for the two lipoproteins. The phenolic antioxidants, probucol, Trolox and butylated hydroxytoluene (BHT), at 2 μmol/L, protected HDL and LDL to the same extent. Estradiol (E2, solid bars) at 2 μmol/L, was much more effective as an antioxidant for HDL than for LDL.*

Figure 5. All steroids were tested at a concentration of 2 μmol/L, and the extent of oxidation was measured by assaying TBARS activity as in Figure 4. The results were expressed as percent of TBARS content. TBARS measured in the HDL and LDL preparations following Cu^{2+}-oxidation in the absence of steroids was taken as 100%. As seen in previous experiments, estradiol inhibited HDL oxidation completely but was less effective in protecting LDL. Progesterone (a representative progestin) and the androgens, testosterone and androstenedione, had no antioxidant activity for either of the lipoproteins. As none of the nonestrogenic steroids contain a phenolic ring, the data suggested that the phenolic A ring of estradiol was requisite for the antioxidant activity of the molecule.

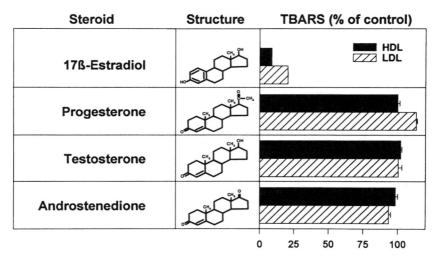

FIGURE 5. *Nonestrogenic steroids do not act as antioxidants for lipoproteins. HDL (solid bars) and LDL (hatched bars) from the same male donor were oxidized as described in Figure 3 in the presence of the steroids indicated (2 μmol/L) and analyzed for lipid peroxidation by measuring TBARS. The TBARS values are presented as percent of control where the control is the TBARS activity of HDL or LDL oxidized in the absence of steroid. The structure of each steroid is illustrated.*

    Donor variability affected the degree of protection from lipid peroxidation conferred on HDL by estradiol-17β. The minimum effective antioxidant concentrations of estradiol-17β for HDL preparations from all donors tested ranged between 12.5 and 100 nmol/L (Figure 2 and data not shown). In contrast, inhibition of lipid peroxidation in LDL preparations from the same donors was not detected with nanomolar concentrations of estradiol. In cycling premenopausal women, estradiol-17β concentrations range between 0.2 and 2 nmol/L. During pregnancy, estradiol reaches concentrations of 35 nmol/L. Therefore, the amount of estradiol shown to be effective in inhibiting lipid peroxidation in HDL in our in vitro system approached physiological levels. Physiological levels of estrogen achieved by estrogen replacement in postmenopausal women were effective in decreasing the susceptibility of LDL to lipid peroxidation.[23,24] If estradiol is more effective as an antioxidant for LDL in vivo, then it is predicted that estradiol is even more potent as an HDL antioxidant in vivo than in our experimental system. Unfortunately, this assertion awaits further testing. Nevertheless, the body of evidence resulting from our studies to date clearly demonstrated an estradiol-dependent selective protection of HDL from lipid peroxidation.

Estrogen Inhibition of HDL Protein Modification

Does the reduction in HDL lipid peroxidation afforded by estradiol result in protection of HDL apoproteins from oxidative modification?

Lipid peroxidation in LDL is accompanied by fragmentation of apoprotein B as well as antigenic changes in the protein.[1,48,49] The antigenic changes are thought to result from conjugation of lipid peroxidation products such as aldehydes to the apoprotein.[50] By contrast, oxidation-dependent modifications of HDL apoproteins are reflected in increased apparent molecular weights of apo A-I and a characteristic pattern of cross-linking of apo A-I and apo A-II.[47,51,52] If the apoprotein modifications in oxidized HDL result from lipid peroxidation, then estradiol, which selectively inhibits lipid peroxidation in HDL, should inhibit apoprotein modification as well. The results of an experiment designed to test this premise are shown in Figure 6. HDL was dialyzed and oxidized for 0, 2, 4, and 6 hours in the absence (−) or presence (+) of estradiol (2 μmol/L) as outlined in Figure 3. The oxidized HDL preparations were separated by sodium dodecyl sulfate polyacrylamide gel electrophoresis (SDS-PAGE) on a 12% gel under nonreducing conditions, and the proteins were stained with Coomassie Blue. Apoproteins A-I and A-II are labeled in the photograph. Cross-linking of the apoproteins was not detectable by Coomassie Blue staining but was detected by Western blotting in HDL preparations oxidized under the same conditions.[47] As indicated in Figure 6, oxidation of HDL in the absence of estradiol resulted in a time-dependent increase in the apparent molecular weight of apo A-I, and the apoprotein became increasingly diffuse in its staining pattern. The exposure of HDL to estradiol during the dialysis and oxidation inhibited both the increase in molecular weight and the diffusion of apo A-I. The inhibition was seen most dramatically after 6 hours of oxidation. Apo A-II decreased in mass with increased time of oxidation. This was most likely due to cross-linking of apo A-II to apo A-I. Inclusion of estradiol during the oxidation partially prevented the disappearance of apo A-II. This impact of estradiol on apo A-II was most notable after 6 hours of oxidation as well. We also have documented an estradiol-dependent decrease in HDL apoprotein cross-linking during oxidation.[47] From these ex-

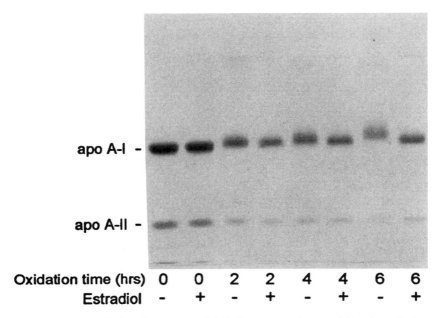

| Oxidation time (hrs) | 0 | 0 | 2 | 2 | 4 | 4 | 6 | 6 |
| Estradiol | - | + | - | + | - | + | - | + |

FIGURE 6. *Estradiol-17β protects HDL from protein modification during oxidation. HDL (1.0 mg protein/ml) was oxidized by exposure to copper acetate (5 μmol/L) for increasing times in the absence (−) and presence (+) of estradiol (2 μmol/L). The samples were separated on a 12% SDS polyacrylamide gel and stained with Coomassie Blue. The major proteins of HDL, apo A-I and apo A-II, are indicated.*

periments, it was concluded that estradiol not only inhibited lipid peroxidation in HDL but also inhibited the modification of HDL apoproteins that accompany HDL oxidation.

Mechanism of Selective Protection of HDL by Estrogen: Hypothesis

The observation that estradiol was a more potent antioxidant for HDL than for LDL suggested that estradiol may become selectively enriched on the HDL particle. This selective enrichment is likely to result from a chemical modification of estradiol on HDL that traps it within the particle. It is my hypothesis that estradiol becomes esterified on the HDL particle making it more hydrophobic and less able to exchange from the particle. The capacity of HDL to carry free cholesterol is limited by the surface area of the particle and this may also be the case for estradiol. After esterification, cholesterol is carried in the core of HDL greatly expanding the mass of total cholesterol in the particle. In a parallel manner, fatty acid esterification of estradiol is predicted to increase the mass of estradiol on an HDL particle. The esterification of estradiol is presumed to occur through the action of lecithin:cholesterol acyltransferase (LCAT). LCAT is responsible for the majority of cholesterol esterification in plasma and functions with apo A-I as its cofactor.[53] Therefore, LCAT-mediated estradiol esterification should occur primarily on HDL. Estradiol fatty acid esters have been identified in human plasma and ovarian follicular fluid.[54,55] The estradiol esters found in follicular fluid are esterified with a variety of fatty acids at the C-17 position. This esterification of the hydroxyl group at the C-17 position would generate a more hydrophobic molecule while leaving the C-3 position phenolic hydroxyl group available for hydrogen abstraction, the reaction necessary for estradiol to serve as a phenolic chain-breaking antioxidant.

Indirect support for my hypothesis that esterification of estradiol results in a selective enrichment of the antioxidant estradiol in HDL involves studies with vitamin E. Esterification of estradiol would yield a molecule with characteristics similar to those of the most potent naturally occurring phenolic antioxidant, vitamin E (α-tocopherol); that is, it would have a phenolic group at one end of the molecule and a long hydrophobic acyl chain at the other (see Figure 7). Others have

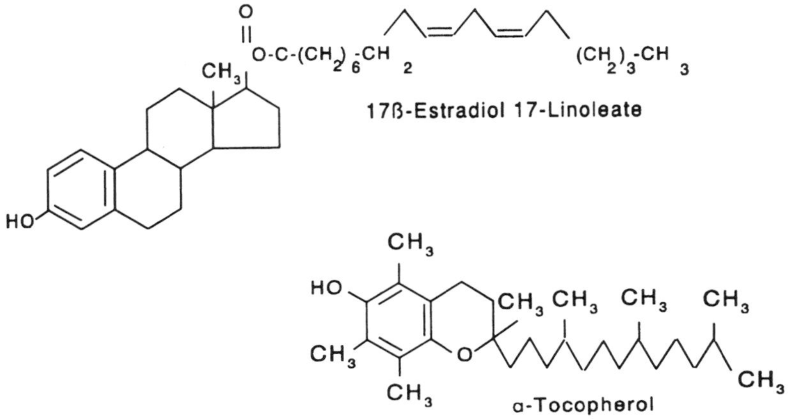

FIGURE 7. *Estradiol-17β 17-linoleate shares structural features with the potent antioxidant, α-tocopherol. Estradiol-17β 17-linoleate (upper structure), a representative estradiol fatty acid ester, shares a phenolic ring at one end of the molecule and a long acyl chain at the other end with α-tocopherol, a representative of the potent vitamin E antioxidants.*

shown that more α-tocopherol is carried in HDL than in the other lipoproteins[56] in spite of the fact that it exchanges more readily from HDL to other lipoproteins.[57] This observation suggests a selective interaction between α-tocopherol and HDL similar to that which I propose for estradiol and HDL. As shown in Figure 4, Trolox (a water-soluble analogue of α-tocopherol) does not selectively protect HDL. However, the speculation that estradiol may be esterified on HDL led to reexamination of vitamin E as a possible model for estradiol esters as lipoprotein antioxidants. The results are shown in Figure 8. As indicated by the hatched bars, HDL and LDL underwent comparable degrees of lipid peroxidation during a 4-hours exposure to copper acetate. Although micromolar concentrations of α-tocopherol were required to inhibit oxidation of both HDL and LDL (solid bars), like estradiol and unlike the other antioxidants tested, α-tocopherol selectively protected HDL from oxidation; that is, lower concentrations were

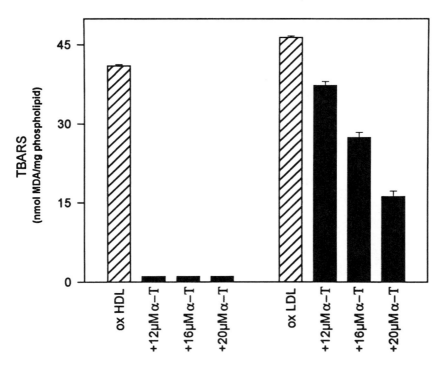

FIGURE 8. α-Tocopherol, like estradiol, selectively protects HDL from lipid peroxidation. HDL and LDL from the same male donor were oxidized as described in Figure 3 in the absence (oxHDL, oxLDL, hatched bars) and presence of increasing concentrations of α-tocopherol (+α-T, solid bars). Lipid peroxidation was assessed by measuring TBARS.

required for the protection of HDL under conditions in which the control lipoproteins were oxidized to the same extent.

Further support for the proposed esterification of estradiol on lipoproteins comes from recent work by Shwaery and his colleagues in which estradiol (10 nmol/L) was added to plasma for 4 hours at 37°C followed by isolation of LDL. Under the conditions of this experiment, the LDL was found to be less susceptible to oxidation (G. T. Shwaery, J. A. Vita, and J. F. Keaney, Jr., personal communication). Furthermore, the estradiol associated with the isolated LDL had been modified such that its mobility on high-pressure liquid chromatography (HPLC) differed from that of estradiol. Moreover, the new compound was susceptible to saponification suggesting that it had been esterified. This esterification of estradiol associated with LDL was most likely mediated by LCAT. LCAT esterification of LDL cholesterol has been observed; however, because the cofactor for LCAT, apo A-I, is found on HDL, the majority of cholesterol in plasma is esterified on the HDL particle. Therefore, in a parallel manner, significantly more estradiol esterification in plasma is predicted to occur on HDL than on LDL. The preferential esterification of estradiol on HDL would result in specific enrichment of estradiol esters in HDL and a selective antioxidant protection of HDL. This hypothesis awaits further testing.

Overview of the Role of Estradiol as a Selective Antioxidant for HDL

HDL is known to be protective against atherosclerosis. One mechanism of its antiatherogenic action appears to be the protection of LDL from oxidation. Oxidation of LDL is a major contributing factor in the onset and progression of atherosclerosis. Recent studies suggest that lipid peroxides are transferred from oxidized LDL to HDL.[38] Several hydrolytic enzymes associated with HDL are thought to inactivate the transferred lipid peroxides. These enzymes include platelet activating factor acetylhydrolase (PAF-AH) and paraoxonase.[58,59] I propose that estradiol, functioning as a selective antioxidant for HDL, works in concert with these other mechanisms. A scheme for the protection of HDL from oxidation is outlined in Figure 9. Illustrated is the surface of an HDL particle containing phospholipids (1) and cholesterol (3). Lipid-soluble antioxidants such as α-tocopherol (2) protect by scavenging radicals. These antioxidants function in men and women and levels are determined by dietary intake. Estradiol (4) also inhibits oxidation and is selectively en-

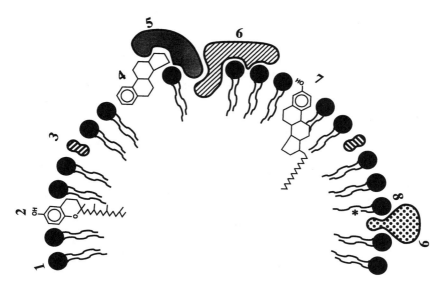

FIGURE 9. *Hypothetical mechanism for selective antioxidant protection of HDL by estradiol. Schematic of the surface of HDL where it is hypothesized that LCAT (5) with its cofactor, apo A-I (6), esterifies estradiol (4), resulting in an estradiol fatty acid ester (7) with higher affinity for the particle. Further antioxidant protection for HDL is conferred by α-tocopherol (2) and the esterases, PAF-acetylhydrolase and paraoxonase (9), which inactivate reactive lipid species (8) through hydrolysis. 1, phospholipid; 3, cholesterol.*

riched on the HDL particle through the action LCAT (5) and its cofactor, apo A-I (6). This action produces an estradiol fatty acid ester (7) that is less likely to be exchanged away from the HDL particle and functions as a chain-breaking antioxidant. This protection would occur only in women. Estrogen levels are cyclic in premenopausal women and determined by estrogen replacement dose and route of administration in postmenopausal women. The enrichment of estradiol on the HDL particle through its esterification may blunt the cyclic patterns of estradiol seen in plasma over the course of the menstrual cycle providing consistent protection of the HDL particle. Finally, if lipid peroxidation does occur in the HDL particle or if lipid peroxides (8) are transferred from LDL, the hydrolytic enzymes PAF-AH and paraoxonase (9) inactivate the damaging species through hydrolysis. These enzymes would function in both men and women.

There appears to be a link between chronic inflammatory conditions, such as rheumatoid arthritis, and atherogenesis in humans.[60] Furthermore, genetic evidence predicts a common pathway mediating inflammatory gene expression, atherogenesis, and oxidative stress in mice.[61] Therefore, lipoproteins may be oxidized to a greater extent under the conditions prevailing during an inflammatory response and antioxidants may be particularly important at these times of physiological stress. Very recent data indicate that during inflammation and other acute phase responses, the PAF-AH and paraoxonase antioxidant mechanisms fail.[62] During these physiological crises, the added protection afforded women by estradiol functioning as a phenolic antioxidant may make a critical difference in the ability of HDL to prevent LDL oxidation. In addition, estradiol is predicted to prevent the deleterious effects of oxidation on the function of HDL in reverse cholesterol transport and to prevent accelerated clearance of oxidatively modified HDL from the circulation.

Summary

In a recent review, Rose and Bode listed the properties of an ideal free radical scavenger.[63] It is of interest to examine estradiol as a representative estrogen in light of their characterization. First, an antioxidant must be present in adequate amounts in the body. Estrogens are present in low-nanomolar concentrations; however, our data suggest that antioxidant effects on HDL are seen at concentrations close to physiological levels.[47] Furthermore, the hypothesized enrichment in the lipoproteins, especially HDL, would serve to ensure effective local concentrations. Second, the molecule must be versatile, ie, it must be oxidized readily. The characteristic phenolic A ring of all estrogens predicts that they fill this requirement (see Figure 1). Third, an antioxidant must be suitable to be compartmentalized (to accumulate in compartments where a need for protection exists). Again, the specific association hypothesized for the interaction between estrogens and HDL would satisfy this requisite property. And fourth, the antioxidant must be available (synthesized de novo or in the diet). Estradiol is synthesized in the premenopausal female and, to a significantly lesser extent, in the male. Thus, the concept of estrogens having protective effects aside from their receptor-mediated effects on lipid metabolism, ie, as phenolic, chain-breaking antioxidants, is worthy of consideration and further testing.

The data presented here suggest that estradiol is a potent chain-breaking antioxidant for HDL at concentrations approaching circulating levels in premenopausal women. Estradiol also protects LDL but only at micromolar concentrations. The selective protection of HDL is not seen with nonestrogenic steroids, and it is not characteristic of other phenolic antioxidants with the exception of α-tocopherol. The selective antioxidant effect on HDL is presumed to reflect a specific interaction between estradiol and the HDL particle. The hypothesis has been presented that this specific interaction involves LCAT-mediated fatty acid esterification of estradiol on the HDL particle. The antioxidant protection of HDL conferred by estrogen should preserve the beneficial functions of HDL including its multiple roles in reverse cholesterol transport and its protection of LDL from oxidation.

Other estrogens have been shown to protect LDL from oxidation in vitro at pharmacological concentrations.[18-22] It is anticipated that any estrogen with a phenolic A ring will act as a lipoprotein antioxidant and that estrogens that can be esterified (by virtue of the C-17 position hydroxyl group) will selectively protect HDL. Therefore, in considering estrogen compounds for use in oral contraceptives and estrogen replacement therapy, estrogens with potent antioxidant properties as well as high receptor affinities should be selected for testing.

References

1. Steinberg D, Parthasarathy S, Carew TE, et al. Beyond cholesterol: Modifications of low-density lipoprotein that increase its atherogenicity. *N Engl J Med* 1989;320:915–924.
2. Witztum JL. The oxidation hypothesis of atherosclerosis. *Lancet* 1994;344:721–724.
3. Stocker R. Lipoprotein oxidation: Mechanistic aspects, methodological approaches and clinical relevance. *Curr Opin Lipidol* 1994;5:422–433.
4. Walzem RL, Watkins S, Frankel EN, et al. Older plasma lipoproteins are more susceptible to oxidation: A linking mechanism for the lipid and oxidation theories of atherosclerotic cardiovascular disease. *Proc Natl Acad Sci USA* 1995;92:7460–7464.
5. Hoffman RM, Garewal HS. Antioxidants and the prevention of coronary heart disease. *Arch Intern Med* 1995;155:241–246.
6. Sasahara M, Raines EW, Chait A, et al. Inhibition of hypercholesterolemia-induced atherosclerosis in the nonhuman primate by probucol. I. Is the extent of atherosclerosis related to resistance of LDL to oxidation. *J Clin Invest* 1994;94:155–164.
7. Kleinveld HA, Demacker PNM, Stalenhoef AFH. Comparative study on the effect of low-dose vitamin E and probucol on the susceptibility of LDL to oxidation and the progression of atherosclerosis in Watanabe heritable hyperlipidemic rabbits. *Arterioscler Thromb* 1994;14:1386–1391.

8. Fruebis J, Steinberg D, Dresel HA, et al. A comparison of the antiatherogenic effects of probucol and of a structural analogue of probucol in low density lipoprotein receptor-deficient rabbits. *J Clin Invest* 1994; 94:392–398.
9. Morel DW, de la Llera-Moya M, Friday KE. Treatment of cholesterol-fed rabbits with dietary vitamins E and C inhibits lipoprotein oxidation but not development of atherosclerosis. *J Nutr* 1994;124:2123–2130.
10. Lafont AM, Chai Y-C, Cornhill JF, et al. Effect of alpha-tocopherol on restenosis after angioplasty in a model of experimental atherosclerosis. *J Clin Invest* 1995;95:1018–1025.
11. Steinberg D. Clinical trials of antioxidants in atherosclerosis: Are we doing the right thing?. *Lancet* 1995;346:36–38.
12. Stampfer MJ, Hennekens CH, Manson JE, et al. Vitamin E consumption and the risk of coronary disease in women. *N Engl J Med* 1993;328: 1444–1449.
13. Rimm EB, Stampfer MJ, Ascherio A, et al. Vitamin E consumption and the risk of coronary heart disease in men. *N Engl J Med* 1993;328: 1450–1456.
14. Sugioka K, Shimosegawa Y, Nakano M. Estrogens as natural antioxidants of membrane phospholipid peroxidation. *FEBS Lett* 1987;210: 37–39.
15. Custódio JBA, Dinis TCP, Almeida LM, et al. Tamoxifen and hydroxytamoxifen as intramembraneous inhibitors of lipid peroxidation. Evidence for peroxyl radical scavenging activity. *Biochem Pharmacol* 1994; 47:1989–1998.
16. Wiseman H. Tamoxifen and estrogens as membrane antioxidants: Comparison with cholesterol. *Methods Enzymol* 1994;234:590–602.
17. Ruiz-Larrea MB, Leal AM, Liza M, et al. Antioxidant effects of estradiol and 2-hydroxyestradiol on iron-induced lipid peroxidation of rat liver microsomes. *Steroids* 1994;59:383–388.
18. Maziere C, Auclair M, Ronveaux M, et al. Estrogens inhibit copper and cell-mediated modification of low density lipoprotein. *Atherosclerosis* 1991;89:175–182.
19. Rifici VA, Khachadurian AK. The inhibition of low-density lipoprotein oxidation by 17-β estradiol. *Metabolism* 1992;41:1110–1114.
20. Negre-Salvayre A, Pieraggi MT, Mabile L, et al. Protective effect of 17 beta-estradiol against cytotoxicity of minimally oxidized LDL to cultured bovine aortic endothelial cells. *Atherosclerosis* 1993;99:207–217.
21. Wiseman H, Paganga G, Rice-Evans C, et al. Protective actions of tamoxifen and 4-hydroxytamoxifen against oxidative damage to human low-density lipoproteins: A mechanism accounting for the cardioprotective action of tamoxifen?. *Biochem J* 1993;292:635–638.
22. Parthasarathy S, Morales AJ, Murphy AA. Antioxidant: A new role for RU-486 and related compounds. *J Clin Invest* 1994;94:1990–1995.
23. Sack MN, Rader DJ, Cannon RO, III. Oestrogen and inhibition of oxidation of low-density lipoproteins in postmenopausal women. *Lancet* 1994;343:269–270.
24. Guetta V, Panza JA, Waclawiw MA, et al. Effect of combined 17β-estradiol and vitamin E on low-density lipoprotein oxidation in postmenopausal women. *Am J Cardiol* 1995;75:1274–1276.
25. Keaney JF Jr., Shwaery GT, Xu A, et al. 17β-estradiol preserves endothelial vasodilator function and limits low-density lipoprotein oxidation in hypercholesterolemic swine. *Circulation* 1994;89:2251–2259.

26. The writing group for the PEPI trial. Effects of estrogen or estrogen/
    progestin regimens on heart disease risk factors in postmenopausal
    women. The Postmenopausal Estrogen/Progestin Interventions (PEPI)
    trial. *JAMA* 1995;273:199–208.
27. Pieters MN, Schouten D, Van Berkel TJC. In vitro and in vivo evidence
    for the role of HDL in reverse cholesterol transport. *Biochim Biophys
    Acta* 1994;1225:125–134.
28. Rothblat GH, Mahlberg FH, Johnson WJ, et al. Apolipoproteins,
    membrane cholesterol domains and the regulation of cholesterol efflux.
    J Lipid Res 1992;33:1091–1097.
29. Jonas A. Lecithin-cholesterol acyltransferase in the metabolism of high-
    density lipoproteins. *Biochim Biophys Acta* 1991;1084:205–220.
30. Gwynne JT, Strauss III JF. The role of lipoproteins in steroidogenesis
    and cholesterol metabolism in steroidogenic glands. *Endocr Rev* 1982;
    3:299–329.
31. Bowry VW, Stanley KK, Stocker R. High density lipoprotein is the major
    carrier of lipid hydroperoxides in human blood plasma from fasting
    donors. *Proc Natl Acad Sci USA* 1992;89:10316–10320.
32. Hahn M, Subbiah MTR. Significant association of lipid peroxidation
    products with high density lipoproteins. *Biochem Mol Biol Int* 1994;
    33:699–704.
33. Hessler JR, Robertson AL Jr., Chisolm GM. LDL-induced cytotoxicity
    and its inhibition by HDL in human vascular smooth muscle and
    endothelial cells in culture. *Arterioscler Thromb Vasc Biol* 1979;32:
    213–229.
34. Ohta T, Takata K, Horiuchi S, et al. Protective effect of lipoproteins
    containing apoprotein A-I on Cu^{2+}-catalyzed oxidation of human low
    density lipoprotein. *FEBS Lett* 1989;257:435–438.
35. Parthasarathy S, Barnett J, Fong LG. High-density lipoprotein inhibits
    the oxidative modification of low-density lipoprotein. *Biochim Biophys
    Acta* 1990;1044:275–283.
36. Navab M, Imes SS, Hama SY, et al. Monocyte transmigration induced
    by modification of low density lipoprotein in cocultures of human aortic
    wall cells is due to induction of monocyte chemotactic protein 1 syn-
    thesis and is abolished by high density lipoprotein. *J Clin Invest* 1991;
    88:2039–2046.
37. Mackness MI, Abbott C, Arrol S, et al. The role of high-density lipopro-
    tein and lipid-soluble antioxidant vitamins in inhibiting low-density li-
    poprotein oxidation. *Biochem J* 1993;294:829–834.
38. Watson AD, Navab M, Hough GP, et al. Biologically active phospho-
    lipids in MM-LDL are transferred to HDL and are hydrolyzed by HDL
    associated esterases. *Circulation* 1994;90:I-353
39. Christison JK, Rye KA, Stocker R. Exchange of oxidized cholesteryl lin-
    oleate between LDL and HDL mediated by cholesteryl ester transfer
    protein. *J Lipid Res* 1995;36:2017–2016.
40. Nagano Y, Arai H, Kita T. High density lipoprotein loses its effect to
    stimulate efflux of cholesterol from foam cells after oxidative modifi-
    cation. *Proc Natl Acad Sci USA* 1991;88:6457–6461.
41. Salmon S, Maziere C, Auclair M, et al. Malondialdehyde modification
    and copper-induced autooxidation of high-density lipoprotein decrease
    cholesterol efflux from human-cultured fibroblasts. *Biochim Biophys
    Acta* 1992;1125:230–235.

42. Morel DW. Reduced cholesterol efflux to mildly oxidized high density lipoprotein. *Biochem Biophys Res Commun* 1994;200:408–416.
43. Senault C, Mahlberg FH, Renaud G, et al. Effect of apoprotein cross-linking on the metabolism of human HDL$_3$ in rat. *Biochim Biophys Acta* 1990;1046:81–88.
44. Guertin F, Brunet S, Gavino V, et al. Malondialdehyde-modified high-density lipoprotein cholesterol: Plasma removal, tissue distribution and biliary sterol secretion in rats. *Biochim Biophys Acta Lipids Lipid Metab* 1994;1214:137–142.
45. Steinbrecher UP, Parthasarathy S, Leake DS, et al. Modification of low density lipoprotein by endothelial cells involves lipid peroxidation and degradation of low density lipoprotein phospholipids. *Proc Natl Acad Sci USA* 1984;81:3883–3887.
46. Puhl H, Waeg G, Esterbauer H. Methods to determine oxidation of low-density lipoproteins. *Methods Enzymol* 1994;233:425–441.
47. Banka CL, Curtiss CL. Estradiol selectively protects high density lipo-protein from oxidative modification. Submitted 1995.
48. Yla-Herttuala S, Palinski W, Rosenfeld ME, et al. Evidence for the presence of oxidatively modified low density lipoprotein in atherosclerotic lesions of rabbit and man. *J Clin Invest* 1989;84:1086–1095.
49. Noguchi N, Niki E. Apolipoprotein B protein oxidation in low-density lipoproteins. *Methods Enzymol* 1994;233:490–494.
50. Palinski W, Ord VA, Plump AS, et al. ApoE-deficient mice are a model of lipoprotein oxidation in atherogenesis. Demonstration of oxidation-specific epitopes in lesions and high titers of autoantibodies to malon-dialdehyde-lysine in serum. *Arterioscler Thromb* 1994;14:605–616.
51. Francis GA, Mendez AJ, Bierman EL, et al. Oxidative tyrosylation of high density lipoprotein by peroxidase enhances cholesterol removal from cultured fibroblasts and macrophage foam cells. *Proc Natl Acad Sci USA* 1993;90:6631–6635.
52. McCall MR, van den Berg JJM, Kuypers FA, et al. Modification of LCAT activity and HDL structure: New links between cigarette smoke and coronary heart disease risk. *Arterioscler Thromb* 1994;14:248–253.
53. Banka CL, Bonnet DJ, Black AS, et al. Localization of an apolipoprotein A-I epitope critical for activation of lecithin-cholesterol acyltransferase. *J Biol Chem* 1991;266:23886–23892.
54. Larner JM, Pahuja SL, Shackelton CH, et al. The isolation and characterization of estradiol-fatty acid esters in human ovarian follicular fluid. *J Biol Chem* 1993;268:13893–13899.
55. Janocko L, Hochberg RB. Estradiol fatty acid esters occur naturally in human blood. *Science* 1983;222:1334–1336.
56. Traber MG, Ingold KU, Burton GW, et al. Absorption and transport of deuterium-substituted $2R,4'R,8'R$-α-tocopherol in human lipoproteins. *Lipids* 1988;23:791–797.
57. Traber MG, Lane JC, Lagmay NR, et al. Studies on the transfer of tocopherol between lipoproteins. Lipids 1992;27:657–663.
58. Stafforini DM, Zimmerman GA, McIntyre TM, et al. The platelet activating factor acetylhydrolase from human plasma prevents oxidative modification of low density lipoprotein. *Trans Am Assoc Phys* 1993; 106:44–63.
59. Mackness MI, Arrol S, Durrington PN. Paraoxonase prevents accumulation of lipoperoxides in low-density lipoprotein. *FEBS Lett* 1991; 286:152–154.

60. Wolfe F, Mitchell DM, Sibley JT, et al. The mortality of rheumatoid arthritis. *Arthritis Rheum* 1994;37:481–494.
61. Liao F, Andalibi A, Qiao J-H, et al. Genetic evidence for a common pathway mediating oxidative stress, inflammatory gene induction, and aortic fatty streak formation in mice. *J Clin Invest* 1994;94:877–884.
62. Van Lenten BJ, Hama SY, de Beer FC, et al. Anti-inflammatory HDL becomes pro-inflammatory during the acute phaseresponse. Loss of protective effect of HDL against LDL oxidation in aortic wall cell co-cultures. *J Clin Invest* 1995;96:2758-2767.
63. Rose RC, Bode AM. Biology of free radical scavengers: An evaluation of ascorbate. *FASEB J* 1993;7:1135–1142.

Chapter 13

Antioxidant Effects of Estrogen Administered to Postmenopausal Women

Richard O. Cannon III, MD

During the past decade, accumulating evidence suggests that oxidative modification of low-density lipoproteins (LDL) greatly increases its atherogenicity.[1] After oxidation, LDL is recognized by receptors on macrophages and smooth muscle cells leading to enhanced intracellular uptake of LDL without feedback regulation, and the conversion of tissue macrophages and smooth muscle cells to lipid-rich foam cells, the earliest histological feature of the atherosclerotic plaque. Oxidatively modified LDL also promotes the expression of chemo-attractant peptides and endothelial cell-surface receptors that attract circulating monocytes, promoting their entry into the vessel wall and conversion into tissue macrophages.[2] Animal studies indicate that administration of potent antioxidants such as probucol may retard the progression of atherosclerosis,[3] and epidemiological studies suggest that chronic use of the antioxidant vitamin E may significantly reduce cardiovascular events in men and women.[4,5]

Several groups have examined the antioxidant properties of estrogen,[6–18] which shares chemical structural similarity with lipophilic antioxidants such as probucol and vitamin E (α tocopherol); all have hydroxyphenol groups with the hydrogen atom of the hydroxy group, and its single electron easily donated to lipid peroxyl free radicals, thus terminating chain propagation of oxidation along fatty acids of lipoprotein membrane phospholipids.[19,20] For example, Rifici and Kachadurian[13] examined the antioxidant effect of estradiol-17β, the most abundant and potent estrogen secreted by the ovaries of reproductive-aged women, and other estrogens on

From: Forte TM, (ed). *Hormonal, Metabolic, and Cellular Influences on Cardiovascular Disease in Women*. Armonk, NY: Futura Publishing Company, Inc.; © 1997.

copper-catalyzed and mononuclear cell-mediated oxidation of LDL as measured by the production of lipoprotein oxidation products. In 1 μM estradiol, the onset of LDL oxidation after the addition of copper was delayed by >50% compared with untreated LDL. At this concentration, estriol was less protective of LDL oxidation, and estrone had no antioxidant activity in their study.

Antioxidant Effect of Estradiol-17β

We found that the acute administration of estradiol-17β into brachial arteries of 18 postmenopausal women significantly delayed the onset and maximum rate of copper-catalyzed oxidation of LDL isolated from the ipsilateral brachial venous blood after 20 minutes infusion compared with baseline samples (Figure 1).[16] The plasma level of estradiol achieved in the brachial venous plasma in this study was within the physiological range (436 ± 186 pg/mL; ~1 nM concentration). After estradiol-17β administration for 3 weeks to 12 of these subjects using a transdermal preparation (0.1 mg daily) to avoid changes in plasma lipid levels, LDL was protected from oxidation by a similar degree as noted in the acute infusion study, but

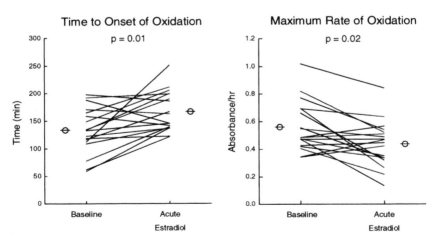

FIGURE 1. *The time to onset of copper-catalyzed LDL oxidation (left) and maximum rate of oxidation (right) is shown at baseline and after intra-arterial infusion of estradiol-17β at 20 ng/mL per minute for 20 minutes, achieving a forearm venous concentration of 436 ± 186 pg/mL (mean ± SD) in 18 postmenopausal women. Reproduced with permission from Reference 16.*

at a plasma level (126 ± 43 pg/mL) approximately one-third of that achieved during the acute study (Figure 2). For all patients, there was weak correlation between the times to onset of copper-catalyzed LDL oxidation (lag times) and the plasma estradiol levels at baseline ($r = 0.46$, $P = 0.053$); no significant correlations were noted between LDL peroxidation lag times and plasma lipid levels or patient's age. There was no correlation between the LDL peroxidation lag times and the plasma estradiol levels after acute infusion ($r = 0.29$, $P = 0.22$) or after 3 weeks of transdermal administration of estradiol-17β ($r = 0.29$, $P = 0.35$). As expected, no alteration in plasma lipid levels were observed due to the transdermal route of estrogen delivery. After discontinuation of estradiol, the lag time and maximum rate of LDL oxidation returned to baseline within 1 month.

The plasma levels of estradiol-17β achieved in both the acute and chronic phases of this study were approximately 1,000-fold lower than concentrations used in in vitro studies. When we added 1 nM estradiol-17β directly to plasma from estrogen-deficient women and let stand for ≤48 hours, no change in copper-catalyzed LDL peroxidation lag times was noted compared with paired plasma samples without estradiol (seven experiments, unpublished observation). This suggests that the antioxidant effects of estradiol may not be the result of additional direct protection of LDL from oxidant

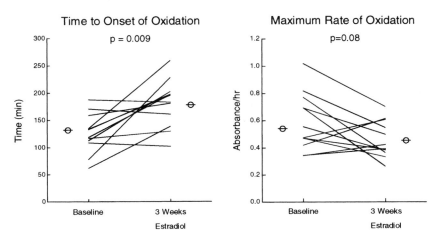

FIGURE 2. *The time to onset of copper-catalyzed LDL oxidation (left) and the maximum rate of oxidation (right) is shown at baseline and after 3-week administration of estradiol-17β using a patch preparation which delivered 0.1 mg estradiol daily, achieving a plasma concentration of 126 ± 43 pg/mL in 12 postmenopausal women. Reproduced with permission from Reference 16.*

stress, but instead be mediated by the release of antioxidant substances from the vessel wall.

Antioxidant Effects of Estradiol-17β and Vitamin E

We also investigated the possibility that estradiol-17β and vitamin E might act synergistically to protect LDL from oxidation when administered to postmenopausal women.[17] In a previous study with 19 hypercholesterolemic middle-aged men and women, we found that vitamin E (800 IU), beta carotene (30 mg), and vitamin C (1 gm) daily for 1 month delayed the onset of copper-catalyzed LDL oxidation by 71%, with a significant correlation between the prolongation in the LDL peroxidation lag times and the increase in vitamin E ($r = 0.72$, $P < 0.001$), but not beta carotene or vitamin C, plasma levels on treatment compared with baseline values.[21] Nineteen postmenopausal women, 15 of whom had total cholesterol plasma levels <240 mg%, were randomized to treatment with either estradiol-17β (transdermal patch preparation 0.1 mg daily) for 3 weeks, vitamin E (800 IU) daily for 6 weeks or a combination of the two treatments with the estrogen patch administered during the final 3 weeks of vitamin E administration. All subjects received monotherapy (estradiol or vitamin E) and combined therapy (estradiol and vitamin E) with a 1-week washout period between the two treatment phases of the study. After 3 weeks of estradiol administration in nine subjects, plasma levels of estradiol increased from 12 ± 3 pg/mL at baseline to 130 ± 56 pg/mL, with no change in plasma lipid levels from baseline values due to the transdermal route of estradiol delivery in this study.

After 6 weeks of vitamin E administration in 10 subjects, plasma levels of vitamin E increased from 1.8 ± 0.7 mg/dL at baseline to 3.0 ± 1.6 mg/dL with unchanged plasma lipid levels compared with baseline values. Estradiol administration as monotherapy resulted in a 17% ± 29% increase in the lag time to onset of copper-catalyzed LDL oxidation compared with baseline values, and vitamin E prolonged the onset of LDL oxidation by 29% ± 44% (Figure 3). After 6 weeks of vitamin E and 3 weeks of estradiol (combined therapy), plasma levels of vitamin E increased from 1.8 ± 0.7 mg/dL at baseline to 2.5 ± 0.7 mg/dL and estradiol levels increased from 17 ± 3 pg/mL at baseline to 128 ± 61 pg/mL, plasma levels similar to those achieved during the respective monotherapies. As was true for each monotherapy, combined therapy produced no change in lipid levels

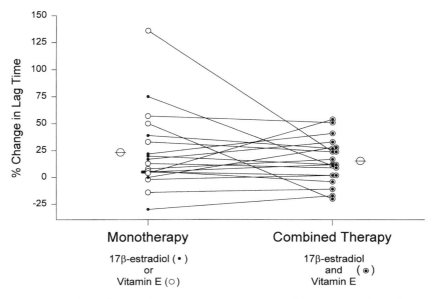

FIGURE 3. *The relative change in time to onset of copper-catalyzed LDL oxidation from pretreatment values is shown during monotherapy with either estradiol-17β (patch preparation 0.1 mg daily for 3 weeks) or vitamin E (800 IU daily for 6 weeks) and during combined therapy with both treatments to 19 postmenopausal women. Reproduced with permission from Reference 17.*

compared with baseline values. After combined therapy, there was a 16% ± 20% (*P* = 0.01) increase in the lag time to onset of LDL oxidation compared with pretreatment measurements (Figure 3). No difference in the effect on LDL oxidation was found between monotherapy with estradiol and combined therapy in 9 subjects (17% ± 29% versus 17% ± 18%, *P* = 0.78), between monotherapy with vitamin E and combined therapy in 10 subjects (29% ± 44% versus 15% ± 24%, *P* = 0.29), and between the two monotherapies regarded as one group and combined therapy in all 19 subjects (23% ± 37% versus 16% ± 20%, *P* = 0.38).

Unlike our experience with antioxidant vitamin administration to hypercholesterolemic subjects,[21] in this study, there was no correlation between the change in LDL peroxidation lag times and the change in vitamin E plasma levels on treatment (*r* = 0.017). However, in agreement with our previous chronic estrogen study,[16] there was no correlation between the change in LDL peroxidation lag times and the change in plasma estradiol levels on treatment (*r* =

0.14). Thus, in this study, combined administration of estradiol and vitamin E protected LDL in postmenopausal women from oxidation but with no synergism noted compared with either therapy given alone. It is possible, however, that vitamin E administration to hypercholesterolemic postmenopausal women would have yielded greater protection of their LDL from oxidation compared with the effect of vitamin E on the LDL of the mostly normocholesterolemic women noted in this study.

Antioxidant Effects of Tamoxifen and Conjugated Equine Estrogen

We recently studied the effect of tamoxifen, a nonsteroidal antiestrogen commonly used in the treatment in breast cancer in postmenopausal women, on susceptibility of LDL to oxidation.[22] Several clinical trials of tamoxifen in patients with breast cancer have reported significant reduction in LDL concentrations[23,24] and significantly fewer cardiovascular events on tamoxifen compared with no treatment.[25,26] In vitro studies indicate that tamoxifen and its metabolite 4-hydroxytamoxifen protect human LDL against lipid peroxidation at suprapharmacological (micromolar) concentrations.[27] In our study, 24 postmenopausal women received tamoxifen (20 mg), conjugated equine estrogen (0.625 mg), and placebo (double-blinded) in random order taken once daily for 2 months at a time (conjugated equine estrogen was taken 3 out of every 4 weeks during that time period). A 1-month washout period followed each 2-month treatment period. At the end of each treatment period, subjects returned for LDL isolation and determination of plasma drug or hormone concentrations. Tamoxifen and conjugated equine estrogen lowered LDL levels by 19% ± 18% and by 13% ± 14%, respectively (both $P = 0.001$ compared with placebo). Conjugated equine estrogen increased HDL levels by 13% ± 20% ($P = 0.003$ compared with placebo); tamoxifen did not affect HDL levels. Parameters of LDL oxidizability differed from placebo only during the tamoxifen treatment period: the lag time to onset of LDL oxidation was 20% ± 35% longer during the tamoxifen treatment period compared with placebo ($P = 0.01$; Figure 4). The effect of conjugated equine estrogen on LDL oxidation was no different from placebo. No correlation was found between the prolongation of LDL peroxidation lag times and either the reduction in LDL levels on tamoxifen compared with placebo ($r = -0.01$) or the plasma tamoxifen concentrations during that treatment period ($r = 0.17$). The antioxidant effect of tamoxifen was

Time to Onset of LDL Oxidation   Maximum Rate of Oxidation

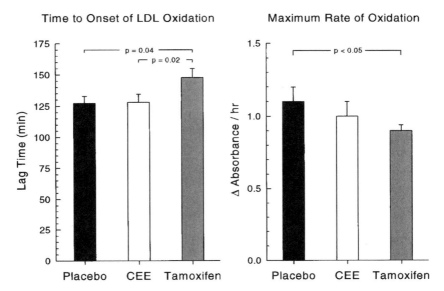

FIGURE 4. *The time to onset of copper-catalyzed LDL oxidation (left) and maximum rate of oxidation (right) is shown during the placebo, conjugated equine estrogen (CEE), and tamoxifen phases of the study when administered to 24 women, with each treatment period lasting 2 months followed by a 1-month washout period. Reproduced with permission from Reference 22.*

achieved at plasma levels (154 ± 140 ng/mL) ~100-fold lower than concentrations that delayed LDL peroxidation in vitro.[27]

Because of the long half-life of tamoxifen (7 days), we tested for the possibility of a carry-over effect of this drug on subsequent treatment periods. In the 13 subjects who received placebo before tamoxifen, there was a 32% ± 27% increase in the lag time to onset of copper-catalyzed LDL oxidation ($P < 0.001$) and a 28% ± 21% in the reduction in the maximum rate of oxidation ($P = 0.002$) on tamoxifen treatment compared with placebo values. In the other 11 subjects who received tamoxifen before placebo, the lag times to onset of LDL oxidation on tamoxifen and on placebo were similar (136 ± 41 minutes versus 135 ± 34 minutes). The carry-over effect of tamoxifen was not related to its plasma concentration because no tamoxifen was detected by our assay after completion of the subsequent placebo treatment period. The protective effect of tamoxifen on the development of breast cancer in women considered at risk is currently being investigated in an NIH-sponsored placebo-controlled trial. Whether or not tamoxifen also protects against the development of cardiovascular disease in this trial will be of considerable interest.

In view of the significant carry-over effect of tamoxifen that might have affected conjugated equine estrogen antioxidant effects, we compared those subjects (n=9) who received conjugated equine estrogen and placebo before the tamoxifen treatment period. The lag time to onset of LDL oxidation was similar between treatment with conjugated equine estrogen and placebo (117 ± 22 minutes versus 124 ± 20 minutes, $P = 0.61$) in these women. The absence of an antioxidant effect may merely reflect the small number of analyzable data in this study; larger numbers of women may be required to show a positive effect of conjugated equine estrogen on LDL oxidation. Subbiah et al. show that micromolar concentrations of the equine estrogen equilin, which comprises approximately one-third of the hormonal composition of conjugated equine estrogen, is a more potent antioxidant than micromolar concentrations of estradiol-17β.[15] On the other hand, Rifici and Kachadurian showed that estrone (which comprises of approximately two-thirds of the hormonal composition of conjugated equine estrogen) in micromolar concentrations is a weaker antioxidant than estradiol-17β.[13] Although estrone can be converted to estradiol in the liver, estradiol levels achieved with conjugated equine estrogen preparations are less than one-half the concentrations achievable with oral or transdermal estradiol preparations. The relevance of these in vitro studies of relative estrogenic antioxidant potencies using micromolar concentrations of hormones to postmenopausal women in whom nanomolar concentrations of estrogenic hormones are achieved with conventional dosages of commercially available estrogenic preparations is unknown.

Oxidized Low-Density Lipoproteins and Vasomotor Function

In addition to its importance in atherogenesis, oxidized LDL may also affect endothelium-dependent vasomotor function. Hypercholesterolemic subjects have impaired endothelium-dependent vasodilation associated with reduced nitric oxide (NO) bioavailability.[28–31] Studies performed on animal arterial tissue in vitro have provided insight into the mechanisms of this abnormal endothelial function. Thus, Mangin et al. showed that oxidatively modified LDL, but not native LDL, reduced the vasorelaxant response of arterial rings to acetylcholine.[32] Shimokawa et al. showed that the pertussis toxin-sensitive, Gi-protein-dependent signal transduction pathway linked to adenylyl cyclase (used by acetylcholine and other agonists) is impaired in tissue from hypercholesterolemic animals with early atherosclerosis, which could reduce NO synthase activity and NO production.[33] Alternatively, enhanced production and release of superoxide anions from the endothelial cells in hypercholesterolemia could reduce the bioavailability of NO by conversion to compounds devoid of vasodilator effects.[34,35]

Keaney et al.[18] investigated the effects of estradiol on LDL oxidation in the endothelium-dependent vasomotor function in three groups of cholesterol-fed miniature swine. Two groups of animals underwent oophorectomy, with one group treated with estradiol-17β delivered by a pump device for 16 weeks. The control group underwent sham operation with ovaries left intact. The plasma estradiol level achieved by the pump infusion was similar to that of the sham-operated control animals. There were no differences in plasma lipid levels among the three groups on the high-fat, high-cholesterol diet. Rings from coronary arteries of the untreated oophorectomized animals had reduced relaxation to the endothelium-dependent vasodilators bradykinin and substance P compared with the sham-operated control animals and the oopherectomized animals that received estradiol. The responses to the endothelium-independent vasodilator nitroglycerin were similar among the three groups of animals. The estradiol-treated animals had time to onset of copper-catalyzed oxidation of LDL comparable with the sham-operated controls and significantly greater than the time to onset of oxidation of LDL from the oophorectomized untreated animals, with significant correlations between the time of onset of LDL oxidation and the extent of vascular relaxation in response to bradykinin ($r = 0.62$, $P < 0.03$) and substance P ($r = 0.61$, $P < 0.03$).

We previously had shown that intra-arterial infusion of estradiol-17β acutely potentiated the endothelium-dependent microvascular dilator response to acetylcholine, but not the endothelium-independent response to nitroprusside, in the forearms of postmenopausal women using venous occlusion strain gauge plethysmography.[36,37] We then administered estradiol to 33 postmenopausal women, using a transdermal patch preparation in order not to affect lipoprotein plasma levels.[37] Resting forearm blood flow, vascular resistance, and blood pressure after 3 weeks of estrogen treatment were unchanged from pretreatment measurements. The forearm blood flow response to serial concentrations of the endothelium-dependent vasodilator acetylcholine was not enhanced after 3 weeks administration of estradiol compared with pretreatment measurements, despite an increase in plasma estradiol levels from 16 ± 11 pg/mL at baseline to 120 ± 57 pg/mL at follow-up. There was also no difference in the forearm microvascular dilator responses to serial doses of the endothelium-independent vasodilator sodium nitroprusside compared with pretreatment baseline values. As discussed previously, this concentration of estradiol achieved with 3 weeks of transdermal estradiol administration significantly prolonged the peroxidation lag times of LDL from postmenopausal women compared with pretreatment values.[16] This absence of improvement in systemic microvascular dilator function despite antioxidant effects was consistent with our previous study with hypercholesterolemic subjects: despite protection of their LDL from peroxidation using a combination of antioxidant vitamins for 1 month, we found that the forearm blood flow responses to the endothelium-dependent vasodilator acetylcholine and the endothelium-independent vasodilator sodium nitroprusside likewise were unchanged compared with pretreatment measurements.[19]

The different vasomotor effects of acute and chronic estradiol-17β administration may be due to the lower plasma levels achieved with chronic estrogen administration. Repeat intra-arterial infusion of estradiol in eight women while receiving transdermal estradiol, increased forearm venous estradiol levels to 268 ± 105 pg/mL, with potentiation of the vasodilator response to acetylcholine to a similar degree as that observed in the initial study after acute administration of estradiol. The lack of improved systemic microvascular dilator function with chronic estrogen replacement therapy may account for the absence of blood pressure lowering effects with chronic estrogen replacement therapy in the normotensive participants of the postmenopausal estrogen/progestin interventions (PEPI) trial[38] or in hypertensive postmenopausal women.[39]

Larger arteries may respond differently than the microcirculation to chronic estrogen administration. Lieberman et al.[40] reported that oral estradiol-17β administration to 13 postmenopausal women for 9 weeks enhanced flow-mediated brachial artery dilator responses measured by ultrasound during postischemic hyperemia, indicative of improved endothelium-dependent vasodilator function, without potentiation of the vasodilator response to nitroglycerin. As in our study, no hormonal effects on blood pressure were noted.

Low-Density Lipoproteins Oxidation and Hemostasis

Oxidized LDL may unfavorably affect endothelium-dependent hemostasis. In the Framingham Offspring Study, reproductive-aged women had lower plasma levels of plasminogen-activator inhibitor (PAI-1) and higher levels of tissue plasminogen activator (t-PA) compared with men of comparable age or postmenopausal women not taking estrogen.[41] However, postmenopausal women on estrogen replacement therapy had PAI-1 and t-PA levels similar to reproductive-aged women. The mechanism of estrogen's apparently favorable hemostatic effects is unknown. Oxidatively modified LDL depresses endothelial release of t-PA, and both oxidatively modified LDL and lipoprotein (a) promote synthesis of PAI-1 by increased transcription of PAI-1 mRNA.[42,43] Thus estrogen's effect on t-PA and PAI-1 may in part be due to antioxidant protection of LDL and reduction in lipoprotein (a) plasma levels.

Future Directions

Although many studies have shown antioxidant effects of estrogen on LDL in vitro and in LDL from postmenopausal women on estrogen therapy (using in vitro assays), many questions remain. For example, how do nanomolar plasma concentrations of estrogen achieved in postmenopausal women receiving conventional preparations administered at conventional dosages, protect LDL from oxidation when micromolar concentrations are required in vitro? Is the antioxidant effect of estrogen a direct effect of the lipophilic hormone, which becomes incorporated into the phospholipid shell of the lipoprotein, analogous to vitamin E? Or does estrogen provoke the release of substances from the vessel wall or elsewhere that mediate estrogen's antioxidant effect? Are there relative differences in antioxidant potential of different estrogenic compounds commonly used as hormone replacement therapy in postmenopausal women? Do progestin compounds attenuate or negate estrogen's antioxidant effect? Do compounds that have antioxidant potential, but do not alter plasma lipid levels (such as transdermally delivered estradiol-17β) provide the same long-term cardiovascular benefit as compounds that favorably alter lipid levels, but may have little or no antioxidant potential (such as conjugated equine estrogen)? Does estrogen's antioxidant effect account for other biological responses to the hormone, such as augmentation of endothelium-dependent vasodilation and profibrinolytic hemostatic effects?

In the future, much effort will undoubtedly be devoted to unraveling the mechanism and biological importance of estrogen's antioxidant effect, in addition to addressing the most clinically important question of all: is the antioxidant effect of a compound important in preventing or delaying the progression of atherosclerosis and its clinically important sequelae.

References

1. Steinberg D, Parasarathy S, Carew TE, et al. Beyond Cholesterol. Modifications of low-density lipoprotein that increase its atherogenicity. *N Engl J Med* 1989;320:915–924.
2. Berliner JA, Territo MC, Savanian A, et al. Minimally modified low density lipoprotein stimulates monocyte endothelial interactions. *J Clin Invest* 1990;85:1260–1266.
3. Carew TE, Schwenke DC, Steinberg D. Antiatherogenic effect of probucol unrelated to its hypocholesterolemic effect: Evidence that antioxidants in vivo can selectively inhibit low density lipoprotein degradation in macrophage-rich fatty streaks slowing the progression of atherosclerosis in the WHHL rabbit. *Proc Natl Acad Sci USA* 1987; 84:7725–7729.
4. Stampfer MJ, Hennekens CH, Manson JE, et al. Vitamin E consumption and the risk of coronary disease in women. *N Engl J Med* 1993;328: 1444–1449.
5. Rimm EB, Stampfer MJ, Ascherio A, et al. Vitamin E consumption and the risk of coronary heart disease in men. *N Engl J Med* 1993;328: 1450–1456.
6. Yagi K, Komura S. Inhibitory effect of female hormones on lipid peroxidation. *Biochem Int* 1986; 13:1051–1055.
7. Sugioka K, Shimosegawa Y, Nakano M. Estrogens as natural antioxidants of membrane phospholipid peroxidation. *FEBS Lett* 1987;210:37–39.
8. Yoshino K, Komura S, Watanabe I, et al. Effect of estrogens on serum and liver lipid peroxide levels in mice. *J Clin Biochem Nutr* 1987;3:233–240.
9. Nakano M, Sugioka K, Naito I, et al. Novel and potent biological antioxidants on membrane phospholipid peroxidation: 2-hydroxy estrone and 2-hydroxy estradiol. *Biochem Biophys Res Commun* 1987;142: 919–924.
10. Mukai K, Daifuku K, Yokoyama S, et al. Stopped-flow investigation of antioxidant activity of estrogens in solution. *Biochim Biophys Acta* 1990; 1035:348–352.
11. Huber LA, Scheffler E, Poll T, et al. 17β-Estradiol inhibits LDL oxidation and cholesterol ester formation in cultured macrophages. *Free Rad Res Comm* 1990;8:167–173.
12. Maziere C, Auclair M, Ronveaux M-F, et al. Estrogens inhibit copper and cell-mediated modification of low density lipoprotein. *Atherosclerosis* 1991;89:175–182.
13. Rifici VA, Khachadurian AK. The inhibition of low-density lipoprotein oxidation by 17β-estradiol. *Metabolism* 1992;41:1110–1114.
14. Negre-Salvayre A, Pieraggi M-T, Mabile L, et al. Protective effect of 17β-estradiol against the cytotoxicity of minimally oxidized LDL to cultured bovine aortic endothelial cells. *Atherosclerosis* 1993;99:207–217.
15. Subbiah MTR, Kessel B, Agrawal M, et al. Antioxidant potential of specific estrogens on lipid peroxidation. *J Clin Endocrin Metab* 1993; 77:1095–1097.

16. Sack MN, Rader DJ, Cannon RO. Oestrogen and inhibition of oxidation of low-density lipoproteins in postmenopausal women. *Lancet* 1994; 343:269–270.

17. Guetta V, Panza JA, Waclawiw MA, et al. Effect of combined 17β-estradiol and vitamin E on low-density lipoprotein oxidation in post-menopausal women. *Am J Cardiol* 1995;75:1274–1276.

18. Keaney JF, Shwaery GT, Xu A, et al. 17β-estradiol preserves endothelial vasodilator function and limits low-density lipoprotein oxidation in hy-percholesterolemic swine. *Circulation* 1994;89:2251–2259.

19. Niki E. Antioxidants in relation to lipid peroxidation. *Chem Phys Lipids* 1987;44:227–253.

20. Esterbauer H, Wag G, Puhl H. Lipid peroxidation and its role in ath-erosclerosis. *Br Med Bull* 1993;49:566–576.

21. Gilligan DG, Sack M, Guetta V, et al. Effect of antioxidant vitamins on low density lipoprotein oxidation and impaired endothelium-dependent vasodilation in patients with hypercholesterolemia. *J Am Coll Cardiol* 1994;24:1611–1617.

22. Guetta V, Lush RM, Figg WD, et al. Effects of the antiestrogen tamox-ifen on low-density lipoprotein concentrations and oxidation in post-menopausal women: Potential mechanisms for cardiovascular benefit. *Am J Cardiol* 1995;76:1072–1073.

23. Rossner S, Wallgren A. Serum lipoproteins and proteins after breast cancer surgery and the effects of tamoxifen. *Atherosclerosis* 1984;52: 339–346.

24. Love RR, Wiebe DL, Newcomb PA, et al. Effects of tamoxifen on car-diovascular risk factors in postmenopausal women. *Ann Intern Med* 1991;115:860–864.

25. Henderson BE, Paganini-Hill A, Ross RK. Estrogen replacement ther-apy and protection from acute myocardial infarction. *Am J Obstet Gy-necol* 1988;159:312–317.

26. McDonald CC, Stewart HJ for the Scottish Breast Cancer Committee. Fatal myocardial infarction in the Scottish adjuvant tamoxifen trial. *Br Med J* 1991;303:435–437.

27. Wiseman H, Paganga G, Rice-Evans C, et al. Protective action of ta-moxifen and 4-hydroxytamoxifen against oxidative damage to human low-density lipoprotein: A mechanism accounting for the cardioprotec-tive action of tamoxifen? *Biochem J* 1993;392:635–638.

28. Drexler H, Zeiher AM, Meinertz T, et al. Correction of endothelial dys-function in coronary microcirculation of hypercholesterolemic patients by L-arginine. *Lancet* 1991;338:1546–1550.

29. Creager MA, Girerd XJ, Gallagher SH, et al. L-arginine improves en-dothelium-dependent vasodilation in hypercholesterolemic humans. *J Clin Invest* 1992;90:1248–1252.

30. Casino PR, Kilcoyne CM, Quyyumi AA, et al. Role of nitric oxide in the endothelium-dependent vasodilation of hypercholesterolemic patients. *Circulation* 1993;88:2541–2547.

31. Quyyumi AA, Dakak N, Andrews NP, et al. Nitric oxide in the human coronary circulation. Impact of risk factors for coronary atherosclero-sis. *J Clin Invest* 1995;95:1747–1755.

32. Mangin EL, Kugiyama K, Nguy JH, et al. Effects of lysolipids and oxi-datively modified low density lipoprotein on endothelium-dependent re-laxation of rabbit aorta. *Circ Res* 1993;72:161–166.

33. Shimokawa H, Flavahan NA, Vanhoutte PM. Loss of endothelial pertussis toxin-sensitive G protein function in atherosclerotic porcine coronary arteries. *Circulation* 1991;83:652–660.
34. Ohara Y, Peterson TE, Harrison DG. Hypercholesterolemia increases superoxide anion production. *J Clin Invest* 1993;91:2546–2551.
35. Minor RL, Myers PR, Guerra R, et al. Diet-induced atherosclerosis increases the release of nitrogen oxides from rabbit aorta. *J Clin Invest* 1990;86:2109–2116.
36. Gilligan DM, Badar DM, Panza JA, et al. Acute vascular effects of estrogen in postmenopausal women. *Circulation* 1994;90:786–791.
37. Gilligan DM, Badar DM, Panza JA, et al. Effects of estrogen replacement therapy on peripheral vascular function in postmenopausal women. *Am J Cardiol* 1995;75:264–268.
38. The Writing Group for the PEPI Trial. Effects of estrogen or estrogen/progestin regimen on heart disease risk factors in postmenopausal women. The Postmenopausal Estrogen/Progestin Interventions (PEPI) Trial. *JAMA* 1995;273:199–208.
39. Lip GYH, Beevers M, Churchill D, et al. Hormone replacement therapy and blood pressure in hypertensive women. *J Hum Hypertens* 1994; 8:491–494.
40. Lieberman EH, Gebhard MD, Uehata A, et al. Estrogen improves endothelium-dependent, flow-mediated vasodilation in postmenopausal women. *Ann Intern Med* 1994;121:936–941.
41. Gebara OCE, Mittleman MA, Sutherland P, et al. Association between increased estrogen status and increased fibrinolytic potential in the Framingham Offspring Study. *Circulation* 1995;91:1952–1958.
42. Kugiyama K, Sakamoto T, Misumi I, et al. Transferable lipids in oxidized low-density lipoprotein stimulate plasminogen activator inhibitor-1 and inhibit tissue-type plasminogen activator release from endothelial cells. *Circ Res* 1993;73:335–343.
43. Etingin OR, Hajjar DP, Hajjar KA, et al. Lipoprotein (a) regulates plasminogen activator inhibitor-1 expression in endothelial cells. *J Biol Chem* 1991;266:2459–2465.

Chapter 14

Estrogen Treatment and Human Lipoprotein Metabolism

Frank M. Sacks, MD, Hannia Campos, PhD, Helena Judge, BA, and Brian W. Walsh, MD

Estrogen has multiple effects on lipoprotein concentrations in plasma that are likely to contribute to the reduction in cardiovascular disease in women who receive hormonal replacement therapy. We review the underlying mechanisms for the changes in lipoprotein levels, and discuss the clinical significance of the estrogen-induced changes in metabolism.

VLDL and LDL Metabolism

Overview

Plasma lipoprotein particles that have apolipoprotein B-100 (apo B-100) as their principal protein component, very low-density lipoprotein (VLDL), intermediate density lipoprotein (IDL), and low-density lipoprotein (LDL), participate in a complex set of metabolic pathways. Apo B-100 is synthesized by hepatocytes and assembled with lipids and other apoproteins to form VLDL, which are secreted into the circulation. Originally, it was thought that VLDL is converted in the circulation by endothelial lipoprotein lipase to progressively smaller particles to become LDL and that all, or nearly all, of LDL was derived from VLDL. During the past 10–15 years, many lines of evidence demonstrate considerable complexity in the metabolism of apo B containing lipoproteins.[1-11] Kinetic studies of

Research was supported by a grant from the National Heart, Lung, and Blood Institute.

VLDL metabolism found that large and small VLDL can be removed from plasma.[1,2] Small VLDL and LDL can be secreted directly into the circulation as well as arise from the dilipidation of larger size particles.[1,3-5] The metabolism of lipoprotein particles in the LDL range also exhibits a complex polydispersity.[3-8] Metabolic rates of light and dense LDL differ from each other, and they may not have an exclusive precursor-product relation. Therefore, there are multiple pathways of entry and removal for plasma VLDL and LDL that must be considered. These pathways are key in regulating steady-state plasma lipoprotein concentrations, and they are affected in a complex way by estrogen.

Clinical Significance of Metabolism Studies

Plasma concentrations of the lipoproteins are convenient measurements used for predicting risk of cardiovascular disease. However, plasma concentrations represent a static description of a dynamic metabolic system. Steady-state plasma concentrations of a lipoprotein class result from production and clearance rates, which themselves are often the sum of multiple pathways of production and multiple routes for clearance.

The functional state of a lipoprotein particle is likely to be more relevant to atherosclerosis than the plasma concentration. For example, the clearance rate of a lipoprotein particle in plasma is influenced greatly by lipoprotein receptor activity. When receptor-mediated lipoprotein uptake is optimal, clearance is rapid, and the time that a particle spends in the circulation is relatively short. VLDL and LDL are normally taken up by high-affinity receptors in the liver and steroidogenic tissues that have special requirements for cholesterol. Abnormal slower routes of uptake are by nonreceptor-mediated mechanisms, such as through vascular endothelium, and by macrophage scavenger receptors. Both lead to cholesterol deposition in the vascular intima and atherosclerosis. These slow uptake pathways increase in importance when receptor mediated uptake is diminished.[12-14]

A long residence time in plasma itself may result in modification of VLDL or LDL, thereby conferring abnormal properties that are associated with atherosclerosis (Figure 1). These processes include cholesterol-ester enrichment of VLDL by the action of cholesterol ester transfer protein, depletion of high-density lipoprotein (HDL) by the same mechanism, depletion of antioxidants within the lipoprotein particles, and perhaps direct oxidative modification of VLDL and LDL in plasma. These modifications result in particles that have enhanced ath-

VLDL and LDL Metabolism
Significance of the residence time
A long residence time may be atherogenic

- Permits undesirable changes to occur to the lipoprotein particles
  - Cholesterol ester enrichment
  - Depletion of natural antioxidants
  - Oxidation of lipoprotein lipids
  - Reduced affinity for LDL receptors
- These changes channel the particle to slow cellular uptake pathways, e.g. arterial wall, rather than to LDL receptors in liver and steroidogenic tissues.
- Reduction in VLDL and LDL residence times by estrogen may be anti-atherogenic

FIGURE 1.

erogenicity.[15–17] Cholesterol-ester-rich VLDL causes cholesterol accumulation in macrophages and is found in diet-induced atherosclerosis in animal models.[17–20] Oxidatively modified VLDL and LDL are recognized by cellular receptors that promote cholesterol deposition and other atherosclerotic processes in vascular intima.[13,14,21] In summary, a long residence time for a lipoprotein class in plasma could enhance the action of several abnormal metabolic pathways that promote atherosclerosis. We propose that an intervention that decreases residence time is likely to be antiatherogenic whether or not plasma concentrations of the lipoprotein are affected. These considerations are critical to interpreting the metabolic perturbations caused by estrogen in the lipoprotein pathways, and explaining the protective effect of estrogen against atherosclerosis.

Effect of Estrogen

VLDL and Triglycerides

Oral estrogen treatment raises plasma VLDL triglyceride (Figure 2). Hepatic triglyceride production increases,[22,23] whereas the

Effects of Estrogen on VLDL Metabolism

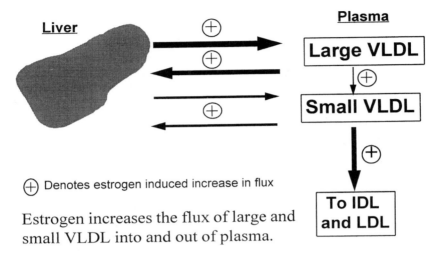

⊕ Denotes estrogen induced increase in flux

Estrogen increases the flux of large and small VLDL into and out of plasma.

FIGURE 2.

clearance of triglyceride, and the activity of lipoprotein lipase, appear to be unaffected.[22-26] There are few studies of estrogen on human VLDL-apo B metabolism. Estrogen increases VLDL-apo B levels.[9] Several mechanisms for these actions have been identified. Estrogen increases VLDL-apo B levels by increasing production by the liver of VLDL particles of all sizes but particularly of large VLDL particles.[10,11] In three premenopausal women, a supraphysiological dose of ethinyl estradiol increased VLDL-apo B synthesis by 86% without affecting clearance.[27] Such large increases in the synthesis of VLDL apo B and of VLDL triglyceride[22,23] may reflect a pharmacological action of oral estrogens. Walsh et al.[10] studied the effect of micronized estradiol, 2 mg daily, compared with placebo in nine postmenopausal women, using a primed continuous infusion of a nonradioactive isotope of leucine to endogenously label apo B. Estradiol increased VLDL apo B production by 50%; most of the effect was on large VLDL, an 82% increase. There was a trend for the fractional catabolic rate of VLDL-apo B also to be increased. Walsh and Sacks[11] compared apo B metabolism in users and nonusers of contemporary low-dose oral contraceptives. As with postmenopausal use of estrogen, estrogen use in oral contraceptives increased the plasma level and production rate of the large, triglyceride rich VLDL subfraction (Sf60–400), by three- and fivefold, respectively, and small VLDL (Sf20–60) levels and production rates were two- and threefold higher. There were no significant differences in fractional catabolic rates for VLDL between users and nonusers. Estrogen had a greater effect in oral contraceptive users than in the postmeno-pausal women, consistent with the higher potency of the estrogen for contraceptive compared to postmenopausal use.

Studies of hepatocytes in culture showed that estrogen increases VLDL secretion.[28] In rats and mice, estrogen increases hepatocyte apo B messenger ribonucleic acid (mRNA) transcription.[29] Estrogen therefore appears to have direct effects on hepatic apo B metabolism that could explain the increase in the VLDL-apo B production rate into plasma.

Clinical Correlation

In summary, the underlying mechanism for the increase in plasma VLDL-apo B and triglyceride levels caused by estrogen is an increase in VLDL secretion into plasma, preceded by increased apo B gene tran-scription. Clearance of VLDL particles from plasma tends to be ac-celerated, decreasing the plasma residence time. This estrogenic mechanism is quite different than that responsible for primary hyper-triglyceridemia, or that associated with obesity or diabetes (Figure 3). In these clinical conditions, lipolysis of VLDL is impaired, clearance of VLDL and triglycerides is diminished, and the residence time is in-creased. The impairment in catabolism may be compounded by in-creased VLDL-apo B or triglyceride production. VLDL remnants form and become enriched in triglyceride and cholesterol ester.[1,4,14,30,31] These remnant particles promote lipid accumulation and are consid-ered to be atherogenic in macrophages.[17–20]

HDL levels are decreased in primary hypertriglyceridemia, or that due to obesity or diabetes, rather than increased as occurs with estrogen treatment. Low-HDL levels may result from the coexisting defect in VLDL catabolism because HDL forms in part from the as-sociation of apolipoproteins, phospholipids, and cholesterol re-leased from VLDL during lipolysis in plasma.[32] These changes in VLDL and HDL are in the direction of increased atherogenicity, the opposite of lipoprotein changes with estrogen.

LDL Metabolism

We investigated the effect of oral estradiol, 2 mg, on LDL me-tabolism in postmenopausal women using endogenous labeling with

Contrast between hypertriglyceridemia due to estrogen and endogenous hypertriglyceridemia

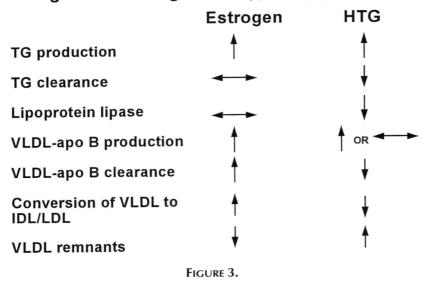

FIGURE 3.

trideuterated leucine (Figure 4). Estrogen treatment decreased LDL levels by increasing the rate of its catabolism by 36%.[10] This increase in clearance exceeds a lesser increase in LDL production[10] by conversion of VLDL.

Erickson et al.[33] found a similar effect on LDL metabolism in men with prostate cancer treated with large doses of synthetic estrogens. Recently, Wolfe and Huff[34] confirmed that estrogen replacement therapy increased the LDL fractional catabolic rate, measured by the disappearance curve of autologous radio-iodinated LDL. In estrogen-treated baboons, LDL-apo B production and clearance were increased with the acceleration of clearance predominating.[35] VLDL particles pass through a subfraction intermediate in density and size between VLDL and LDL, appropriately termed, IDL. Our preliminary work indicates that estrogen increases the flux (number of particles per time) of VLDL through the IDL fraction to LDL, thereby increasing LDL flux. There is little direct LDL production by the liver.

Estrogen increases LDL receptor activity. Estrogen upregulates LDL receptors in vitro in rat hepatocytes[36] and in porcine granulosa cells.[37] Angelin et al.[38] studied liver biopsy specimens from two men who were receiving estrogen treatment for prostate cancer. Com-

Evidence for increased LDL-receptor mediated clearance of LDL by estrogen

Human Studies

- Postmenopausal women
  - LDL fractional catabolic rate increased by physiological estrogen replacement.
- Elderly men with prostate cancer
  - LDL FCR increased by massive doses of estrogen
  - ^{125}I-LDL binding activity increased in liver membranes from biopsy specimens

Rodent Models

- Specific binding of ^{125}I-LDL increased in liver membranes
- Increased LDL receptor gene transcription and mRNA levels
- Increased LDL receptor protein translation and levels

FIGURE 4.

pared with liver biopsies from healthy subjects, the biopsies from estrogen-treated patients showed LDL receptor activity was increased threefold, HMG coenzyme A (CoA) reductase activity was increased twofold, and microsomal unesterified cholesterol concentration was 30% lower. Estrogen appears to increase LDL receptor synthesis. Hepatocytes of estrogen-treated rats and mice, compared with untreated animals, have a higher transcription rate of the LDL receptor gene, higher LDL receptor mRNA levels, increased mRNA translation rates, and increased LDL receptor protein mass in the rat.[29] These experiments indicate multiple points of action by estrogens on LDL receptor synthesis. Therefore, an increase in LDL receptor activity, preceded by increased LDL receptor gene transcription and receptor synthesis is the likely cause of the accelerated clearance of LDL from the circulation.

LDL Subclass Metabolism

LDL is composed of a heterogeneous group of particles that differ in size, density and functional characteristics.[39–41] One classification system determines the predominant type of LDL particles based on size. LDL subclass Pattern A (predominant LDL species of large sizes $\geq$260 A) is prevalent in women and is associated with a low rate of cardiovascular disease compared with the alternate LDL type, Pattern B, (predominant LDL species of small size <260 A). Within Pattern A, there is an LDL subclass I pattern (predominant LDL species >271 A) and subclass II pattern (predominant LDL size 260-271A). The clinical significance of this subclassification of Pattern A is unknown, and it cannot be assumed that the larger the LDL the lower the cardiovascular risk. For example, in atherosclerosis models in monkeys, dietary cholesterol produces very large, cholesterol-rich LDL particles that are considered responsible for the atherosclerosis.[42]

Estrogens affect the predominant type of LDL particles in plasma. Campos et al.[43] found that postmenopausal hormonal replacement therapy with conjugated equine estrogens, 0.625 and 1.25 mg, decreased the relative amount and the size of LDL subclass I particles compared with subclass II particles, but only in the women who were classified as having a predominant LDL subclass I band (Figure 5). Estrogen treatment did not convert any women to an LDL subclass pattern B, nor did it increase the relative quantity of the LDL subclass III particles (<260 A). This is an important consideration, because small LDL III particles, which constitute the Pattern B designation, are associated with coronary heart disease in men. These findings are consistent with those of Granfone et al.[44] in post-

Effect of estrogen on LDL size distribution in women with LDL Subclass I

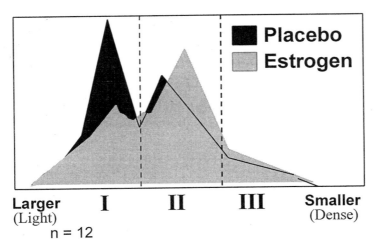

FIGURE 5.

menopausal women treated with ethinyl estradiol and de Graaf et al.[45] in premenopausal women taking oral contraceptives, both showing a relative shift to a smaller average size LDL particle. Our unpublished work indicates that estrogen decreased light (d = 1.019–1.035) LDL-apo B but not dense (d = 1.035–1.063) LDL apo B concentrations. These findings suggest that the shift in LDL particle size distribution is caused by a decrease in large LDL rather than by an increase in small LDL particles.

Functional characteristics of LDL particles are also affected by estrogen. The affinity of LDL for the LDL receptor was reduced after estrogen treatment.[33] This could result from the shift in particle size because the reduction in the larger size particles with higher affinity leaves smaller size particles with lower affinity.[40,46,47] Our preliminary data on the metabolism of LDL subclasses suggest that estrogen increased the clearance rate of light LDL subfraction more than the dense fraction thereby increasing the proportion of LDL in the dense region. Our proposed model of the effects of estrogen on LDL subclass metabolism, derived from published work and our preliminary observations, is shown in Figure 6.

Unifying Mechanism for the Effects of Estrogen on VLDL and LDL Metabolism

Estrogen has multiple actions on VLDL and LDL metabolism: increased triglyceride synthesis, increased apo B production, increased LDL production, and increased LDL receptors (Figure 7). We hypothesize that these actions may be linked. O'Sullivan et al.[48] provide evidence from a case report that estrogen decreases β-oxidation of fatty acids by the liver. A 19-year-old woman being treated with estrogen for ovarian agenesis showed a dose-dependent reduction in lipid oxidation in the fasting and postprandial states, measured by indirect calorimetry. Inhibition of fatty acid oxidation promotes triglyceride synthesis. The increased intrahepatic triglyceride in turn may enhance the synthesis of VLDL particles by protecting newly translated apo B from degradation. An increase in VLDL synthesis depletes cellular cholesterol used in the assembly of VLDL particles. The hepatocyte, to restore normal cholesterol levels, increases cholesterol biosynthesis as well as upregulates LDL receptor activity. In this view, the primary effect of estrogen is the stimulation of VLDL production preceded by redirection of fatty acids from β-oxidation to triglyceride synthesis.

Proposed model of LDL subclass metabolism

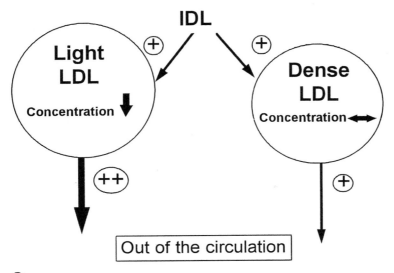

⊕ Denotes increase in flux by estrogen

FIGURE 6.

Effects of estrogen on VLDL and LDL metabolism: Proposed unifying mechanism

Inhibition of beta-oxidation of fatty acids?

↓

Stimulation of triglyceride synthesis

↓

Stimulation of apo B and VLDL production

↓

Depletion of microsomal cholesterol for use in VLDL assembly

↓

Upregulation of LDL receptors

↓

Increased LDL uptake from plasma

FIGURE 7.

HDL Metabolism

Commonly prescribed doses of oral postmenopausal estrogens increase plasma HDL levels, measured either by the cholesterol component, or by apolipoprotein A-I (apo A-I), the principal protein component (Figure 8). The magnitude of the increases is ~15%.[9] The predominant effect of estrogen is on the larger size HDL2 rather than the smaller HDL3 subfraction. This is clearly shown by Silliman et al.,[49] who studied women in late pregnancy when serum estradiol levels are extremely high. The HDL particles during pregnancy became much larger shifting the distribution to the largest, HDL2b, subfraction. Walsh et al.[50] found that oral estradiol treatment of postmenopausal women significantly increased the levels of HDL-2 apo A-I by 37% and HDL-3 apo A-I by 11%. Kinetic studies found that HDL apo A-I is produced at a more rapid rate during estrogen treatment and accounted for the increase in HDL-apo A-I levels.[50] The apo A-I clearance rate was unchanged. Schaefer et al.[27] found that the production of total HDL protein was increased by ethinyl estradiol treatment of premenopausal women.[27] In baboons, Kushwaha et al.[51] also found increases in plasma apo A-I production.

In vitro experiments in cultured cells support the conclusions from in vivo metabolism studies that estrogen increases apo A-I production. Estrogen increases apo A-I synthesis in cultured human

Effects of estrogen on HDL metabolism

- Apo A-I production rate increased in postmenopausal women
- HDL protein production rate increased in premenopausal women
- HDL size increased
- Apo A-I secretion increased in liver cells (HepG2)
- Apo A-II levels not increased by estrogen in postmenopausal women
- Probable selective increase in LpA-I not LpAI/AII particles
- Hepatic lipase decreased
- CETP unchanged

FIGURE 8.

hepatoma cells,[52] increased apo A-I transcription and translation rates in rat and mouse liver.[29] Transcription was stimulated more so than translation, suggesting multiple points of regulation of hepatic apo A-I synthesis. In contrast, intestinal apo A-I mRNA synthesis was not affected by estrogen.[29]

We found that postmenopausal estrogen replacement increased plasma HDL-apo A-I concentrations much more than it increased plasma HDL-apolipoprotein A-II (apo A-II).[10] We hypothesized that estrogen selectively increases the subspecies of HDL that contains apo A-I but not apo A-II.[53,54] This subspecies, but not the subspecies of HDL that contains both apo A-I and apo A-II, is higher in women than in men and increases in girls during puberty.[55] Brinton et al.[56] recently reported that estrogen increased the flux of apo A-I but not apo A-II. Thus the combined evidence makes it likely that estrogen has a selective effect on the HDL particles that contain apo A-I but not apo A-II, which are likely to be the antiatherogenic particles.

Estrogen diminishes hepatic lipase activity, which is thought to facilitate the catabolism of HDL particles.[25,26] Although this could inhibit the clearance rate of HDL particles, it appears that the stimulation of HDL production is the dominant metabolic change caused by estrogen. Cholesterol ester transfer protein, which transfers cholesterol ester from HDL to VLDL and LDL in exchange for triglyceride, is not affected by postmenopausal estrogen replacement[57] and does not appear to explain the triglyceride enrichment of HDL during estrogen treatment.[10]

Lipoprotein(a)

Estrogens lower lipoprotein(a) [Lp(a)] levels. Sacks et al.[57] studied the effect of two doses of conjugated estrogens, 0.625 and 1.25 mg daily on Lp(a) levels in postmenopausal women. Lp(a) levels decreased by 14% and 16% on the two doses, respectively. Soma et al.[58] found that hormonal replacement therapy with conjugated estrogens 1.25 mg daily plus medroxyprogesterone acetate 10 mg daily for 10 days per month, both relatively physiological doses, lowered Lp(a) levels by ~50%. Kim et al.[59] and Lobo et al.[60] found that conjugated estrogen treatment, with and without concomitant MPA, lowered Lp(a) levels. Henriksson et al.[61] found estrogen treatment of men with prostate cancer lowered Lp(a). Nabulsi et al.[62] reported that Lp(a) levels in postmenopausal women who were receiving hormonal replacement therapy with estrogen were 13% lower than in a comparison group of women who were not taking hormones.

There are no published studies on the mechanism by which estrogen lowers Lp(a). Our preliminary results using endogenous labeling of apo (a) with trideuterated leucine indicate reduced production of apo (a) with no change in clearance. This is consistent with other Lp(a) metabolism studies that show that changes in Lp(a) levels are caused by changes in the production rate.[63–66] Although Lp(a) has apo B-100 and could theoretically be affected by upregulation of LDL receptors by estrogen, it appears that the apo (a) protein interferes with recognition of apo B by LDL receptors.

Summary and Conclusions

Estrogen has many and complex effects on lipoprotein metabolism (Figure 9). Estrogen increases the production of VLDL triglycerides and apo B, raising triglyceride and VLDL levels. Although both VLDL and triglycerides are risk factors for the development of cardiovascular disease, the responsible mechanisms for the estrogenic effect are not the same as in genetic hypertriglyceridemia or with obesity or diabetes. In these high-risk patients, clearance of VLDL and triglycerides from plasma is impaired; this can lead to

Composite view: effects of estrogen on lipoprotein metabolism

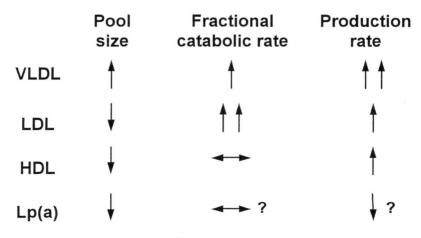

FIGURE 9.

atherogenic remnant formation. In fact, clearance of VLDL may well be accelerated with estrogen. This could be an instance where an increase in a risk factor, the triglyceride level, may paradoxically reflect an anti-atherogenic state. This illustrates that plasma lipoprotein concentrations provide an incomplete picture, and, at times, a misleading one with regard to inferring cardiovascular risk in certain groups of individuals.

The results of metabolism studies also suggest that the underlying mechanisms for the decrease in LDL and increase in HDL are protective. Enhanced clearance of LDL by upregulated LDL receptors directs plasma LDL to normal, physiological removal sites, rather than entry and accumulation in vascular intima. Increased clearance reduces the time a particle spends in the circulation, limiting the adverse effect of oxidative processes. For HDL, an increase in the production rate into plasma of HDL particles with apo A-I, increases the flux of particles that can participate in cholesterol removal from cells and in reverse cholesterol transport.

The question arises as to why evolution favored multiple actions of estrogen that protects against atherosclerosis, a disease of aging persons. Each of the effects on lipoprotein metabolism increases the efficiency of lipid transport between tissues. These actions of estrogen, a reproductive hormone, could be beneficial during pregnancy or lactation to deliver fatty acids to adipose tissue for storage or to the developing fetus.

References

1. Packard CJ, Munro A, Lorimer AR, et al. Metabolism of apolippprotein B in large triglyceride-rich very low density lipoproteins of normal and hypertriglyceridemic subjects. *J Clin Invest* 1984;74:2178–2192.
2. Howard BV, Egusa G, Beltz WF, et al. Compensatory mechanisms governing concentration of plasma low density lipoprotein. *J Lipid Res* 1986;2711–2720.
3. Teng B, Sniderman AD, Soutar AK, et al. Metabolic basis of hyperapobetalipoproteinemia. *J Clin Invest* 1986;77:663-672.
4. Beltz WF, Kesaniemi YA, Miller NH, et al. Studies on the metabolism of apo B in hypertriglyceridemic subjects using simultaneous administration of tritiated leucine and radioiodinated VLDL. *J Lipid Res* 1990; 31:361–374.
5. Marzetta CA, Foster DM, Brunzell JD. Conversion of plasma VLDL and IDL precursors into various LDL subpopulations using density gradient ultracentrifugation. *J Lipid Res* 1990;31:975–984.
6. Vega GL, Grundy SM. Kinetic heterogeneity of LDL in primary hypertriglyceridemia. *Arteriosclerosis* 1986;6:395–406.

7. Fisher WR, Zech LA, Bardalaye P, et al. The metabolism of apo B in subjects with hypertriglyceridemia and polydisperse LDL. *J Lipid Res* 1980;21:760–774.
8. Hara H, Howard BV. Characterization of LDL binding in TR 715-19 cells. *Atherosclerosis* 1990;83:155–165.
9. Sacks FM, Walsh BW. Sex hormones and lipoprotein metabolism. An extensive review of the effects of estrogen and progestins on VLDL, and LDL metabolism. *Curr Opin Lipidol* 1994;5:236–240.
10. Walsh BW, Schiff I, Rosner B, et al. Effects of postmenopausal estrogen replacement on the concentrations and metabolism of plasma lipoproteins. *N Engl J Med* 1991;325:1196–1204.
11. Walsh BW, Sacks FM. The effect of low dose oral contraceptives on very low density and low density lipoprotein metabolism. *J Clin Invest* 1993;91:2126–2132.
12. Kesaniemi YA, Witztum JL, Steinbrecher UP. Receptor-mediated catabolism of low density lipoproteins in man. *J Clin Invest* 1983; 71:950–959.
13. Packard CJ, Boag DE, Clegg R, et al. Effects of 1,2-cyclohexanedione modification on the metabolism of very low density lipoprotein apolipoprotein B: Potential role of receptors in intermediate density lipoprotein catabolism. *J Lipid Res* 1985;26:1058–1067.
14. Spady DK, Huettenger M, Bilheimer DW, et al. Role of receptor-independent low density lipoprotein transport in the maintenance of tissue cholesterol balance in the normal and WHHL rabbit. *J Lipid Res* 1987;28:32–41.
15. Hoff HF, Hoppe G. Structure of cholesterol-containing particles accumulating in atherosclerotic lesions and the mechanisms of their derivation. *Curr Opin Lipidol* 1995;6:317–325.
16. Bruce C, Tall AR. Cholesteryl ester transfer proteins, reverse cholesterol transport, and atherosclerosis. *Curr Opin Lipidol* 1995;6:306–311.
17. Tabas I. The stimulation of the cholesterol esterification pathway by atherogenic lipoproteins in macrophages. *Curr Opin Lipidol* 1995; 6:260–268.
18. Bradley WA, Gianturco SH. Triglyceride-rich lipoproteins and atherosclerosis: Pathophysiological considerations. *J Intern Med* 1994; 236(suppl 736):33–39.
19. Sacks FM, Breslow JL. Very low density lipoproteins stimulate cholesterol ester formation in U937 macrophages. Heterogeneity and biologic variation among normal humans. *Arteriosclerosis* 1987;7:35–46.
20. Zilversmit DB. Atherogenesis: A postprandial phenomenon. *Circulation* 1979;60:473–485.
21. Navab M, Berliner JA, Watson AD, et al. The Yin and Yang of oxidation in the development of the fatty streak. A review based on the 1994 George Lyman Duff Memorial Lecture. *Arterioscler Thromb Vasc Biol* 1996;16:831–42.
22. Glueck CJ, Fallat RW, Scheel D. Effects of estrogenic compounds on triglyceride kinetics. *Metabolism* 1975;24:537–545.
23. Kissebah AH, Harrigan P, Wynn V. Mechanism of hypertriglyceridemia associated with contraceptive steroids. *Horm Metab Res* 1973;5:184–190.
24. Taskinen M-R. Lipoprotein lipase in hypertriglyceridemias. In: Borensztajn J (ed). *Lipoprotein Lipase* Chicago: Evener Publishers, 1987: 201–228.

25. Tikkanen MJ, Kuusi T, Nikkila EA, et al. Very low density lipoprotein triglyceride kinetics during hepatic lipase suppression by estrogen. *FEBS Lett* 1985;181:160–164.
26. Tikkanen MJ, Nikkila EA, Kuusi T, et al. HDL-2 and hepatic lipase: Reciprocal changes produced by estrogen and norgestrel. *J Clin Endocrinol Metab* 1982;54:1113–1117.
27. Schaefer EJ, Foster DM, Zech LA, et al. The effects of estrogen administration on plasma lipoprotein metabolism in premenopausal females. *J Clin Endocrinol Metab* 1983;57:262–267.
28. Miller KW, Lane MD. Estradiol-induced alteration of very-low-density lipoprotein assembly. *J Biol Chem* 1984;259:15277–15286.
29. Srivastava RAK, Baumann D, Schonfeld G. In vivo regulation of LDL receptors by estrogen differs at the post-transcriptional level in rat and mouse. *Eur J Biochem* 1993;216:527–538.
30. Bradley WA, Gianturco SH. Triglyceride-rich lipoproteins and atherosclerosis: Pathophysiological considerations. *J Intern Med* 1994; 236(suppl 736):33–39.
31. Brunzell JD, Hazzard WR, Porte D Jr, et al. Evidence for a common, saturable, triglyceride removal mechanism for chylomicrons and very low density lipoprotens in man. *J Clin Invest* 1973;52:1578–1585.
32. Eisenberg S. High density lipoprotein metabolism. *J Lipid Res* 1984; 25:1017–1058.
33. Erickson M, Berglund L, Rudling M, et al. Effects of estrogen on LDL metabolism in males. *J Clin Invest* 1989;84:820–10.
34. Wolfe BM, Huff MW. Effects of continuous low-dosage hormonal replacement therapy on lipoprotein metabolism in postmenopausal women. *Metabolism* 1995;44:410–417.
35. Kushwaha RS, Foster DM, Barrett PH, et al. Effect of estrogen and progesterone on metabolism of apoprotein B in baboons. *Am J Physiol* 1990;258:E172–E183.
36. Windler E, Kovanen PT, Chao YS, et al. The estradiol-stimulated lipoprotein receptor of rat liver. *J Biol Chem* 1980;255:10464.
37. Veldhuis JD, Gwynne JT, Azini P, et al. Estrogen regulates LDL metabolism by cultured swine granulosa cells. *Endocrinology* 1985;117:1321.
38. Angelin B, Olivecrona H, Reihner E, et al. Hepatic cholesterol metabolism in estrogen-treated men. *Gastroenterology* 1992;103:1657–1663.
39. Krauss RM, Burke DJ. Identification of multiple subclasses of plasma LDL in normal humans. *J Lipid Res* 1982;23:97–104.
40. Austin MA, Breslow JL, Hennekens CH, et al. LDL subclass patterns and risk of myocardial infarction. *JAMA* 1988;260:1917–1921.
41. Fisher WR. Heterogeneity of plasma LDL. *Metabolism* 1983;32: 283–291.
42. Rudel LL, Parks JS, Johnson FS, et al. LDL in atherosclerosis. *J Lipid Res* 1986;27:465–474.
43. Campos H, Sacks FM, Walsh BW, et al. Differential effects of estrogen on low density lipoprotein subclasses in healthy postmenopausal women. *Metabolism* 1993;42:1153–1158.
44. Granfone A, Campos H, McNamara JR, et al. Effects of estrogen replacement on plasma lipoproteins and apolipoproteins in postmenopausal, dyslipidemic women. *Metabolism* 1992;41:1193–1198.
45. de Graaf J, Swinkels DW, Demacker PN, et al. Differences in the LDL subfraction profile between oral contraceptive users and controls. *J Clin Endocriol Metab* 1993;76:197–202.

46. Kleinman Y, Eisenberg S, Oschry Y, et al. Defective metabolism of hypertriglyceridemic LDL in cultured human skin fibroblasts. *J Clin Invest* 1985;75:1796.
47. Kinoshita M, Krul ES, Schonfeld G. Modification of the core lipids of LDL produces selective alterations in the expression of apoB-100 epitopes. *J Lipid Res* 1990;31:701–708.
48. O'Sullivan AJ, Hoffman DM, Ho KK. Estrogen, lipid oxidation, and body fat. Letter. *N Engl J Med* 1995;333:669–670.
49. Silliman K, Tall AR, Kretchmer N, et al. Unusual HDL subclass distribution during late pregnancy. *Metabolism* 1993;42:1592–1599.
50. Walsh BW, Li H, Sacks FM: Effects of postmenopausal hormone replacement with oral and transdermal estrogen on HDL metabolism. *J Lipid Res* 1994;35:2083–2093.
51. Kushwaha RS, Foster DM, Murthy VN, et al. Metabolic regulation of high-density lipoproteins by estrogen and progesterone in the baboon. *Metabolism* 1990;39:544.
52. Archer TK, Tam Sp, Deeley RG. Kinetics of estrogen-dependent modulation of apolipoprotein A-I synthesis in human hepatoma cells. *J Biol Chem* 1986;261:5067–5074.
53. McVicar JP, Kunitake ST, Hamilton RL, et al. Characteristics of human lipoproteins isolated by immunoaffinity chromatography. *Proc Natl Acad Sci USA* 1984;81:1356–1360.
54. Cheung MC, Albers JJ. Characterization of lipoprotein particles isolated by immunoaffinity chromatography. *J Biol Chem* 1984;259:12201–12209.
55. Ohta T, Hattori H, Murakami M, et al. Age and sex related differences in lipoproteins containing apo A-I. *Arteriosclerosis* 1989;9:90–95.
56. Brinton EA. Oral estrogen replacement therapy in postmenopausal women selectively raises levels and production rates of lipoprotein A-I and lowers hepatic lipase activity without lowering the fractional catabolic rate. *Arterioscler Thromb Vasc Biol* 1996;16:431–440.
57. Sacks FM, McPherson R, Walsh BW. Effect of postmenopausal estrogen replacement on plasma Lp(a) lipoprotein concentrations. *Arch Intern Med* 1994;154:1106–1110.
58. Soma MR, Osnago-Adda I, Paoletti, et al. The lowering of lipoproten(a) induced by estrogen plus progesterone replacement therapy in postmenopausal women. 1993;153(12):1462–1468.
59. Kim CJ, Jang HC, Cho DH, et al, Effects of hormone replacement therapy on lipoprotein(a) and lipids in postmenopausal women. *Arterioscler Thromb* 1994;14:275–281.
60. Lobo RA, Pickar JH, Wild RA, et al. Metabolic impact of adding medroxyprogesterone acetate to conjugated estrogen therapy in postmenopausal women. *Obstet Gynecol* 1994;84:987–995.
61. Henriksson P, Angelin B, Berglund L. Hormonal regulation of serum Lp(a) levels. Opposite effects after estrogen treatment and orchidectomy in males with prostatic carcinoma. *J Clin Invest* 1992;89(4):1166–1171.
62. Nabulsi AA, Folsom AR, White A, et al. Association of hormone-replacement therapy with various cardiovascular risk factors in postmenopausal women. *N Engl J Med* 1993;328(15):1115–1117.
63. Krempler F, Kostner GM, Bolzano K. Turnover of lipoprotein (a) in man. *J Clin Invest* 1980;65:1483–1490.
64. Rader DJ, Cain W, Ikewaki K, et al. The inverse association of plasma lipoprotein (a) concentrations with apolipoprotein (a) isoform size is

not due to difference in Lp(a) catabolism but to differences in production rate. *J Clin Invest* 1994;93:2758–2763.

65. Rader DJ, Cain W, Zech LA, et al. Variation in lipoprotein (a) concentrations among individuals with the same apolipoprotein (a) isoform is determined by the rate of lipoprotein (a) production. *J Clin Invest* 1993;91:443–447.

66. Morrisett JM, Gaubatz JW, Nava MN, et al. Metabolism of apo(a) and apoB100 in human lipoprotein (a). In: Catapano AL, Gotto AM, Smith LC, Paoletti R, eds. *Drugs Affecting Lipid Metabolism.* Amsterdam: Kluwer Academic Publishers; 1993;161–167.

Chapter 15

Triglyceride as a Risk Factor For Cardiovascular Disease in Women and Men

Melissa A. Austin, PhD
and John E. Hokanson, MPH

Plasma triglyceride has long been implicated as a risk factor for coronary heart disease. The first case-control studies in men[1] and women[2] showed that fasting triglyceride levels were increased among coronary heart disease (CHD) cases compared with controls subjects. The earliest prospective study of triglyceride and ischemic heart disease (IHD) demonstrated increased incidence of IHD among men in the cohort with elevated triglyceride levels at baseline compared with men with lower triglyceride levels.[3] The authors speculated that the triglyceride association may not have been independent of other plasma lipid levels. Gordon et al.[4] extended these observations to women, showing that triglyceride was associated with incident disease among women in the Framingham Study, but this association was not independent of other lipids.

In the decades after these studies, an extensive literature developed examining the role of triglyceride as a risk factor for cardiovascular disease. In a review of these studies, Austin noted that most studies showed a relation between triglyceride and CHD.[5] However, a number of studies found that this association did not remain statistically significant after controlling for other lipid risk factors, especially high-density lipoprotein cholesterol (HDL-C). In reviewing this and other evidence, the National Institutes of Health Consensus Development Panel on Triglyceride, HDL and Coronary Heart Dis-

This study was supported by National Heart, Blood, and Lung Institute grants HL-30086 and HL-45913. This work was performed during Dr. Austin's tenure as an Established Investigator of the American Heart Association.

From: Forte TM, (ed). *Hormonal, Metabolic, and Cellular Influences on Cardiovascular Disease in Women.* Armonk, NY: Futura Publishing Company, Inc.; © 1997.

ease concluded that, "For triglyceride, the data are mixed, although strong associations are found in some studies, the evidence for a causal relation (with CHD) is still incomplete"[6]. Similarly, recent data from the Lipid Research Clinics (LRC) follow-up study demonstrated that triglyceride was related to 12-year CHD mortality in both men and women,[7] but this relation was no longer statistically significant after adjustment for covariates. Thus, the role of triglyceride as a risk factor for CHD remains to be fully elucidated.

This chapter will focus on three types of studies that have examined the relation between triglyceride and cardiovascular disease. First, the semiquantitative techniques of meta-analysis will be applied to population-based, prospective studies of triglyceride and cardiovascular disease (CVD), resulting in estimates of the strength of the association among women and men, and evaluating the effects of other risk factors, especially HDL-C.[8,9] Second, recent clinical studies that have investigated postprandial lipoproteins in relation to coronary artery disease, and triglyceride-rich lipoproteins and atherosclerosis severity will be considered. Finally, ongoing genetic studies of the familial forms of hypertriglyceridemia and 20-year cardiovascular disease mortality will be described.

Epidemiological Studies

Meta-Analysis of Triglyceride and Cardiovascular Disease

Published studies from the literature were selected for the meta-analysis based on several criteria.[8] First, only studies using a prospective study design were selected, ensuring that elevations in plasma triglyceride preceded the onset of disease. Second, only studies using population-based samples of study subjects were selected, so that relative risk estimates are as applicable as possible to the general population. Because the results from the LRC follow-up study[7] were based on a sample enriched with hyperlipidemic subjects, the relative risks for this analysis were adjusted for ascertainment (hyperlipidemic vs. random sample) based on results kindly provided by Dr. M. H. Criqui (personal communication). To exclude the possibility of postprandial effects, only studies evaluating fasting triglyceride levels were included. Each study cohort was included only once in the analysis, the publication reporting the longest follow-time was used. Both fatal and nonfatal cardiovascular endpoints were included, although most studies focused on myocardial infarction or CHD death. Finally, only Caucasian study subjects were included in the analysis, because little data are currently available on other ethnic groups.

As shown in Tables 1 and 2, a total of 17 studies conforming to these selection criteria were identified,[3,7,10–26] 16 in men and 5 in women. Study subjects ranged in age from 15 to 81 years old in all the studies. Of the studies in men, six were from the USA, six from Scandinavian countries, and one each from France, Germany, Italy, and the United Kingdom. A total of 46,413 men were included in these studies, and 2,445 cardiovascular events were reported. Of the studies in women, three were from the USA and two from Scandinavia. A total of 10,684 women were studied, and 439 cardiovascular events were reported. Average follow-up time was 8.4 years in men and 11.4 years in women.

The meta-analysis was performed separately for men and women using the techniques described by Greenland.[9] Briefly, relative risk (RR) estimates were determined for each individual study by calculating β, the estimated slope from logistic regression analysis, representing the natural logarithm of the RR for the association between triglyceride and CVD. The β for each study was then standardized to a 1 mmol/L increase in triglyceride. To determine the statistical significance of the association and to calculate confidence intervals (CI), the variance of β was computed next. The β value for each study then was weighted by the inverse of the variance, reflecting both the sample size and follow-up time of study. Finally, the weighted β values were averaged and converted to the summary RR value, so that the larger the study and the longer the follow-up time, the greater its contribution to the summary RR. These procedures resulted in the univariate summary RR for the association between triglyceride and CVD. To further determine the effect of covariates on this estimate, the same procedures were used to estimate the multivariate summary RR using the six studies that included HDL-C as a covariate.[7,10,18,22,24,25] Of these studies, four also included adjustment for age, four for total cholesterol, two for low-density lipoprotein cholesterol (LDL-C), four for smoking, six for body mass index, and five for blood pressure. To maximize the potential effects of the potential confounders on the multivariate summary RR, all these covariate adjustments were included in the analysis.

As shown in Table 1, univariate RR estimates for cardiovascular disease associated with a 1 mmol/L increase in triglyceride ranged from 1.07 to 1.98 for men. In 13 of the 16 studies, this association was statistically significant, as shown by the lower bounds of the 95% confidence intervals exceeding 1.0. The univariate summary RR was 1.32 (95% CI 1.26–1.39), indicating a 32% increase in disease

TABLE 1

Population-Based Prospective Studies of Triglyceride and Cardiovascular Disease in Men

Study[a]	Study subjects[b]		Follow-up time (yrs)	Outcome[c] (no. of events)	Univariate relative risk[d]	Multivariate relative risk[d,e]
	Sample size	Age range				
Cardiovascular Health Center (3)	1,711	50–75	5	CHD death (56)	1.31 (0.78, 2.19)	—
Western Collaborative Group Study (10, 11)	2,966	39–59	8.5	CHD (257)	1.36 (1.13, 1.62)	0.98 (0.82, 1.17)
Stockholm Prospective Study (12)	3,486	15–79	14.5	MI death (321)	1.72 (1.35, 2.25)	—
Men Born in 1913 Study (13)	834	50	9	MI (44)	1.55 (1.01, 2.37)	—
Suomi-Salama Life Insurance Cohort (14)	1,648	50–53	7	CV death (75)	1.23 (1.03, 1.48)	—
Paris Prospective Study (15)	6,999	43–53	11.4	CHD death (157)	1.13 (1.04, 1.22)	—
Uppsala Primary Preventive Study (17)	2,322	45–53	7–10	MI (106)	1.72 (1.41, 2.10)	—
Framingham Heart Study (18)	2,536	30–74	14	CHD (374)	1.20 (0.84, 1.71)	1.12 (0.89, 1.41)
North Karelia Project (19)	4,057	30–59	7	MI (211)	1.66 (1.21, 2.29)	—

Study	No.	Age	Follow-up	Endpoint (events)	RR (95% CI)	RR (95% CI)
Cardiovascular Epidemiology Study (20)	294	50–75	4.5	CHD death (21)	1.07 (0.82, 1.40)	—
Normative Aging Study (21)	1,427	21–81	3–5	IHD (44)	1.98 (1.25, 3.11)	—
Caerphilly and Speedwell Collaborative Heart Disease Studies (22)	4,860	45–63	4.2	IHD (251)	1.46 (1.31, 1.84)	1.32 (1.08, 1.60)
Reykjavik Study (stage IV) (23)	1,332	45–72	8.6	MI (104)	1.39 (1.09, 1.77)	—
Prospective Cardiovascular Münster Study (24)	4,407	40–64	6	CAD (186)	1.33 (1.15, 1.52)	1.13 (0.96, 1.32)
Rome Occupational Groups (25, 26)	3,395	46–65	10	CHD death (98)	1.97 (1.58, 2.47)	0.98 (0.61, 1.62)
Lipid Research Clinics Follow-up Study (7)	4,129	≥30	12	CHD death (140)	1.49 (1.18, 1.89)	1.34 (0.93, 2.43)
Summary					1.32 (1.26, 1.39)	1.14 (1.05, 1.28)

[a] References numbers in parentheses.

[b] Includes only Caucasian study subjects.

[c] Fatal and nonfatal events unless indicated. CAD, coronary artery disease; CHD, coronary heart disease; CV, cardiovascular; IHD, ischemic heart disease; MI, myocardial infarction.

[d] Associated with a 1 mmol/L increase in triglyceride; 95% C.I. in parentheses.

[e] —, not calculated because HDL adjustment not reported.

TABLE 2

Population-Based Prospective Studies Included of Triglyceride and Cardiovascular Disease in Women

| Study[a] | Years of study | Study subjects[b] | | Follow-up time (yrs) | Outcome[c] (no. of events) | Univariate relative risk[d] | Multivariate relative risk[d,e] |
		Sample size	Age range				
Stockholm Prospective Study (12)	1961–1975	2,738	15–74	14.5	MI death (51)	1.94 (1.08, 4.40)	—
Study of Women in Gothenburg (16)	1968–1981	1,462	38–60	12	CHD death (75)	2.05 (1.33, 3.09)	—
Framingham Heart Study (18)	1972–1986	2,969	30–74	14	CHD (238)	1.69 (1.35, 2.10)	1.48 (1.08, 2.01)
Cardiovascular Epidemiology Study (20)	1974–1979	319	50–75	4.5	CHD death (14)	1.70 (1.12, 2.59)	—
Lipid Research Clinics Follow-up Study (7)	1972–1987	3,376	≥30	12	CHD death (61)	1.80 (1.18, 2.77)	1.13 (0.41, 2.42)
Summary						1.76 (1.50, 2.07)	1.37 (1.13, 1.66)

[a] Reference numbers in parentheses.
[b] Includes only Caucasian study subjects.
[c] Fatal and nonfatal events unless indicated; CHD, coronary heart disease; MI, myocardial infarction.
[d] Associated with a 1 mmol/L increase in triglyceride.
[e] —, not calculated because HDL cholesterol adjustment not reported.

risk associated with triglyceride. The narrow confidence interval is the result of including >46,000 men in the analysis. Note that because only prospective studies were analyzed, by definition, triglyceride elevations preceded the onset of disease. Among the five prospective studies in women, individual RR estimates for triglyceride ranged from 1.69 to 2.05 (Table 2), all of which were statistically significant. The summary univariate RR was higher for women than men, 1.76 (95% CI 1.50–2.07), although the confidence interval is somewhat wider due to the smaller sample size (~10,800 women). Thus, a 1 mmol/L increase in triglyceride was associated with a 76% increase in risk of incident cardiovascular disease in women.

It has long been noted that triglyceride is a more potent risk factor in Scandinavian countries than in other countries,[5] and meta-analysis allows a quantitative comparison of RR risk values in different geographic locations. Among men, RR values were 1.49 for studies conducted in Scandinavia, 1.25 for studies conducted in other European countries, and 1.34 for studies conducted in the USA (all $P < 0.05$). Among studies in women, RR values were also higher in Scandinavian countries than in the USA, 2.02 and 1.71, respectively. Thus, in both men and women, univariate RRs are indeed higher for studies conducted in Scandinavian countries compared with studies conducted elsewhere.

As expected, multivariate RR estimates with adjustment for HDLC were attenuated. For men, the multivariate RR for triglyceride ranged from 0.98 to 1.32, and the RR remained statistically significant for only one study (Table 1). However, the summary RR of 1.14 was statistically significant, with a 95% confidence interval of 1.05–1.28. In women, the multivariate adjusted RRs in women remained statistically significant in one study, but not the other (Table 2). Again, the summary estimate was higher for women than men, with a value of 1.37 (95% CI 1.13–1.66). Thus, even after adjustment for HDL-C, a statistically significant increase in risk of incident cardiovascular disease was associated with triglyceride for both men and women. Importantly, studies conducted in Scandinavia, in which univariate RRs are highest, are not included in these multivariate RRs because HDL-C adjustments were not reported. Thus, the multivariate RRs reported here for triglyceride are likely to be conservative.

This analysis appears to suggest that triglyceride may have a larger impact on CVD risk in women than men. However, when the data are standardized to age and gender specific variances of triglyceride in the general population (derived from the Lipid Research Clinics Prevalence Study[27]), the relative risk values were similar for men and women. Specifically, the univariate RR standardized to one standard deviation was 1.40 (95% CI 1.34–1.47) for men and 1.51 (95% CI 1.29–1.77) for women. The multivariate standardized RRs were 1.17 (95% CI 1.11–1.23) for men and 1.26 (95% CI 1.03–1.53) for women.

To summarize, based on all the available data from population-based, prospective studies, meta-analysis shows that increases in plasma triglyceride are associated with a significant increase in risk of incident cardiovascular disease among both men and women. In men, an increase of 1 mmol/L was associated with a 32% increase in risk of disease. A higher, 76% increased risk, was found in women. Based on data from studies that reported adjustment for HDL-C and other risk factors, multivariate RR estimates were attenuated, but were still statistically significant, representing a 14% increase in risk for men and a 37% increase in risk for women. Importantly, because only population-based studies were included in the analysis, these results provide the best available estimates of triglyceride risk in the general population. Therefore, triglyceride is a risk factor for cardiovascular disease, independent of HDL-C.

However, as demonstrated by the attenuated multivariate RR estimates, a major proportion of the risk of CVD attributable to triglyceride is accounted for by HDL-C, body mass index, blood pressure and possibly other risk factors. Austin et al.[28] have proposed an "atherogenic lipoprotein phenotype" characterized by small, dense LDL, increased triglyceride and lower HDL-C. The insulin-resistance syndrome[29] is characterized by a similar constellation of abnormal lipids, glucose intolerance, and hypertension, as well as insulin resistance itself. These complex metabolic syndromes, which include plasma triglyceride, suggest that the search for "independent" risk factors may mask the multifactorial nature of the pathophysiology involved. Rather, it may be useful to combine these correlated risk factors into a small number of composite variables using multivariate factor analysis[30] to elucidate the underlying disease mechanisms.

The analysis presented here was limited to Caucasian study subjects because very little data are currently available for non-Caucasian ethnic groups. However, a recent paper from the Honolulu Heart Program investigated the joint effects of HDL-C, triglyceride and total cholesterol on 18-year risk of atherosclerotic disease (including angina, aortic aneurysm, definite CHD, or thromboembolic stroke) in men of Japanese-American ancestry.[31] This study examined 1,646 men who were free of disease in 1970 and ranging in age from 51 to 72 years at that time. With follow-up through 1988, >25,000 person-years were included in the analysis. Age-adjusted incidence per 1,000 person years was computed for subgroups of study subjects using cutpoints of 35 mg/dL for HDL-C, 200 mg/dL for triglyceride, and total cholesterol <200, 200–239, and ≥240 mg/ dL. Among men with HDL <35 mg/dL, incidence rates were increased for those with high triglyceride (>200 mg/dL) in men with total cholesterol >200. Among men with HDL >35 mg/dL, incidence rates were increased among men with total cholesterol <239 mg/dL. These results show again that triglyceride is associated with increased risk of atherosclerosis in specific subgroups, even when HDLC and total cholesterol are taken into account.

Clinical Studies

Postprandial Lipoproteins and Coronary Artery Disease and Triglyceride-rich Lipoproteins and Atherosclerosis Severity

Interestingly, data from a variety of clinical studies corroborate the findings from epidemiological studies. For example, at least two recent studies have investigated the role of postprandial triglyceride-rich lipoproteins in relation to coronary artery disease.[32,33] In the first of these, postprandial response to a fatty meal was evaluated in 61 male subjects with severe coronary artery disease, compared to 40 control subjects.[32] Not only were postprandial triglyceride levels increased at 4, 6, and 8 hours after the meal in cases, but the peak concentration was also delayed. These findings persisted even after adjustment for fasting triglyceride levels. In the second study, 32 young male myocardial infarction survivors underwent angiography twice, 5 years apart.[33] The postprandial triglyceride response was significantly increased among hypertriglyceridemic cases compared with controls. Furthermore, a significant correlation was found between an atherosclerosis progression score and the concentration of Sf 20–60 apolipoprotein (apo) B-48 lipoproteins, reflecting small chylomicrons of intestinal origin.

Also important are the findings from the Monitored Atherosclerosis Progression Study, a double-blind, 2-year, placebo-controlled randomized trial of lovastatin to lower LDL-C among both men and women.[34] The primary endpoint in this study was per-subject change in percent diameter stenosis based on angiographic findings. In this study, cholesterol-rich lipoproteins were associated with lesion progression among subjects with severe lesions at baseline (>50% stenosis). In contrast, triglyceride-rich lipoproteins were related to progression of mild/moderate lesions (<50% stenosis). These findings indicate that triglycerides may have a role in atherogenesis that is distinct from cholesterol.

Genetic Studies

Familial Forms of Hypertriglyceridemia and Coronary Heart Disease

The two familial forms of hypertriglyceridemia, familial "monogenic" hypertriglyceridemia (FHTG) and familial combined hyperlipidemia (FCHL) were first characterized by Goldstein and colleagues[35] based on families of myocardial infarction (MI) survivors in the early 1970s. FHTG is characterized by familial aggregation of elevated plasma triglyceride levels in relatives, but with normal plasma cholesterol values. In contrast, relatives in families with FCHL have elevated triglyceride, elevated cholesterol or both, and these lipid phenotypes can vary over time. These two familial disorders were the most common in families of the MI survivors, with a prevalence of 16% and 32%, respectively. Importantly, *both* disorders were associated with increased risk of coronary heart disease in relatives of the probands.

Brunzell and colleagues further characterized these disorders based on families with familial aggregation of hypertriglyceridemia, regardless of CHD status. Among the 24 FCHL families and 19 FHTG families, the prevalence of MI among hyperlipidemic relatives, normolipidemic relatives and spouse controls were compared.[36] In contrast to the Goldstein studies, hyperlipidemic relatives in FCHL families were at increased risk, whereas relatives in FHTG families were not. On the basis of these findings, FCHL is generally associated with familial risk of CHD, whereas FHTG is not.

However, this conclusion remains to be confirmed prospectively, and the underlying genetic basis of these disorders is not yet understood. To address these and other questions, the "Genetic Epidemiology of Triglyceride Study" (GET Study), currently in progress, will follow-up these families after >20 years since the original family studies were performed. A total of 105 extended kindreds from both FCHL and FHTG families are included, with three primary goals. First, the study will determine whether total mortality and cardiovascular disease mortality is increased among relatives in these two types of families, using married-in spouses as controls. These studies will also allow an evaluation of triglyceride levels at baseline in relation to subsequent mortality. Second, the genetic epidemiology of a variety of lipoprotein-related risk factors are being evaluated based on new blood samples from surviving family members. Because FCHL and FHTG may be heterogeneous, statistical-genetic analyses of these variables may lead to refinement of the lipoprotein phenotypes that characterize these disorders. Finally, a repository of frozen white cells has been created for future DNA marker studies to determine the genetic basis of these common, triglyceride-related familial disorders.

Summary and Conclusions

In conclusion, meta-analysis of data from population-based prospective studies demonstrate that increased plasma triglyceride is associated with a 32% increase in risk of cardiovascular disease in men and a 76% increase in risk among women. After adjustment for HDL-C and other risk factors, these risks were reduced to 14% in men and increased to 37% in women, but remained statistically significant. These results, based on >46,000 men and 10,800 women, show that plasma triglyceride is an independent risk factor for cardiovascular disease. Clinical studies of triglyceride-rich lipoproteins in the postprandial state, and in relation to atherosclerosis severity confirm the importance of understanding triglyceride as a risk factor. However, few studies have included women and non-Caucasian ethnic groups and more data are urgently needed in these populations. Furthermore, better understanding of the familial forms of hypertriglyceridemia, including familial combined hyperlipidemia, will be important in determining how triglyceride may be involved in genetic susceptibility to CHD.

The current treatment recommendations for hypertriglyceridemia reflect the complex relations between triglyceride, HDL-C, and other plasma lipid risk factors. For example, the U.S. National Cholesterol Education Program Adult Treatment Panel II also proposed nonpharmacological therapy for elevated triglycerides, including increased physical activity.[37] In addition, drug therapy may be indicated for individuals with hypertriglyceridemia and other "atherogenic dyslipidemias" such as high total cholesterol or low HDL-C. Despite these recommendations, no clinical trial to date has been designed to directly evaluate whether lowering triglyceride can reduce risk of coronary heart disease. Taken together, the data presented in this chapter clearly demonstrate the necessity for rigorous testing of the impact of treating hypertriglyceridemia on cardiovascular risk by clinical trials.

References

1. Albrink MJ, Man EB. Serum triglycerides in coronary artery disease. *Arch Intern Med* 1959;103:4–8.
2. Patterson D, Slack J. Lipid abnormalities in male and female survivors of myocardial infarction and their first degree relatives. *Lancet* 1972; 1:393–399.
3. Brown DF, Kinch SH, Doyle JT. Serum triglycerides in health and in ischemic heart disease. *N Engl J Med* .1965;273:947–952.
4. Gordon T, Castelli W, Hjortland M, et al. High density lipoprotein as a protective factor against coronary heart disease. The Framingham Study. *Am J Med* 1977;62:707–714.
5. Austin MA. Plasma triglyceride and coronary heart disease. *Arterioscler Thromb* 1991;11:2–14.
6. NIH Consensus Development Panel on Triglyceride, High Density Lipoprotein, and Coronary Heart Disease. Triglyceride, high density lipoprotein, and coronary heart disease. *JAMA* 1993;269:505–510.
7. Criqui MH, Heiss G, Cohn R, et al. Plasma triglyceride level and mortality from coronary heart disease. *N Engl J Med* 1993;328:1220–1225.
8. Hokanson JE, Austin MA. Plasma triglyceride is a risk factor for cardiovascular disease independent of high-density lipoprotein cholesterol. A meta-analysis of population-based prospective studies. *J Cardiovasc Risk* 1996;3:213–219.
9. Greenland S. Quantitative methods in the review of epidemiologic literature. *Epidemiol Rev* 1987;9:1–30.
10. Hulley SB, Rosenman RH, Bawol RD, et al. Epidemiology as a guide to clinical decisions. The association between triglyceride and coronary heart disease. *N Engl J Med* 1980;302:1383–1389.
11. Rosenman RH, Brand RJ, Jenkins CD, et al. Coronary heart disease in the Western Collaborative Group Study. Final follow-up experience of 8 1/2 years. *JAMA* 1975;233:872–877.
12. Bottinger LE, Carlson LA. Risk factors for death for males and females. A study of the death pattern in the Stockholm Prospective Study. *Acta Med Scand* 1982;211:437–442.
13. Wilhelmsen L, Wedel H, Tibblin G. Multivariate analysis of risk factors for coronary heart disease. *Circulation* 1973;48:950–958.
14. Pelkonen R, Nikkilä EA, Koskinen S, et al. Association of serum lipids and obesity with cardiovascular mortality. *BMJ* 1977;2:1185–1187.
15. Cambien F, Jacqueson A, Richard JL, et al. Is the level of serum triglyceride a significant predictor of coronary death in "normocholesterolemic" subjects? The Paris Prospective Study. *Am J Epidemiol* 1986; 124:624–632.
16. Bengtsson C, Bjorkelund C, Lapidus L, et al. Association of serum lipid concentrations and obesity with mortality in women: 20 year follow-up of participants in prospective population study in Gothenburg, Sweden. *Br Med J* 1993 307:1385–1388.
17. Åberg H, Lithell H, Selinus I, et al. Serum triglcyerides are a risk factor for myocardial infarction but not for angina pectoris. Results from a 10-year follow-up of Uppsala Primary Preventive Study. *Atherosclerosis* 1985;54:89–97.

18. Wilson P, Larson G, Castelli W. Triglycerides, HDL-cholesterol and coronary artery disease: A Framingham update on the interactions. *Can J Cardiol* 1994;10 (suppl B):5B-9B.
19. Salonen JT, Puska P. Relation of serum cholesterol and triglycerides to the risk of acute myocardial infarction, cerebral stroke and death in eastern Finnish male population. *Int J Epidemiol* 1983;12:26–31.
20. Heyden S, Heiss G, Hames CG, et al. Fasting triglycerides as predictors of total and CHD mortality in Evans County, Georgia. *J Chronic Dis* 1980;33:275–282.
21. Glynn RJ, Rosner B, Silbert JE. Changes in cholesterol and triglyceride as predictors of ischemic heart disease. *Circulation* 1982;66:724–731.
22. Bainton D, Miller NE, Bolton CH, et al. Plasma triglyceride and high density lipoprotein cholesterol as predictors of ischaemic heart disease in British men. The Caerphilly and Speedwell Collaborative Heart Disease Studies. *Br Heart J* 1992;68:60–66.
23. Sigurdsson G, Baldursdottir, Sigvaldason H, et al. Predictive value of apolipoproteins in a prospective survey of coronary artery disease in men. *Am J Cardiol* 1992;69:1251–1254.
24. Assmann G, Schulte H. Relation of high-density lipoprotein cholesterol and triglyceride to incidence of atherosclerotic coronary artery disease (the PROCAM experience). *Am J Cardiol* 1992;70:733–727.
25. Menotti A, Spagnolo A, Scanga M, et al. Multivariate prediction of coronary disease deaths in a 10 year follow-up of an Italian occupational male cohort. *Acta Cardiol* 1992;47:311–320.
26. Menotti A, Scanga M, Morisi G. Serum triglycerides in the prediction of coronary artery disease (an Italian experience). *Am J Cardiol* 1994;73:29–32.
27. Lipid Research Clinics. *Population Study Data. Book The Prevalence Study.* Vol. 1, 1980. Bethesda, MD: US Dept of Health and Human Services publication NIH 80-157.
28. Austin MA, King M-C, Vranizan KM, et al. Atherogenic lipoprotein phenotype. A proposed genetic marker for coronary heart disease risk. *Circulation* 1990;82:495–506.
29. Reaven G. Role of insulin resistance in human disease. *Diabetes* 1988;39:1595–1607.
30. Edwards KL, Austin MA, Newman B, et al. Multivariate analysis of the insulin resistance syndrome. *Arterioscler Thromb* 1994;1940–1945.
31. Burchfiel CM, Laws A, Benfante R, et al. Combined effects of HDL-C, triglyceride ad total cholesterol on 18 year risk of atherosclerotic disease. *Circulation* 1995;92:1430–1436.
32. Patsch JR, Miesenböck G, Hopferwieser T, et al. Relation of triglyceride metabolism and coronary artery disease. Studies in the postprandial state. *Arterioscler Thromb* 1992;12:1336–1345.
33. Karpe F, Steiner G, Uffelman K, et al. Postprandial lipoproteins and progression of coronary atherosclerosis. *Atherosclerosis* 1994;106:8397.
34. Hodis HN, Mack WJ, Azen SP, et al. Triglyceride- and cholesterol-risk lipoproteins have a differential effect on mild/moderate and severe lesion progression as assessed by quantitative coronary angiography in a controlled trial of lovastatin. *Circulation* 1994;90:42–49.
35. Goldstein JL, Schrott HG, Hazzard WR, et al. Hyperlipidemia in coronary heart disease. II. Genetic analysis in 176 families and delineation of a new inherited disorder, combined hyperlipidemia. *J Clin Invest* 1973;52:1544–1568.

36. Brunzell JD, Schrott HG, Motulsky AG, et al. Myocardial infarction in the familial forms of hypertriglyceridemia. *Metabolism* 1976; 25:313–320.
37. Expert panel on detection, evaluation, and treatment of high cholesterol in adults (Adult Treatment Panel II). Summary of the second report of the National Cholesterol Education Program (NCEP) expert panel on detection, evaluation, and treatment of high cholesterol in adults (Adult Treatment Panel II). *JAMA* 1993;269:3015–2023.

Chapter 16

Women, Diabetes, Lipoproteins, and the Risk for Coronary Heart Disease
Studies in Four Ethnic Groups

Barbara V. Howard, PhD,
Linda D. Cowan, PhD,
Steven M. Haffner, MD, Oscar Go, PhD,
Jeunliang L. Yeh, PhD,
and David C. Robbins, MD

Epidemiological studies suggest that diabetes is generally associated with an increased risk for coronary heart disease (CHD) that is greater in women than in men. Review of the population data in four ethnic groups reveals that diabetes is associated with a more adverse lipoprotein profile in women than in men. Mechanisms for the greater lipoprotein changes may include the insulin resistance that accompanies noninsulin-dependent diabetes mellitus (NIDDM) and diabetes-associated changes in sex hormones. These findings highlight the need for increased care of diabetic women and for further research into the mechanisms of the accelerated atherosclerosis in diabetes.

Introduction

The focus during the past 50 years on the impact of CHD in men has tended to obscure the magnitude of this major health problem in women. CHD is the primary cause of death in women, exceeding by far the combined rate of death from malignancies and other

From: Forte TM, (ed). *Hormonal, Metabolic, and Cellular Influences on Cardiovascular Disease in Women*. Armonk, NY: Futura Publishing Company, Inc.; © 1997.

causes.[1] Although the age of onset of CHD is somewhat later in women than in men, it is sometimes accompanied by significantly more morbidity and poorer prognosis in women.

Diabetes has been shown to be a significant independent risk factor for CHD. Although the prevalence rates for some important risk factors such as cigarette smoking, elevated cholesterol levels, and hypertension appear to be declining in the United States, the rate of NIDDM, the most common form of diabetes, is steadily increasing.[2] Further, in most ethnic groups, the prevalence rates for NIDDM are higher in women than in men.[2] Thus, diabetes is becoming a major risk factor for CHD in the United States, especially in women. This chapter will provide a brief survey of the available population data on the effect of diabetes on CHD risk in women and examine the role of diabetic dyslipidemia in heightening CHD risk in diabetic women.

Diabetes as a Risk Factor for CHD

Numerous studies have shown that individuals with diabetes have higher rates of CHD. Other CHD risk factors associated with diabetes, such as hypertension and dyslipidemia, are responsible for some of the increased risk; after adjustment for these risk fac-

				TABLE 1		
		Gender and CHD Risk in NIDDM				
	Method of diagnosis of				Relative risk	
Study[a]	NIDDM	Endpoint	Ages		Women	Men
Framingham[3]	Medical history	CVD	45–74		3.3	1.7
Evans County[4]	Medical history	CHD	>22		2.8	1.0
Rancho Bernardo[5]	Self report or fasting glucose	IHD	40–79		3.5	2.4
Tecumseh[10]	Self report	CHD	>40		3.0	3.0
Chicago Workers[6]	GTT	CHD	35–64		4.7	3.8
Rochester, MN[7]	GTT	CHD	>30		3.2	2.7
NHANES I[9]	Self report	CVD	40–77		2.2	2.6
Strong Heart[8]	GTT	CHD	45–74		4.6	1.8

CVD, cardiovascular disease; CHD, coronary heart disease; IHD, ischemic heart disease; GTT, glucose tolerance test.

[a] References are noted as superscripts.

tors, however, diabetes continues to show a consistent, independent effect on CHD risk.

Table 1 summarizes data from several population-based studies
that have examined rates of CHD in individuals with diabetes. The
majority of the studies suggest that NIDDM increases the risk of CHD
in women to a greater extent than in men. The Framingham Study first
reported that women and men had virtually an equal prevalence of
CHD if the subjects were diabetic, whereas nondiabetic women had
significantly less CHD than nondiabetic men.[3] The relative risk, after
adjustment for age, blood pressure, smoking, plasma cholesterol, and
left ventricular mass was 3.3 in women and 1.7 in men. In urban and
rural whites in Evans County, GA, the increased risk for CHD-related
deaths in diabetic women, when adjusted for age, blood pressure, cholesterol, triglycerides, and smoking, was greater than for diabetic men.[4]
The Rancho Bernardo Study also showed that diabetes, after adjustment for age, cholesterol, blood pressure, smoking, obesity, and exogenous sex hormones, had a greater effect on CHD risk in women than
in men in a follow-up of a middle-class retirement community.[5] The
Chicago Heart Association Detection Project in Industry, which compared self-reported diabetics with nondiabetics among employed white
men and women, revealed a relative risk of diabetes versus no diabetes
for developing CHD that was higher in diabetic women than in diabetic
men after adjustment for age, cholesterol, blood pressure, smoking,
electrocardiogram abnormalities, and education.[6] Similarly, in a Rochester, MN follow-up of a cohort of white participants in whom diabetes
was diagnosed via glucose tolerance test, diabetic women showed a
greater relative risk for CHD compared with nondiabetics than did
men.[7] Finally, examination of 4,500 American Indians from three geographic communities in The Strong Heart Study showed a prevalence
ratio of diabetics to nondiabetics of CHD in diabetic women more than
twice that of diabetic men.[8]

A few studies, however, suggest that diabetes does not increase
the risk of CHD in women more than in men. Among these is an
analysis of mortality among participants in the First National Health
and Nutrition Examination Survey (NHANES I), which showed an
increased risk for cardiovascular disease that was similar in men and
women after adjustment for age, smoking, blood pressure, cholesterol, and body mass index (BMI).[9] Further, the Tecumseh Study,
which followed 90% of the population of Tecumseh, MI, for 18 years,
showed no difference in the relative risk of CHD-related death in
diabetic men and women after controlling for blood pressure, cholesterol, relative weight, and smoking.[10]

This survey reveals that the majority of the studies in the literature suggest that diabetes exerts a greater adverse effect on CHD

risk in women than in men. The most recent consensus conference of the American Diabetes Association on the detection and management of lipid disorders recommended that women with diabetes should be approached clinically as having a risk of CHD that is at least equal to diabetic men.[11]

Effect of Diabetes on Lipoproteins

Because the great majority of individuals with diabetes in the United States have NIDDM, the discussion of lipoproteins as a contributor to the CHD risk in diabetes will focus exclusively on studies of NIDDM.

NIDDM is accompanied by a characteristic dyslipidemia that includes increased triglyceride concentrations and decreased high-density lipoprotein cholesterol (HDL-C); sometimes increased total cholesterol and low-density lipoprotein (LDL) concentrations are observed as well.[12] Dyslipidemia undoubtedly plays a major role in the development of CHD in those with NIDDM. Data from the Prospective Cardiovascular Munster Study (PROCAM), a follow-up of >50,000 men and women in Germany, showed that diabetic women were significantly more likely to have hypercholesterolemia and/or low HDL than were diabetic men.[13] This observation was repeated in studies from the Rancho Bernardo cohort, in which diabetic women had greater increases in total and LDL cholesterol (LDL-C) and greater decreases in HDL-C than did diabetic men.[14]

We recently examined the serum lipoproteins in diabetic African American and white men and women in the NHANES II survey.[15] Data were available from 439 African Americans and 3,738 whites between the ages of 20 and 74 who were classified as having NIDDM based on the results of oral glucose tolerance tests and a medical history of diabetes. The differences in plasma lipoprotein levels between diabetics and nondiabetics by race and gender are shown in Figure 1. In whites, the data suggest that diabetes is associated with a greater increase in total cholesterol in women than in men, except in the oldest decade. In both white and African American women, diabetes appeared to be associated with greater decreases in HDL, except in the oldest decade. On the other hand, multivariate analysis adjusted for age, BMI, skin folds, smoking, and alcohol consumption showed no significant diabetes by gender interaction for any lipid measure in either whites or African Americans (Table 2).

In the San Antonio Heart Study, 3,302 Mexican Americans and 1,877 non-Hispanic whites, ages 25–64, were recruited from San

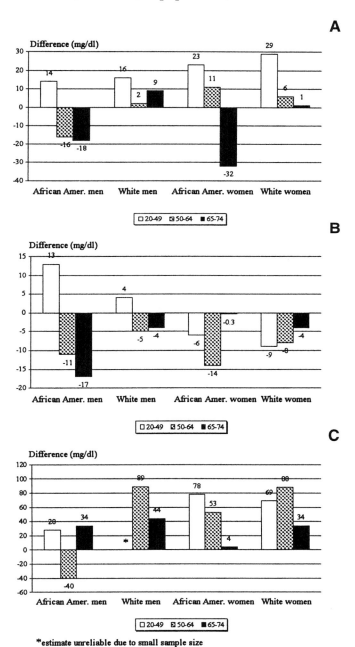

FIGURE 1. *Differences in plasma lipoprotein levels in diabetic versus non-diabetic African Americans and whites by gender: NHANES II. A: total cholesterol; B: HDLC; C: total triglycerides.*

TABLE 2

Significance of Diabetes by Gender Interaction in Multivariate Analyses in Four Ethnic Groups

Variable	White[a]	African American[a]	Mexican American[b]	American Indian[c]		
				Arizona	Oklahoma	South/North Dakota
Total cholesterol	NS	NS	0.004	NS	NS	NS
LDL cholesterol			0.002	0.046	NS	NS
HDL cholesterol	NS	NS	NS	0.039	0.017	0.006
Total triglycerides	NS	NS	NS	NS	NS	NS

Values are P values for diabetes by gender interaction; NS = P > 0.05.
[a] Model included age, body mass index (BMI), skin folds, smoking, and alcohol consumption.
[b] Model included age, BMI, and skin folds.
[c] Model included age, smoking, percent body fat, and waist/hip ratio.

Antonio, Texas, census tracts that represented various income levels. The examination included a glucose tolerance test, anthropometric measurements, and measures of lipoprotein concentrations.[16] Data on Mexican Americans in this study showed that diabetes in women was associated with a greater increase in LDL and a greater decrease in HDL-C (Figure 2). In a multivariate analysis adjusting for age, BMI, and skin folds, there were significant diabetes by gender interactions for both total and LDL-C (Table 2).

Data on American Indians in the Strong Heart Study were obtained during clinical examinations of 4,549 participants between the ages of 45 and 74, who represented 13 tribes in three geographic areas across the United States. Fasting blood samples were obtained from all participants, and an oral glucose tolerance test was performed on all except persons on insulin or taking antidiabetic medication.[17,18] Results of the study indicated that diabetes was associated with greater decreases in HDL in both men and women in all three geographic areas (Figure 3), and in the model adjusting for age, smoking, percent body fat, and waist/hip ratio, the diabetes by gender interaction was significant for the HDL changes (Table 2). There were also gender differences in the effect of diabetes on LDL-C in Arizona.

Discussion

These epidemiological studies suggest that diabetes is generally associated with an increased relative risk for CHD that is greater in

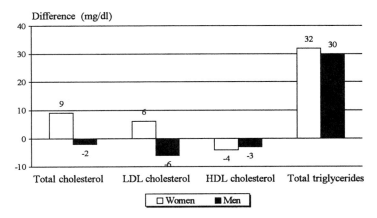

FIGURE 2. *Differences in plasma lipoprotein levels in diabetic versus non-diabetic Mexican Americans by gender: The San Antonio Heart Study.*

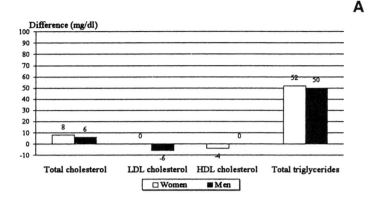

Women, 156 nondiabetic, 663 diabetic; men, 120 nondiabetic, 343 diabetic

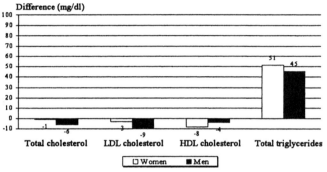

Women, 337 nondiabetic, 359 diabetic; men, 368 nondiabetic, 201 diabetic

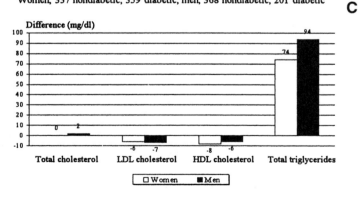

Women, 366 nondiabetic, 352 diabetic; men, 316 nondiabetic, 231 diabetic

FIGURE 3. *Differences in plasma lipoprotein levels in diabetic versus non-diabetic American Indians by gender: The Strong Heart Study. A: Arizona; B: Oklahoma; C: South/North Dakota.*

women than in men—a finding that has implications for both direct patient care and future research. First, clinicians whose patients include diabetic women not only must strive to control their diabetes, but also must be ready to intervene should any of the other known CHD risk factors appear in these patients. In the research arena, this finding emphasizes the need for further investigational attention in order to understand the many complex changes unique to diabetic women that may be responsible for this phenomenon.

This chapter has emphasized NIDDM-related dyslipidemia and examined its possible role in explaining the gender differences in CHD risk in those with diabetes. The data suggest that diabetic women in many cases have more adverse lipoprotein changes than do diabetic men. This observation was first made in populations of middle-aged to elderly whites in Europe[13] and in a retirement community in the United States.[14] In the univariate analysis of the NHANES II data for whites,[15] there appeared to be gender differences in the diabetes-associated changes in lipoproteins, but the gender differences were not significant in the multivariate analysis that was adjusted for other factors known to influence lipoprotein concentrations. One possible explanation is the lower age distribution for the NHANES sample compared with the above-mentioned studies of older individuals.

More data are needed to examine diabetes-induced changes in lipoproteins in African Americans. The only population-based data available to date are from the NHANES II cohort, in which the number of African Americans who received glucose tolerance tests was not large.[15] Univariate analysis suggested gender differences in the effect of diabetes on lipoproteins; the fact that these were not statistically significant in the multivariate analysis may be due to the small sample size.

The data on gender differences in effects of diabetes and lipoproteins on CHD for Mexican Americans are based on the population-based sample from the San Antonio Heart Study in which the diabetes by gender interaction was highly significant for total cholesterol and LDL-C. Thus, Mexican American women with diabetes have greater increases in LDL-C than do their male counterparts— a change that would contribute to increased atherogenicity.

Significant gender differences also were seen in data in American Indians, as presented in The Strong Heart Study of 4,500 participants. The significant gender by diabetes interaction was most consistent with HDL; diabetic women had greater decreases in HDL, a lipoprotein change that is significantly associated with CHD in this population.

A number of mechanisms may explain the greater adverse effect of diabetes on plasma lipoproteins in women. Nondiabetic women, especially those who are premenopausal, generally have a lipoprotein profile that is less atherogenic than that of nondiabetic men of comparable ages. Nondiabetic women have lower levels of LDL-C and very low-density lipoprotein cholesterol (VLDL-C), and higher concentrations of HDL-C.[19] This difference is believed to be caused in part by the influence of estrogen, a hormone that is known to lower LDL and raise HDL,[20] whereas androgens are associated with higher LDL and lower HDL.[21] At least one recent study suggests that the sex hormone balance may change in NIDDM.[22] Estrogen concentrations are lower in pregnant diabetic women than in pregnant nondiabetic women[23] and androgen concentrations have been shown to be higher in women with NIDDM compared with nondiabetic controls.[24] The association of diabetes with a more androgenic hormone profile could thus result in greater changes in lipoproteins in diabetic women compared to nondiabetic women.

A second mechanism that may be related closely to the observations on hormonal changes in diabetes is the insulin resistance that accompanies NIDDM. Insulin resistance, accompanied by hyperinsulinemia and central adiposity, is present in most individuals with NIDDM and appears to precede or exacerbate the development of this disorder.[25] The insulin resistance syndrome is closely associated with a characteristic dyslipidemia that consists of elevated VLDL, lower HDL, and changes in composition of the LDL particle (and sometimes LDL elevations).[12] Insulin resistance is also reported to be associated with hyperandrogenicity and lower estrogen concentrations.[26] Thus, insulin resistance may reverse the usually favorable lipoprotein profile in women by raising triglyceride levels; lowering HDL-C concentrations; and, through accompanying hormonal changes, increasing the concentration and composition of LDL-C. This combination of worsening insulin resistance and hormonal changes in women with diabetes thus could explain the adverse effects on their lipoprotein profiles relative to nondiabetic women.

In closing, it must be pointed out that, although this chapter has focused on lipoproteins, a variety of other mechanisms may exist for the increased CHD risk in diabetic women. CHD is accelerated by multiple factors, many of which are known to change in diabetes. Individuals with diabetes have higher blood pressure, higher platelet reactivity, higher concentrations of several clotting factors, and changes in cardiac function.[27] Further, many other lipoprotein compositional changes occur in diabetes that were not measured in the studies presented here but that may contribute to the diabetes-associated CHD risk.[12] Some of these changes may disproportionately affect diabetic women, as recently reported by

Haffner and colleagues, who showed that diabetic women had greater rates of hypertension than did diabetic men.[28] Recent data also suggest that diabetic women have a greater decrease in LDL size than do diabetic men.[29]

Further work is needed to completely understand the reasons why diabetes increases CHD risk and why this risk is often higher in women.

References

1. Harlan WR. Cardiovascular disease care for women: Service utilization, disability, and costs from the National Medical Care Utilization and Expenditure Survey. In: Eaker ED, Packard B, Wenger NK, Clarkson TB, Tyroler HA, eds. *Coronary Heart Disease in Women*. New York: Haymarket Doyma Inc; 1986:55–61.
2. Kenny SJ, Aubert RE, Geiss LS. Prevalence and incidence of non-insulin-dependent diabetes. In: *Diabetes in America*, 2nd ed. National Institutes of Health, National Institute of Diabetes and Digestive and Kidney Diseases, NIH Publication No. 95-1468; 1995:47–68.
3. Kannel WB, McGee DL. Diabetes and glucose tolerance as risk factors for cardiovascular disease: The Framingham Study. *Diabetes Care* 1979; 2:120–126.
4. Heyden S, Heiss G, Bartel AG, et al. Sex differences in coronary mortality among diabetics in Evans County, Georgia. *J Chron Dis* 1980; 33:265–273.
5. Barrett-Connor E, Wingard DL. Sex differential in ischemic heart disease mortality in diabetics: A prospective population-based study. *Am J Epidemiol* 1983;118:489–496.
6. Pan WH, Cedres LB, Liu K, et al. Relationship of clinical diabetes and asymptomatic hyperglycemia to risk of coronary heart disease mortality in men and women. *Am J Epidemiol* 1986;123:504–516.
7. Elveback LR, Connolly DC, Melton LJ III. Coronary heart disease in residents of Rochester, Minnesota. VII. Incidence, 1950 through 1982. *Mayo Clin Proc* 1986;61:896–900.
8. Howard BV, Lee ET, Cowan LD, et al. Coronary heart disease prevalence and its relation to risk factors in American Indians: The Strong Heart Study. *Am J Epidemiol* 1995;142:254–268.
9. Kleinman JC, Donahue RP, Harris MI, et al. Mortality among diabetics in a national sample. *Am J Epidemiol* 1988;128:389–401.
10. Butler WJ, Ostrander LD, Carman WJ, et al. Mortality from coronary heart disease in the Tecumseh Study: Long-term effect of diabetes mellitus, glucose tolerance and other risk factors. *Am J Epidemiol* 1985; 121:541–547.
11. American Diabetes Association. 1993 Detection and management of lipid disorders in diabetes. *Diabetes Care* 1993;16:828–839.
12. Howard BV. Pathogenesis of diabetic dyslipidemia. *Diabetes Rev* 1995; 3:423–432.

13. Assman G, Schulte H. Relation of high-density lipoprotein cholesterol and triglycerides to incidence of atherosclerotic coronary heart disease (the PROCAM experience). *Am J Cardiol* 1992;70:733–737.
14. Barrett-Connor E, Grundy SM, Holdbrook JJ. Plasma lipids and diabetes mellitus in an adult community. *Am J Epidemiol* 1982;115:657–663.
15. Cowie CC, Howard BV, Harris MI. Serum lipoproteins in African Americans and Whites with non-insulin dependent diabetes in the US population. *Circulation* 1994;90:1185–1193.
16. Stern MP, Rosenthal M, Haffner SM, et al. Sex difference in the effects of sociocultural status on diabetes and cardiovascular risk factors in Mexican Americans: The San Antonio Heart Study. *Am J Epidemiol* 1984;120:834–851.
17. Lee ET, Welty TK, Fabsitz R, et al. The Strong Heart Study—A study of cardiovascular disease in American Indians: Design and methods. *Am J Epidemiol* 1990;132:1141–1155.
18. Howard BV, Welty TK, Fabsitz RR, et al. Risk factors for coronary heart disease in diabetic and nondiabetic Native Americans. The Strong Heart Study. *Diabetes* 1992;41(suppl 2):4–11.
19. U.S. Department of Health and Human Services. *The Lipid Research Clinics Population Studies Data Book. Volume 1: The Prevalence Study.* US DHHS, Public Health Service, National Institutes of Health.
20. Knopp RH, Zhu X, Bonet B. Effects of estrogens on lipoprotein metabolism and cardiovascular disease in women. *Atherosclerosis* 1994;110(suppl):S83-S91.
21. Whitehead M. Progestins and androgens. *Fertil Steril* 1994;62(suppl 2):161S-167S.
22. Birkeland KI, Hanssen KF, Torjensen PA, et al. Level of sex hormone-binding globulin is positively correlated with insulin sensitivity in men with Type 2 diabetes. *J Clin Endocrinol Metab* 1993;76:275–278.
23. Montelongo A, Lasunción MA, Pallardo LF, et al. Longitudinal study of plasma lipoproteins and hormones during pregnancy in normal and diabetic women. *Diabetes* 1992;41:1651–1659.
24. Anderson J, Mårin P, Lissner L, et al. Testosterone concentrations in women and men with NIDDM. *Diabetes Care* 1994;17:405–411.
25. Reaven GM. Role of insulin resistance in human disease. *Diabetes* 1988;37:1595–1607.
26. Peiris AN, Aiman EJ, Drucker WD, et al. The relative contributions of hepatic and peripheral tissue to insulin resistance in hyperandrogenic women. *J Clin Endocrin Metab* 1989;68:715–720.
27. Bierman EL. Atherogenesis in diabetes. *Arterioscler Thromb* 1991;12:647–656.
28. Haffner SM, Valdez RZ, Morales PA, et al. Greater effect of glycemia on incidence of hypertension in women than in men. *Diabetes Care* 1992;15:1277–1284.
29. Haffner SM, Mykkänen L, Valdez RA, et al. LDL size and subclass pattern in a biethnic population. *Arterioscler Thromb* 1993;13:1623–1630.

Chapter 17

Cardiovascular Risk Factors During First Five Years Postmenopause in Nonhormone Replacement Therapy Users

Lewis H. Kuller, MD, DrPH,
Elaine N. Meilahn, DrPH,
Holly Lassila, DrPH, Karen Matthews, PhD,
and Rena Wing, PhD

Previous publications of the Healthy Women Study (HWS) have explored the characteristics of women during the peri- to the postmenopausal period and the determination of level of changes in specific risk factors.[1-8] Several other papers from the HWS have described the behavioral and psychosocial attributes and their changes during the peri- to postmenopausal period.[9-12] Other papers have focused on the determinants of the use of hormone replacement therapy (HRT), baseline, and risk factor changes among women who did and did not use HRT.[1,8,11]

This chapter focuses on changes in risk factors from premenopausal to first through fifth postmenopausal years among nonhormone users at all visits, the correlation of risk factors from premenopause to five years postmenopausal, and determinants of change in risk factors from premenopause to fifth postmenopausal years.

Methods

The HWS is a longitudinal investigation of 541 initially premenopausal women, age 42–50 at baseline, recruited from driver

From: Forte TM, (ed). *Hormonal, Metabolic, and Cellular Influences on Cardiovascular Disease in Women.* Armonk, NY: Futura Publishing Company, Inc.; © 1997.

license lists within selected zip codes in Allegheny County, Pennsylvania.[1] The primary goal of this study was to evaluate the changes in biological and behavioral characteristics of women during the peri- to the postmenopause. The eligibility was determined first by a telephone interview. Eligible women had to be premenopausal, having had menstrual bleeding within the past 3 months, no surgical menopause, diastolic blood pressure <100, and no medication known to influence the biological risk factors, or psychotropic medications. The women also could not be taking oral contraceptives or HRT at the time of recruitment.

Approximately 90% of the women contacted agreed to the initial telephone interview, and 60% of eligible women participated in the study. Detailed descriptions of the eligible and ineligible women, including reasons for ineligibility, have been published previously.[1,9,13]

After recruitment to the study, the women completed a baseline clinical examination that included measurements of lipoproteins, apoproteins, blood pressure, height, weight, behavioral attributes, psychological characteristics, and menstrual and reproductive history. The women had a second clinical evaluation ~3 years after recruitment. The perimenopause was defined as 3 months of amenorrhea. A subsample of women had a perimenopausal examination. Women were classified as postmenopausal either by 12 months of amenorrhea and FSH ≥ 720 ng/mL or a combination of 12 months of amenorrhea and HRT or not menstruating for a total of 12 months.[1] A first postmenopausal examination (post) was completed that included the same measurements as the baseline examination. The examination also included measurements of sex-steroid hormones and waist-to-hip ratio.

Examinations were repeated at the second and fifth year postmenopausal. In the intervening years, the women were contacted by mail and telephone to determine health status, changes in risk factors, HRT, and other psychosocial and behavioral attributes. At approximately the fifth post year, carotid ultrasound measurements to evaluate carotid intimal medial thickness and presence of plaque using a technique similar to that for the Cardiovascular Health Study (CHS) were done.[14]

Blood levels of lipoproteins and blood glucose were measured in a Centers for Disease Control (CDC) certified laboratory for total cholesterol and high-density lipoprotein cholesterol (HDL-C) levels. The women fasted for 12 hours before venipuncture for measurement of lipoprotein lipids, apoprotein, and triglycerides. Using sera, HDL-C was measured by heparin manganese precipitation procedure.[15] The HDL-C subfractions, HDL_2-C forms a precipitate after addition of dextran sulfate to the supernatant obtained with heparin manganese chloride.[16] The cholesterol content of the supernatant was measured and the concentration of HDL_2-C was found by subtracting HDL_3-C from the concentration of total HDL-C. Triglycerides were determined enzymatically[17] and low-density lipoprotein cholesterol (LDL-C) was calculated by using the Friedewald equation.

The laboratory is maintained at the required level of proficiency to be included in the CDC/NHLBI Lipid Standardization Program since 1982 and has participated in the Miles-Techinicon Program as a reference methods site for triglycerides since 1987. The coefficients of variation between runs for total cholesterol is 1.3%, for triglycerides 1.7%, for HDL-C 2.1%, and for HDL-C subfractions 6%. Serum glucose is determined by an enzymatic determination. The coefficient of variation is ∼1.8%. The plasma insulin is determined by radioimmune assay in the Diabetes Research Laboratory at Children's Hospital of Pittsburgh.[18]

Statistical Analysis

Analyses were conducted using the SPSS-X statistical package. Frequency distributions of each variable were run and outliers excluded prior to conducting the analyses. Natural log transformation were used on skewed measures having skewness >2.0 and/or kurtosis >1.0. Nonparametric tests were used when the variables were not normally distributed or when groups n were small.

Assumptions of each of the above tests were examined thoroughly and verified. For example, diagnostics were conducted after running multiple regression analysis. Some of the diagnostics included standardized residual statistics and normal probability plots.

Results

There were 541 women initially evaluated between 1983 and 1985. The mean age at baseline examination was 48 years. Ninety-one percent of the women were white. As of June 30, 1995, of the 541 women, 46 had dropped out before their fifth post, 4 had died, and 188 were not yet eligible for a fifth post. Of the 373 active and eligible for the fifth post, 307 (82%) were seen in the clinic, and 34 (9%) had information collected by mail only, including 30 living outside the area. Follow-up data were, therefore, available for 341 (91%)

of the 373 eligible women. Of the 46 women who had dropped out of the study as of June 30, 1995, 32 (70%) did so before their first scheduled post. The number of women in some of the analyses may vary because of differences in length of follow-up in the analysis through August 30, 1995, and changes in protocol over time for inclusion of specific laboratory tests.

The mean elapsed time between the baseline examination and the first post, 1 year amenorrhea, or a combination of amenorrhea and hormone therapy for 12 months was 54 months. The mean age of the women was 52 at their first post, and 57 at their fifth post. Among those who attended the fifth post (n=309), 141 (45.6%) were on HRT. Women who did not attend or have laboratory data for their fifth post were more likely to have been cigarette smokers at baseline, less educated, and not married. There was little difference in baseline risk factors between those who did and did not attend the fifth post (Table 1).

The use of HRT in this study is very different than in previous reports in that most of the women who started on HRT at first post continued on HRT through the fifth post. Of the women who had completed their fifth post, 79 (83%) of the 95 on HRT at first post were still on HRT at fifth post, and 54 (28%) of the 133 on HRT at

TABLE 1

Comparison of Women Attending Clinic at Fifth Postmenopausal Exam

Baseline attribute (premenopausal)	Attended clinic visit		Did not attend or no laboratory data
	HRT	No HRT	
Age	48	48	48
Cigarette smoking (%)	22	36	41
Married	78	73	63
Education—College + (%)	55	54	45
Black (%)	05	12	13
Weight (lbs)	142	152	146
BMI (kg/m^2)	24	26	25
LDL-C (mg%)	108	108	113
HDL-C (mg%)	62	59	56
Percent fat diet	37	38	39
Kilocalorie exercise/week	1,652	1,310	1,235
Alcohol (g/day)	10	09	07

Comparison of women by hormone use at fifth exam (344) as of 4-1-95. n = 131 HRT (38%), 151 No HRT (44%), 62 no attendance (18%).

fifth post began HRT after the first post. The prevalence of HRT use by fifth post was 46% (134 of 288) of women eligible for fifth post.

We have also reported a detailed analysis comparing baseline characteristics of women who were or were not taking postmenopausal HRT. At baseline, women taking HRT were less likely to be cigarette smokers, more likely to be white, thinner and have higher HDLC levels at baseline than those not taking HRT (Table 1). By the time of the fifth post, 10.7% of the women had a hysterectomy.

The distribution and standard deviation of the risk factors at fifth post for 168 women not on HRT is shown in Table 2.

Risk Factor Change

The changes in risk factors for 127 women not on HRT from baseline through the fifth post were greatest for LDL-C between the premenopause and first post (Table 3). The LDL-C increased very little after year two postmenopausal. The HDL-C levels changed very little. The HDL$_2$-C decreased and the HDL$_3$-C increased as has been previously reported in the HWS. Triglyceride levels and insulin in-

---

TABLE 2

Distribution of Risk Factor Levels at Fifth Postmenopausal Examination—Not on Hormone Replacement Therapy

Variable	Risk factor levels[a]
Age (yr)	56 ± 2.0
Percent current smokers	25
BMI (kg/m^2)	28 ± 0.06
Waist-hip ratio	0.78 ± 0.08
Weight (lbs)	161 ± 35
Total cholesterol (mg%)	213 ± 39
LDL-C (mg%)	134 ± 37
HDL-C (mg%)	58 ± 17
HDL$_3$-C (mg%)	45 ± 11
HDL$_2$-C (mg%)	13 ± 10
Triglycerides (mg%)	108 ± 65
Diastolic blood pressure (mm Hg)	72 ± 10
Systolic blood pressure (mm Hg)	117 ± 19
Fasting glucose (mg)	90 ± 25
Kilocalories exercise	1,730 ± 1,368
Alcohol (g/day)	4.7 ± 9.7

n=168 women.

[a] Values are means ± SD.

TABLE 3

Distribution of Change in Cardiovascular Risk Factors: Cohort Not on HRT

Variable	Premenopausal to year one post	Premenopausal to year two post	Premenopausal to year five post	Postmenopausal years 1–5
BMI (kg/m$_2$)	1.1	1.3	1.9	0.8
Weight (lbs)	5.1	6.8	09	3.8
LDL-C (mg%)	20	23	23	2.7
Cholesterol (mg%)	24	24	28	3.2
HDL-C (mg%)	—	−01	−01	−01
HDL2-C (mg%)	−5.0	−8.0	−7.0	−2.8
HDL3-C (mg%)	5.0	6.5	7.0	1.9
SBP (mm Hg)	—	—	5.4	5.8
DBP (mm Hg)	1.1	−1.2	−2.0	−3.1
Glucose (mg)	−2.3	−2.5	0.0	2.1
Triglycerides (mg%)	11	10	23	10.9
Alcohol (g/day)	−1.3	−1.2	−3.5	2.8
Kcalories/exercise	175	135	409	186
Waist-hip				.02

Data are for pre- to fifth postmenopausal; 127 women.

creased throughout the pre- to fifth post. The change in systolic blood pressure was different. Most of the increase occurring in the latter part of the postmenopause, from years two to the fifth post. There was relatively little change in diastolic blood pressure. In the cohort of 127 women not on HRT from baseline through the fifth post, 33% were smoking cigarettes at baseline, 27% at the first post, 26% at the second, and 24% at the fifth post. The women reported a small decrease in alcohol as measured in grams per day and an increase in physical activity (Table 3). Weight gain was the most important determinant of the changes in these risk factors from baseline to fifth post (Table 4). As noted, the increase in weight was relatively constant from premenopause through the fifth postmenopausal year, and averaged ~1 lb/year.

Correlation of Risk Factors Over Time

There was a very high tracking of risk factors and lifestyles over time. The correlations were highest for weight, body mass index (BMI), and waist-to-hip, and lower for blood pressure (both systolic and diastolic) than for lipids. This is probably due to greater within-individual short-term variability of blood pressure measurements. The very high correlation of lipids, especially LDLC (even through the menopause), was somewhat surprising (Table 5).

We next compared the correlations of risk factors for women who had been on HRT from the first through the fifth post. The Spearman Correlation coefficients were high and all were statistically significant ($P \leq 0.05$). The coefficients were stronger for lipids than for blood pressure. The coefficients for lipids were lower than for women who had never been on HRT, whereas the coefficients for blood pressure and weight were similar for hormone and non-hormone users (Table 6).

Discussion

The HWS was designed to test the hypothesis that changes in risk factors during the pre- to the postmenopause were related to decreases in sex-steroid hormone (ie, peri-postmenopause), weight gain, and increasing body fatness and aging. After >8–10 years of follow-up, the evidence is relatively consistent. The increase in LDL-C peri- to postmenopause has been the most striking observation in the HWS, as well as in other similar studies of menopause. The increase in LDL-C from

TABLE 4

Relationship of Weight Change From First to Fifth Postmenopausal Exam and Changes in Cardiovascular Risk Factors

Weight change (lb)	n	Change in risk factor 1–5 postmenopausal examinations					
		LDL-C (mg/dL)	HDL-C (mg/dL)	Triglycerides (mg/dL)	Systolic BP (mm Hg)	Diastolic BP (mm Hg)	Glucose (mg)
Weight gain:							
9.50–48	33	9.3	−2.0	17	9.4	−1.6	4.2
4.0–9.5	31	−2.5	−2.9	26	6.4	−3.5	2.5
1–3.5	29	5.5	0.8	0.7	3.1	−3.2	1.0
Lost weight	33	−1.0	−.25	−2.8	4.1	−1.1	0–.4
Total	126	2.7	−1.0	10.8	5.8	−3.1	2.0

Cardiovascular risk factors and LDL-C, HDL-C, triglycerides, and systolic blood pressure. Data are from nonhormone users.

TABLE 5

Spearman Correlation of Risk Factors by Non-HRT User at Fifth Postmenopausal Examination

Variable	Baseline first	Baseline fifth	First to fifth
	Correlation*		
Weight	0.93	0.89	0.93
Waist-to-hip	—	—	0.68
BMI	0.93	0.88	0.91
SBP	0.60	0.49	0.59
DBP	0.52	0.47	0.48
Cholesterol	0.78	0.70	0.75
HDL-C	0.84	0.77	0.80
LDL-C	0.83	0.65	0.75
Triglycerides	0.73	0.61	0.68
Fasting glucose	0.30	0.33	0.37
Kilocalories of exercise	0.54	0.49	0.55
Alcohol consumption (gms/day)	0.74	0.62	0.71

Table is correlating first and fifth postmenopausal examination data. *$P \leq 0.05$.

TABLE 6

Spearman Correlation Coefficients Baseline to First and Fifth Postmenopausal Examination for Hormone Users

Variable	Baseline first	Baseline fifth	First to fifth
	Correlation*		
Weight	0.88	0.88	0.92
Waist-to-hip	—	—	0.64
BMI	0.93	0.88	0.91
SBP	0.54	0.43	0.66
DBP	0.44	0.50	0.48
Cholesterol	0.63	0.41	0.53
HDL-C	0.76	0.72	0.69
LDL-C	0.66	0.55	0.59
Triglycerides	0.59	0.50	0.53
Fasting glucose	0.40	0.42	0.47
Kilocalories of exercise	0.31	0.45	0.46
Alcohol consumption (gms/day)	0.64	0.64	0.72

*$P \leq 0.05$.

the peri- through the postmenopause is noted in practically all populations that have been studied. The increase is clearly related to menopause and is blunted by the use of estrogen or estrogen/progesterone therapy. Most of the increase in occurred early in the peri- to the postmenopause and is substantially diminished after the first few years. The increase in LDL-C also is related directly to weight gain. Thus, the changes in LDL-C appear to be a function of both the decrease in estrogen production and weight gain.

The significantly high correlation of risk factors during the peri- to postmenopause, in spite of the effects of decreased ovarian function, weight gain, and even use of HRT, is likely a function of both genetic determinants of levels of risk factors such as apolipoprotein apo(e) polymorphism and LDL-C levels as previously reported for both peri- and postmenopausal women[19] and the consistency of lifestyles that affect risk factor levels such as exercise, alcohol intake, dietary cholesterol and saturated fat consumption. These results are significant in that premenopausal women who have higher risk factors (ie, their LDL-C, lower HDL-C compared with other premenopausal women) are likely to also have higher levels during the postmenopause. The high correlation of risk factors over time may also explain our previously reported association of risk factors measured premenopausal, such as systolic blood pressure, BMI, LDL-C, HDL-C, triglycerides, and extent of carotid artery wall thickness and plaque measured 5 years postmenopausal.[20]

The measures of subclinical atherosclerosis, including carotid artery wall thickness and plaque, have been shown to be an independent predictor of clinical cardiovascular disease. In the CHS among older women 65+, the LDLC was also an important determinant of the extent of subclinical vascular disease.[21] The presence of subclinical vascular disease, as compared with no subclinical vascular disease, was an important and independent determinant of the risk of clinical cardiovascular disease, especially myocardial infarction and death among both men and women.[22] Higher LDL-C is a risk factor for coronary heart disease among women.[23]

A basic question has been the inability to relate endogenous hormone levels to the lipoprotein levels, especially the LDL-C. We hypothesized that low-endogenous estrone or estradiol would be associated with higher LDL-C. To date, however, most studies, including previous reports from the HWS,[24] based on the first year after menopause, have failed to document any relation between endogenous hormone levels and LDL-C.[25,26]

Preliminary analysis reported for the HWS showed an inverse relation between blood estradiol levels (n=87) and LDLC levels among nonhormone users after adjustment for BMI and waist-to-hip ratio (regression coefficient -1.57, $P=0.03$). There was no association of estrone and LDL-C levels.[27]

The interrelation between obesity and weight gain and changes in both LDL-C and sex-steroid hormone levels may explain the failure to note a strong relation between endogenous estrogen levels, estrone and estradiol, and LDL-C levels. The low levels of estradiol, especially among older postmenopausal women may further complicate the evaluation of the association between endogenous hormone levels and risk factors, such as LDL-C levels.[28–31] The levels of the hormones represent the production, secretion, and metabolism of hormones.

The epidemiology of HDL-C is very different. The change in HDL-C at menopause is very small, possibly 1 or 2 mg at most.[1] There is, however, a substantial decrease in HDL_2-C and an increase in HDL_3-C. The differences in HDL-C between the men and women are not, apparently, due to estrogens in women, as much as they are to the decrease in HDL-C among men at puberty.[32]

The HDL-C declined among women who gained weight.[5] Also, women with higher waist-to-hip ratio have lower HDL-C. Women not only gain weight through the peri- to postmenopause, but there is a decrease in bone and lean body mass and an increase in percentage of fat, as well as a change in the fat distribution, with an increase in android or upper body obesity, as well as intra-abdominal fat.[33,34] The relation of these changes to HDL-C and, perhaps triglyceride metabolism, needs further evaluation, especially the relation of intra-abdominal fat and HDL-C. The decrease in estradiol at menopause may contribute to the changes in fat distribution including increase in intra-abdominal fat.[35] Similarly, the increase in intra-abdominal fat or total body fat may be related to increases in insulin levels, which would also effect HDL-C, insulin resistance, and diabetes mellitus.

The changes in systolic blood pressure appear to be related primarily to aging and weight change.[36] The increase in systolic blood pressure in contrast to LDL-C occurred in the later years after menopause. The systolic blood pressure, increased with weight gain. The changes in systolic blood pressure were similar for women whether taking or not taking HRT. Clinical trials have also not documented an important effect of HRT on change in blood pressure levels.[37] It is possible that an increase in LDL-C and extent of atherosclerosis in larger arteries peri- to the postmenopause, may contribute to the increasing rigidity of blood vessels and the elevation of systolic blood pressure.

We have previously reported that the extent of carotid artery wall thickness and presence of plaque in the carotid arteries was substantially greater in peri- than postmenopausal women.[20] The measure of carotid artery wall thickness included both intima and medial changes of an artery. Systolic blood pressure or pulse pressure and BMI measured premenopausal were significant predictors of intima medial thickness, measured ~5 years postmenopausal. The changes in pulse pressure baseline to fifth post was also related to carotid artery wall thickness. It is not known whether the change in blood vessel characteristics is the primary determinant of increase in systolic blood pressure and pulse pressure peri- to postmenopausal or whether increase in lipids, LDL-C secondary to peri- to postmenopause, decrease in estrogens, and weight gain is the primary determinant of atherosclerosis, vascular disease, with a subsequent increase in systolic blood pressure that may then further enhance the development of atherosclerosis.

The changes in blood glucose were very modest during the peri- to postmenopause. There was no consistent change in fasting blood glucose between pre- and first- or second-post and a small increase between second to fifth. The changes in blood glucose are similar to systolic blood pressure rather than for LDL-C. The increase in blood glucose was directly related to weight gain. The results are consistent with the genetic and lifestyle (ie, weight gain effects on blood glucose levels), but little effect of peri- to postmenopause (ie, decreased estradiol production by the ovary). Women with diabetes were excluded from the study.

The public health implications of some of these initial findings are important. The increasing LDL-C levels through peri- to postmenopause is clearly associated with atherosclerosis and subsequent risk of cardiovascular disease. Weight gain is very prevalent in this population and is an important determinant of both increasing glucose, triglycerides, and LDL-C levels and decreased HDL-C levels. As noted, even in this well-educated population, smoking was very prevalent (25%) and only 12 (29%) of 42 smokers at baseline, among non-HRT users, had stopped smoking by the fifth post.

The long-term reduction of atherosclerosis or clinical cardiovascular complications in women will depend on preventing the increase in LDL-C during peri- through postmenopause (ie, keeping the average LDL-C ~100–110 mg%) preventing the rise in systolic blood pressure, and substantially reducing the prevalence of cigarette smoking.

There is a very high correlation of risk factors among the women from baseline to 5 years postmenopausal, even with the changes during menopause. For example, among the 113 women not on HRT at baseline through year five who had LDL-C in the highest quartile at baseline premenopausal (mean 154 mg%), 17 (61%) were in the highest quartile at year five, and 8 in the third quartile (29%). Therefore, in spite of the variability of a single measure of LDL-C and regression to the mean of a single measure, the LDL-C at baseline (premenopausal) is a very strong predictor of high LDL-C postmenopausal. These women, as noted, have more carotid atherosclerosis and, at older ages, higher risk of both clinical and subclinical coronary heart disease. Therefore, it is possible to identify very high-risk individuals during perimenopause for more aggressive individualized preventive pharmacological and nonpharmacological therapies.

References

1. Matthews KA, Meilahn E, Kuller LH, et al. Menopause and risk factors for coronary heart disease. *N Engl J Med* 1989;321:641–646.
2. Kuller LH, Meilahn EN, Cauley JA, et al. Epidemiologic studies of menopause: Changes in risk factors and disease. *Exp Gerontol* 1994;29: 495–509.
3. Wing RR, Matthews KA, Kuller LH, et al. Environmental and familial contributions to insulin levels and change in insulin in middle-aged women. *JAMA* 1992;268(14):1890–1895.
4. Wing RR, Matthews KA, Kuller LH, et al. Waist to hip ratio in middle-aged women. *Arterioscler Thromb* 1991;11:1250–1257.
5. Wing RR, Matthews KA, Kuller LH, et al. Weight gain at the time of the menopause. *Arch Intern Med* 1991;151:97–102.
6. Yeh LLL, Bunker CH, Evans RW, et al. Serum fatty acid distributions in postmenopausal women. *Nutr Res* 1994;14:675–691.
7. Meilahn EN, Kuller LH, Matthews KA, et al. Hemostatic factors according to menopausal status and use of hormone replacement therapy. *Ann Epidemiol* 1992;2:445–455.
8. Meilahn EN, Kuller LH, Matthews KA, et al. Variation in plasma fibrinogen levels by menopausal status and use of hormone replacement therapy (The Healthy Women Study). In: Ernst E, Koenig W, Lowe GDO, Meade TW. eds. *Fibrinogen: A "New" Cardiovascular Risk Factor.* Austria: Blackwell-MZV; 1992:338–343.
9. Matthews KA, Wing RR, Kuller LH, et al. Influence of the perimenopause on cardiovascular risk factors and symptoms of middle-aged healthy women. *Arch Intern Med* 1994;154:2349–2355.
10. Matthews KA, Kuller LH, Wing RR, et al. Biobehavioral aspects of menopause: Lessons from the Healthy Women Study. *Exp Gerontol* 1994; 29:337–342.
11. Egeland GM, Kuller LH, Matthews KA, et al. Hormone replacement therapy and lipoprotein changes during early menopause. *Obstet Gynecol* 1990;76:776–782.
12. Matthews KA, Bromberger JT, Egeland GM. Behavioral antecedents and consequences of the menopause. In: Korenman SG, ed. *The Menopause (Proceedings of the Serono Symposium on the Menopause, March 1989, Napa, CA).* Norwell, Mass: Serono Symposia; 1990:1–15.

13. Kuller LH, Meilahn EN, Gutai J, et al. Lipoproteins, estrogens and the menopause. In: Korenman SG, ed. *The Menopause—Biological and Clinical Consequences of Ovarian Failure: Evolution and Management.* Norwell, Mass: Serono Symposia, 1990:179–197.

14. O'Leary DH, Polak JF, Wolfson SK Jr, et al. The use of sonography to evaluate carotid atherosclerosis in the elderly: The Cardiovascular Health Study. *Stroke* 1991;22:1155–1163.

15. Warnick GR, Alberts JJ. A comprehensive evaluation of the heparin-manganese precipitation procedure for estimating high density lipoprotein cholesterol. *J Lipid Res* 1978;19:65–76.

16. Gidez LI, Miller GJ, Burstein M, et al. Analysis of plasma high density lipoprotein subclasses by a precipitation procedure: Correlations with preparative and analytical centrifugation. In: Lippel K, ed. *Report of the High Density Lipoprotein Methodology Workshop, San Francisco, Calif, March 12–14, 1979.* Bethesda, MD: Department of Health, Education, and Welfare publication NIH 79-1661.

17. Bucolo G, David H. Quantitative determination of serum triglycerides by the use of enzymes. *Clin Chem* 1973;19:476–482.

18. Herbert V, Lauk K-S, Gottlieb CW, et al. Coated charcoal immunoassay of insulin. *J Clin Endocrinol Metab* 1965;25:1375–1384.

19. Cauley JA, Eichner JE, Kamboh MI, et al. Apo E allele frequencies in younger (age 42–50) vs older (age 65–90) women. *Genet Epidemiol* 1993;10:27–34.

20. Herzog HC, Sutton-Tyrrell K, Jansen-McWilliams L, et al. Asymptomatic carotid atherosclerosis in women pre and post menopause. Abstract. *Circulation* 1996;93:630.

21. Kuller L, Borhani N, Furberg C, et al. Prevalence of subclinical atherosclerosis and cardiovascular disease and association with risk factors in the Cardiovascular Health Study. *Am J Epidemiol* 1994;139:1164–1179.

22. Kuller LH, Shemanski L, Psaty BM, et al. Subclinical disease as an independent risk factor for cardiovascular disease. *Circulation* 1995;92:720–726.

23. Kannel WB, Wilson PWF. Risk factors that attenuate the female coronary disease advantage. *Arch Intern Med* 1995;155:57–61.

24. Kuller LH, Gutai JP, Meilahn E, et al. Relationship of endogenous sex steroid hormones to lipids and apoproteins in postmenopausal women. *Arteriosclerosis* 1990;10:1058–1066.

25. Longcope C, Herbert PN, McKinlay SM, et al. The relationship of total and free estrogens and sex hormone-binding globulin with lipoproteins in women. *J Clin Endocrinol Metab* 1990;71:67–72.

26. Cauley JA, Gutai JP, Kuller LH, et al. The relation of endogenous sex steroid hormone concentrations to serum lipid and lipoprotein levels in postmenopausal women. *Am J Epidemiol* 1990;132:884–894.

27. Meilahn E, Herzog H, Sutton-Tyrrell K, et al. Endogenous estrogen levels, lipoproteins and carotid artery wall thickness among postmenopausal women. Abstract. *Circulation* 1996;93:630.

28. Cauley JA, Gutai JP, Kuller LH, et al. Reliability and interrelations among serum sex hormones in postmenopausal women. *Am J Epidemiol* 1991;133:50–57.

29. Hankinson SE, Manson JE, London SJ, et al. Laboratory reproducibility of endogenous hormone levels in postmenopausal women. *Cancer Epidemiol Biom Prev* 1994;3:551–56.

30. Hankinson SE, Manson JE, Spiegelman D, et al. Reproducibility of plasma hormone levels in postmenopausal women over a 2–3 year period. *Cancer Epidemiol Biom Prev* 1995;4:649–654.
31. Bolelli G, Muti P, Micheli A, et al. Validity for epidemiological studies of long-term cryoconservation of steroid and protein hormones in serum and plasma. *Cancer Epidemiol Biom Prev* 1995;4:509–513.
32. Berenson GS. Evolution of cardiovascular risk factors in early life: Perspectives on causation. In: Berenson GS, ed. *Causation of Cardiovascular Risk Factors in Childhood*. New York: Raven Press, 1976:1–26.
33. Wing RR, Jeffery RW, Burton LR, Tet al. Change in waist-to-hip ratio with weight loss and its association with change in cardiovascular risk factors. *Am J Clin Nutr* 1992;55:1086–1092.
34. Kaye SA, Folsom AR, Prineas RJ, et al. The association of body fat distribution with lifestyle and reproductive factors in a population study of postmenopausal women. *Int J Obesity* 1990;14:583–591.
35. Schapira DV, Clard RA, Wolff PA, et al. Visceral obesity and breast cancer risk. *Cancer* 1994;74:632–639.
36. Kiani F, Knutsen S. Estrogen replacement therapy and the risk of myocardial infarction. The Adventist Health Study. Abstract. *Am J Epidemiol* 1996;143:No. 273.
37. PEPI Trial Writing Group. Effects of estrogen or estrogen/progestin regimens on heart disease risk factors in postmenopausal women. The Postmenopausal Estrogen/Progestin Interventions (PEPI) trial. *JAMA* 1995;273:199–208.

Chapter 18

Effect of Oral Contraceptive Hormones on Lipoprotein (a) and Other Lipoproteins In Premenopausal Women

Joel D. Morrisett, PhD, Mauro L. Nava,
Maryanne Reilly, RN,
Michael C. Snabes, MD,
and Ronald L. Young, MD

During the past two decades, significant qualitative and quantitative changes have been made in the composition of oral contraceptives (OC). The estrogen dosage has been reduced in response to observed thrombotic complications, and the progestogen dosage has been decreased due to observed disturbances in metabolic pathways related to an increased risk for cardiovascular disease. These reductions in steroid dosage have resulted in a new generation of OC that have somewhat reduced the incidence of adverse side effects yet are still quite efficacious. In addition to these quantitative changes in OC pill composition, there have been qualitative changes as well. New progestogens have been developed in a continuing effort to reduce undesirable side effects even further.[1,2]

It is well established that exogenous steroid hormones can have a profound effect on lipid metabolism. Oral estrogens cause a reduction in hepatic triglyceride lipase that typically degrades high-density lipoprotein (HDL).[3,4] Estrogens also enhance HDL cholesterol (HDL-C) production and hepatic synthesis of apolipoprotein (apo) A-I. However, it is possible that the increase in HDL-C accompanying estrogen treatment is not a pure effect but is partly due to

Supported in part by a grant from Organon, Inc. and a Specialized Center of Research in Atherosclerosis Grant, HL-27341.

From: Forte TM, (ed). *Hormonal, Metabolic, and Cellular Influences on Cardiovascular Disease in Women.* Armonk, NY: Futura Publishing Company, Inc.; © 1997.

estrogen-stimulated removal of cholesterol from the systemic circulation resulting in enhanced reverse cholesterol transport. Reduction in low-density lipoprotein cholesterol (LDL-C) is another beneficial effect of estrogen treatment. This change is probably due to both hepatic and nonhepatic effects. Although estrogens increase very low-density lipoprotein (VLDL) and triglycerides through direct enhancement of their synthesis and secretion, the catabolism of VLDL to LDL is actually decreased, probably due to enhanced uptake of VLDL by the liver.[5] Furthermore, kinetic measurements have shown that the rate of LDL removal is increased by estrogens, an effect probably resulting from the upregulation of LDL receptors both in the liver and in peripheral tissues. In contrast to estrogens, progestins induce hepatic lipase activity, resulting in increased degradation of HDL.[3] This effect appears to be related not only to the progestin dose but also to its androgenic potency. Although the estrogen-stimulated increase in HDL_2 is attenuated by progestin, HDL-C levels remain above base line and then increase again after discontinuation of the progestin. Progestin also leads to reduced total triglyceride levels. Consequently, the elevation of triglycerides with estrogen is mostly eliminated during progestin treatment.

Desogestrel is metabolized rapidly and completely to 3-keto desogestrel.[6,7] This active metabolite has shown relatively strong progestational activity and minimal residual androgenic activity. Metabolic studies have indicated a greater dissociation of the desired progestagenic effects from the undesired androgenic effects of desogestrel than was observed with norgestrel and norethindrone.[8,9] Desogen (Organon, West Orange, NJ) is a monophasic OC tablet that contains desogestrel and ethinyl estradiol, whereas Lo/Ovral (Wyeth-Ayerst, Philadelphia, PA), also a monophasic contraceptive, contains norgestrel and ethinyl estradiol. Accordingly, undesirable changes in the lipid profile that might be induced by these contraceptives was anticipated to be significantly less with Desogen than with Lo/Ovral. The objective of this study was to compare the effect of these two different contraceptive formulations on the levels of lipoproteins in premenopausal women, especially lipoprotein(a) [Lp(a)], which is now accepted widely as a risk factor for cardiovascular disease in women as well as men.

Experimental Methods

Study Design

This was a randomized, open label, single center study in which 100 women were assigned to one of two parallel active treatment groups that received either Desogen or Lo/Ovral during the treatment period. After an initial screening phase, subjects who met the selection criteria were assigned randomly to receive either Desogen (a monophasic OC tablet containing 150 μg desogestrel/30 μg ethinyl estradiol) or Lo/Ovral (a monophasic OC tablet containing 300 μg norgestrel/30 μg ethinyl estradiol). The OC was taken for 21 consecutive days followed by 7 inert-tablet days each cycle for six cycles. In addition to laboratory tests performed during the initial screening phase, these tests were repeated upon entry into the study (0 cycle), after three cycles, and after six cycles on OC. The study subjects were premenopausal women 18–50 years of age, were not pregnant, had three regular menstrual cycles for 3 months immediately preceding study entry, and voluntarily gave informed written consent to participate in the study. Candidates were excluded from the study if OCs were contraindicated for them. They were also excluded if they: had used an injectable hormonal method of contraception within the past 6 months, had contraceptive implants removed or used OCs within 60 days of the screening visit, were breast feeding, had not had three regular menstrual cycles in the past 3 months, were either <80 or >130% of ideal body weight, had taken medications known to alter blood lipid levels within the past 30 days, were hypertensive, had an abnormal pelvic or breast examination, showed evidence of significant cardiovascular, pulmonary, hepatic, renal, or endocrine disease, were consuming more than two alcoholic drinks per day, or had a cervical pap test indicating epithelial, nonepithelial, or glandular cell abnormalities.

Subjects who qualified for the study and consented to participate in it, returned between days 22 and 24 of the next normal menstrual cycle (visit 1). Vital signs and general characteristics were recorded, and blood samples were collected for determination of the lipid profile, sex hormone-binding globulin (SHBG), β-human chorionic gonadotrophin (β-hCG), free and total testosterone, and progesterone. Study subjects returned to the clinic between days 18 and 21 of treatment cycle 3 (visit 2) at which time bleeding diaries were reviewed and new OC medication was issued. Subjects returned on days 18–21 of treatment cycle 6 (visit 3) for a physical examination and blood drawing. Each subject also had a posttreatment visit (visit 4) ~1 month after completion of the study.

Analytical Methods

Lipid and lipoprotein measurements were performed on plasma samples obtained by 4°C centrifugation of venous blood collected after a 12-hour fast into Vacutainer tubes containing EDTA. Total plasma cholesterol[10] and triglycerides[11] were measured enzymatically (Boehringer Mannheim Diagnostics, Indianapolis, IN). HDL-C was determined by measuring cholesterol in the supernatant liquid after precipitation of the plasma with $MgCl_2$ and dextran sulfate.[12] LDL-C levels were calculated according to Friedewald et al.[13] with correction for Lp(a) cholesterol determined by Lp(a) protein $\times$ 1.5. Lp(a) protein levels were determined with an enzyme-linked immunoassay (ELISA) using goat polyclonal anti-apo(a) as the trapping antibody and rabbit polyclonal anti-apo(a) as the detecting antibody.[14] Lp(a) levels reported here in mg/dL represent the total protein component of Lp(a), including apo(a) and apo B. The intra- and interassay coefficients of variation were 4.0% and 9.0%, respectively. For normal Lp(a) protein levels in the range of 1–10 mg/dL, the contribution of plasminogen at physiological concentrations (200 mg/dL) to Lp(a) levels was negligible.

Statistical Methods

Data were obtained for most of the 50 subjects in each group after OC treatment for three cycles. Only limited data for subjects completing six treatment cycles have been collected thus far. If the data for an analyte were distributed normally, parametric analysis was performed with a paired t-test. When the distribution was nonnormal, nonparametric analysis was performed with Wilcoxon's rank sum test. Data set differences of >95% probability ($P < 0.05$) were regarded as significant.[15]

Results

The mean total cholesterol concentration in the women on Desogen rose from 179 to 189 mg/dL (+6%) during the initial 3 months of the study, whereas in subjects on Lo/Ovral, total cholesterol did not change significantly during this period (Tables 1 and 2). HDL-C rose from 60 to 66 mg/dL (+10%) in subjects on Desogen, but decreased from 61 to 56 mg/dL (−8%) in subjects on Lo/Ovral, although this latter change was not statistically significant. These diverging effects are strikingly apparent in Figure 1 (top right). For women on Desogen, this favorable change in HDL-C was reflected in a 13% increase in the mean levels of HDL_2-C and an 8% increase in HDL_3-C. In contrast, women on Lo/Ovral experienced a 17% de-

TABLE 1

Effect of Desogen on Lipid and Apolipoprotein Levels in Premenopausal Women

	0 mon		3 mon		6 mon
TOTAL-C					
Median	174		190		190
Mean[a]	179 ± 30		189 ± 30		187 ± 23
n	50		46		19
P		0.001		NS	
HDL-C					
Median	59		66		66
Mean	60 ± 16		66 ± 14		64 ± 17
n	50		46		19
P		0.004		NS	
HDL$_2$-C					
Median	21		24		24
Mean	23 ± 9		26 ± 10		23 ± 10
n	50		46		19
P		NS		NS	
HDL$_3$-C					
Median	38		40		40
Mean	37 ± 9		40 ± 9		40 ± 9
n	50		46		19
P		0.03		NS	
LDL-C					
Median	100		98		103
Mean	103 ± 30		101 ± 31		101 ± 22
n	50		46		19
P		NS		NS	
TRIG					
Median	75		105		104
Mean	79 ± 30		113 ± 42		110 ± 40
n	50		46		19
P		0.0001		NS	
ApoA-I					
Median	128		154		145
Mean	129 ± 27		155 ± 32		147 ± 34
n	50		46		15
P		0.0001		NS	
Apo B					
Median	76		87		98
Mean	79 ± 18		88 ± 22		96 ± 16
n	50		46		15
P		0.002		NS	
Apo E					
Median	7.7		6.4		6.8
Mean	8.0 ± 2.2		7.0 ± 1.8		6.8 ± 1.1
n	50		44		13
P		0.001		NS	
Lp(a) protein					
Median	6.0		3.7		6.5
Mean	10.1 ± 11.2		9.0 ± 12.5		8.1 ± 7.7
n	50		46		22
P		0.05		0.02	

[a] Values are ± SD.

TABLE 2

Effect of Lo/Ovral on Lipid and Apolipoprotein Levels in Premenopausal Women

	0 mon		3 mon		6 mon
TOTAL-C					
Median	181		188		195
Mean[a]	187 ± 33		191 ± 37		189 ± 20
n	50		34		15
P		NS		NS	
HDL-C					
Median	56		54		58
Mean	61 ± 18		56 ± 16		58 ± 17
n	50		34		15
P		NS		<0.05	
HDL$_2$-C					
Median	20		18		19
Mean	23 ± 11		19 ± 10		20 ± 10
n	50		34		15
P		NS		NS	
HDL$_3$-C					
Median	38		37		39
Mean	38 ± 10		37 ± 9		38 ± 10
n	50		34		15
P		NS		NS	
LDL-C					
Median	100		115		110
Mean	109 ± 31		115 ± 41		112 ± 26
n	50		34		15
P		<0.05		NS	
TRIG					
Median	76		90		80
Mean	89 ± 50		101 ± 59		95 ± 45
n	50		34		15
P		NS		NS	
ApoA-I					
Median	128		126		126
Mean	134 ± 29		131 ± 37		124 ± 23
n	50		32		15
P		NS		0.045	
Apo B					
Median	82		91		84
Mean	82 ± 21		91 ± 23		90 ± 22
n	50		32		15
P		<0.05		NS	
Apo E					
Median	7.2		7.4		7.0
Mean	8.4 ± 4.4		7.3 ± 1.9		6.8 ± 1.6
n	50		29		12
P		NS		NS	
Lp(a) protein					
Median	8.1		5.7		4.0
Mean	12.9 ± 13.1		9.9 ± 10.8		8.4 ± 10.3
n	50		34		16
P		<0.01		NS	

[a] Values are $\pm$ SD.

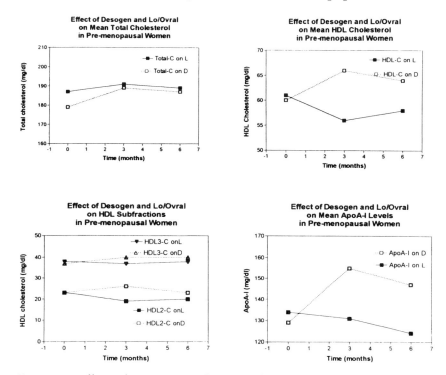

FIGURE 1. *Effect of Desogen and Lo/Ovral on total cholesterol, HDL-C, HDL_2-C, HDL_3-C, and apo A-I over time in premenopausal women.*

crease in HDL_2-C and a 3% decrease in HDL_3-C, although these changes did not reach statistical significance. The above significant increase in HDL-C in women on Desogen is also reflected in a very significant rise of 20% in the levels of their apo A-I, the principle apoprotein of HDL. Apo A-I in subjects on Lo/Ovral did not change significantly during this initial 3-month phase. (Table 1; Figure 1, bottom right).

Some of the largest changes observed in lipid analytes occurred in the triglycerides. For subjects on Desogen, the mean triglyceride level rose from 79 to 113 mg/dL (+43%) over the initial 3-month period (Table 1, Figure 2, top left). In subjects on Lo/Ovral, the mean triglyceride level rose from 89 to 101 mg/dL (+13%), although this latter change was not significant. The increase in triglycerides observed in both groups over the initial 3-month period was attended by a significant 12% decrease for apo E in subjects on Desogen, and an insignificant decrease of 13% in subjects on Lo/Ovral. LDL-C showed no significant change in subjects on Desogen and a 5% in-

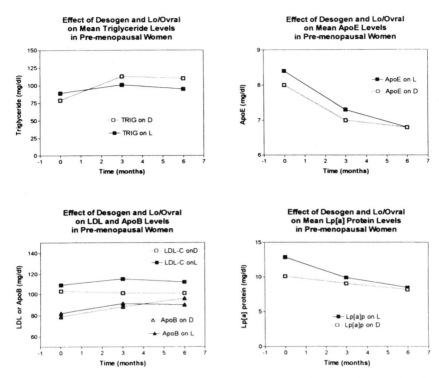

FIGURE 2. *Effect of Desogen and Lo/Ovral on LDL-C, apo A-I over time in premenopausal women.*

crease in subjects on Lo/Ovral during the first 3 months. Nevertheless, both groups of subjects experienced significant increases of 11% in mean apo B levels during the initial 3-month regimen.

The large difference between the median and mean values of Lp(a) in subjects on Desogen or Lo/Ovral indicate the nonnormal distribution of Lp(a) protein levels in both groups. In the Desogen group, the median level decreased from 6.0 to 3.7 mg/dL (−38%) and the mean level from 10.1 to 9.0 mg/dL (−11%). In the Lo/Ovral group, the median level decreased 30% and the mean by 23% (Tables 1 and 2). In both cases, these decrements were significant.

Comparison of lipid and apolipoprotein levels in subjects at 3 and 6 months showed significant changes only for Lp(a) in subjects on Desogen, and in HDL-C and apo A-I in subjects on Lo/Ovral. These results may be due to the achievement of metabolic equilibrium by 3 months with no further change during the following 3 months. Lack of statistical significance could also be do to insufficient population size for the paired comparison tests.

Discussion

During the past 5 years, a number of studies have demonstrated that hormone replacement therapy in postmenopausal women causes a very favorable change in the lipoprotein profile, particularly in the reduction of Lp(a) levels.[16–24] During this same time period, there have been >50 publications describing the effects of contraceptive hormones on lipids and lipoproteins in premenopausal women. However, relatively few of these studies reported the effects of OC on the level of Lp(a), now a well-established independent risk factor for cardiovascular disease in women. From those studies that have examined a possible relation between contraceptive hormone use and Lp(a) levels, somewhat mixed results have been obtained. In a French population, Steinmetz et al.[25] observed no relation between plasma levels of Lp(a) and cholesterol, triglyceride, glucose, inflammatory proteins, obesity, tobacco use, and OC use. In a small group of 13 Chinese women given a triphasic OC for three cycles, Sheu et al. found that Lp(a) levels did not change significantly.[26] Delplanque et al.[27] have measured the levels of Lp(a) in healthy OC users, contraceptive users with thrombosis, and nonusers. They found no significant difference in the Lp(a) levels among these groups. Oyelola et al.[28] have studied the effect of low-dose combination oral or injectable contraceptives on plasma lipoprotein levels in a group of Nigerian women. In subjects using either type of contraception, there were plasma elevations of total cholesterol, LDL-C, apo B, and Lp(a). However, there was no significant difference between these parameters for subjects using the oral versus the injectable contraceptive.

One of the earliest and most definitive studies evaluating the effect of OC on the levels of lipoproteins, including Lp(a), was conducted by März et al.[29] This study compared the effects of OC containing levonorgestrel or desogestrel in premenopausal women. These progestins were given as the Triquilar (Schering Corp, Kenilworth, NJ) and Marvelon (Organon) formulations. These formulations may be compared with Lo/Ovral and Desogen since they contain norgestrel and desogestrel, respectively. In fact, Marvelon and Desogen are identical. Triquilar and Lo/Ovral taken for three cycles cause significant 16% and 13% elevations of triglycerides, respectively. The desogestrel-containing formulations elevate triglyceride to higher levels; Marvelon by 21% and Desogen by 43%. Total cholesterol levels are not significantly changed by the norgestrel-containing formulations. Of the desogestrel-containing contraceptives, only Desogen elevates cholesterol significantly (+5%). Whereas nei-

TABLE 3

Comparison of the Effect of Oral Contraceptives Containing Levonorgestrel or Desogestrel (3 cycles) on Plasma Levels of Lipids and Lipoproteins in Premenopausal Women

	Levonorgestrel		Desogestrel	
	Triquilar[a]	Lo/ovral[b]	Marvelon[a]	Desogen[b]
Triglyceride	+16%*	+13%*	+21%*	+43%
Phospholipids	+7%	—	+8%	—
Cholesterol	NSC	NSC	NSC	+5%*
Lipoprotein (a)	NSC	−30/−23%*	NSC	−30/−11%*

NSC, no significant change; *$P < 0.05$.
[a] März et al. (1985).
[b] Houston study.

ther Triquilar nor Marvelon significantly altered Lp(a) levels,[29] in the present study Lo/Ovral and Desogen decreased median Lp(a) levels by 30% (Table 3). Because Marvelon and Desogen are identical formulations, it is a bit surprising that their effects on triglyceride and Lp(a) levels differ significantly. This difference may be due to different diets and ethnic compositions of the German and American

TABLE 4

Comparison of the Effect of Oral Contraceptives Containing Desogestrel (3 cycles) on Plasma Levels of Lipids and Lipoproteins in Premenopausal Women

	Gracial[a]	Desogen[b]
Total-C	+5%	+5%**
HDL-C	+29%**	+10%**
HDL$_2$-C	+9%	+13%**
HDL$_3$-C	+7%	+8%*
LDL-C	−5%	+2%
TG	+50%**	+43%**
ApoA-I	+17%**	+20%**
Apo B	+15%*	+11%**
Apo E	−35%*	−12%**
Lp (a)	−20%*	−38/−11%*

*$P < 0.05$; **$P < 0.01$.
[a] Kuhl et al. (1993); Frankfurt study.
[b] Houston study.

study populations. The latter contained a significant number of black women who typically have higher Lp(a) levels than white women.

A much more recent study has examined the effect of a biphasic formulation containing 40 μg ethinyl estradiol + 25 μg desogestrel (7 tablets) and 30 μg ethinyl estradiol + 125 μg desogestrel (15 tablets) known as Gracial, and the results of that study[30] are directly comparable with the results we have obtained in the present study with Desogen. (Table 4) Both formulations caused only small elevations in total cholesterol (5%/5%), and modest elevations in HDL$_2$-C (+9%/+13%) and HDL$_3$-C (+7%/+8%). Both contraceptives caused large elevations in triglycerides (+50%/+43%). They also produce similar elevations in apo A-I (+17%/+20%) and apo B (+15%/+11%), but declinations in apo E (−35%/−12%). Lp(a) underwent significant decrease with both Gracial (−20%) and Desogen (−38%).

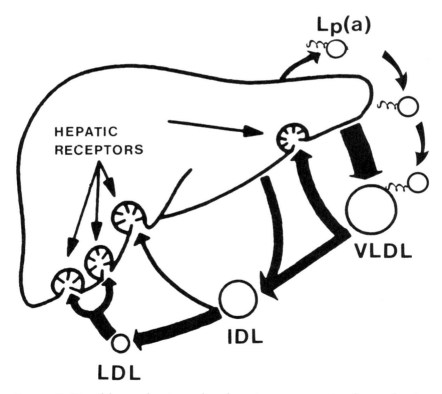

FIGURE 3. *Possible mechanism whereby estrogen may stimulate reduction of plasma Lp(a) levels.*

The observed decrease in Lp(a) caused by OC may have a significant linkage to the concomitant large elevation in triglyceride. Several laboratories have now observed a reciprocal relation between these two species.[31-33] The synchronous perturbation of their levels by estrogen may allow us to gain new insight into their metabolic relation. Estrogen stimulates both the secretion of VLDL and an increased uptake of VLDL remnants by hepatic receptors.[5] Lp(a) is known to associate noncovalently with other apo B-100-containing lipoproteins.[34] Hence elevation of VLDL increases the probability of their association with Lp(a) and the formation of a VLDL-Lp(a) complex. An increased uptake of the complex would cause a net decrease in plasma Lp(a)[35] (Figure 3). An additional or alternative mechanism may also be operating; the increased synthesis and secretion of VLDL, which requires apo B-100, may deplete the pool of apo B, thereby making it less available for the production of Lp(a). The latter mechanism is consistent with our recent observation that Lp(a) is about twofold higher in type IIa than in type IIb hyperlipoproteinemic subjects, and the observation that fibrate induced lowering of triglycerides in type IIb subjects leads to significant elevation of Lp(a).[36]

Acknowledgment

The authors thank John Gaubatz, Karima Ghazzaly, and Charles Etta Rhodes for their technical assistance and Renee Wells for editorial assistance (TTGA).

References

1. Rebar RW, Zeserson K. Characteristics of the new progestogens in combination oral contraceptives. *Contraception* 1991;44(1):1–9.
2. Chez RA. Clinical aspects of three new progestogens: Desogestrel, gestodene, and norgestimate. *Am J Obstet Gynecol* 1989;160(5)(pt 2): 1296–1300.
3. Lobo RA. Clinical review 27: Effects of hormonal replacement on lipids and lipoproteins in postmenopausal women. *J Clin Endocrin Metab* 1991;73(5):925–930.
4. Colvin, PL, Auerbach BJ, Case DL, et al. A dose-response relationship between sex hormone-induced change in hepatic triglyceride lipase and high-density lipoprotein cholesterol in postmenopausal women. *Metabolism* 1991;40(10):1052–1056.

5. Walsh BW, Schiff I, Rosner B, et al. Effects of postmenopausal estrogen replacement on the concentrations and metabolism of plasma lipoproteins. *N Eng J Med* 1991;325:1196–1204.
6. Virnikka L, Ylikorkala O, Vikro R, et al. Metabolism of a new synthetic progestogen org 2969 (13 ethyl-11-methylene-18, 19-di nor-17-alpha-pregn-4-In-20 yn-17 ol) in female volunteers: Distribution and excretion of radioactivity after an oral dose of labeled drug. *Acta Endocrin* 1980;93(3):375–379.
7. Hasenack HG, Bosch AMG, Kaar K. Serum levels of 3-ketodesogestrel after oral administration of desogestrel and 3-ketodesogestrel. *Contraception* 1986;33(6):591–596.
8. Elger W, Beier S. Aktuelle aspekte der Hormonalen Kontrazeption (Actual aspect of hormonal contraception). *Excerpta Med* 1982;9–26.
9. Berarink EW, van Meel F, Turpijn EW, et al. Binding of progestogens to receptor proteins in MCG-7 cells. *J Steroid Biochem* 1983;19:1563–1570.
10. Siedel J, Hagele E, Ziegenhorn J, et al. Reagent for the enzymatic determination of serum total cholesterol with improved lipolytic efficiency. *Clin Chem* 1983;29:1075–1080.
11. Nagele U, Hagele E, Sauer G, et al. Reagent for the enzymatic determination of serum total triglyceride with improved lipolytic efficiency. *J Clin Chem Clin Biochem* 1984;22:165–174.
12. Warnick GR, Benderson J, Albers JJ. Dextran sulfate Mg^{2+} precipitation procedure for quantification of high-density-lipoprotein cholesterol. *Clin Chem* 1982;28:1379–1388.
13. Friedewald WT, Levy RI, Fredrickson DS. Estimation of the concentration of low-density lipoprotein in plasma, without use of the preparative ultracentrifuge. *Clin Chem* 1972;18:499–502.
14. Gaubatz JW, Cushing GL, Morrisett JD. Quantitation, isolation and characterization of human lipoprotein[a]. Plasma lipoproteins. Characterization, cell biology and metabolism. *Methods Enzymol* 1986; 129:167–185.
15. Mathews DE, Farewell VT. *Using and Understanding Medical Statistics.* S. Karger A.G., Basel; 1988:11–19.
16. Lobo RA, Notelovitz M, Bernstein L, et al. Lp(a) Lipoprotein: Relationship to Cardiovascular disease risk factors, exercise, and estrogen. *Am J Obstet Gynecol* 1992;166:1182–1190.
17. Soma MR, Osnago-Gadda I, Paoletti R, et al. The lowering of lipoprotein[a] induced by estrogen plus progesterone replacement therapy in postmenopausal women. *Arch Intern Med* 1993;153:1462–1468.
18. Farish E, Rolton HA, Barnes JF, et al. Lipoprotein(a) and postmenopausal oestrogen. *Acta Endocrinol* 1993;129:225–228.
19. Farish E, Rolton HA, Barnes JF, et al. Lipoprotein (a) concentrations in postmenopausal women taking norethisterone. *JAMA* 1992;267: 2327–2328.
20. Kim CJ, Jang HC, Cho DH, et al. Effects of hormone replacement therapy on lipoprotein(a) and lipids in postmenopausal women. *Arterioscler Thromb* 1994;14(2):275–281.
21. Julius U, Fritsch H, Fritsch W, et al. Impact of hormone replacement therapy on postprandial lipoproteins and lipoprotein(a) in normolipidemic postmenopausal women. *Clin Invest* 1994;72:502–507.
22. Mendoza S, Velazquez E, Osona A, et al. Postmenopausal Cyclic estrogen-progestin therapy lowers lipoprotein[a]. *J Lab Clin Med* 1994; 123:837–841.

23. Caruso MG, Berloco P, Notarnicola M, et al. Lipoprotein(a) serum levels in post-menopausal women treated with oral estrogens administered at different times. *Horm Metab Res* 1994;26:379–382.
24. Shewmon DA, Stock JL, Rosen CJ, et al. Tamoxifen and estrogen lower circulating lipoprotein(a) concentrations in healthy postmenopausal women. *Arterioscler Thromb* 1994;14:1586–1593.
25. Steinmetz J, Tarallo P, Fournier B, et al. Reference values of lipoprotein (a) in a French population. *Presse Med* 1994;23(37):1695–1698.
26. Sheu WH, Hsu CH, Chen YS, et al. Prospective elevation of insulin resistance and lipid metabolism in women receiving oral contraceptives. *Clin Endocrin* 1994;40(2):249-255.
27. Delplanque B, Beaumont V, Lemort N, et al. Lp(a) levels and antiestrogen antibodies in women with and without thrombosis in the course of oral contraception. *Atherosclerosis* 1993;100:183–188.
28. Oyelola OO. fasting plasma lipids, lipoproteins and apolipoproteins in Nigerian women using combined oral and progestin-only injectable contraceptives. *Contraception* 1993;47(5):445–454.
29. März W, Gross W, Gabriele G, et al. A randomized crossover comparison of two low-dose contraceptives: Effects on serum lipids and lipoproteins. *Am J Obstet Gynecol* 1985;153(3):287–293.
30. Kuhl H, März W, Jung-Hoffman C, et al. Effect on lipid metabolism of a biphasic desogestrel-containing oral contraceptive: Divergent changes in apolipoprotein B and E and transitory decrease in Lp(a) levels. *Contraception* 1993;47:69–83.
31. Kostner GM: Interrelation of Lp(a) with plasma triglycerides. *Atheroscler Rev* 1991;22:131–135.
32. Bartens W, Rader DJ, Talley G, et al. Decreased plasma levels of lipoprotein(a) in patients with hypertriglyceridemia. *Atherosclerosis* 1994; 108:149–157.
33. Walek T, von Eckardstein A, Schulte H, et al. Effect of hypertriglyceridemia on lipoprotein(a) serum concentrations. *Eur J Clin Invest* 1995; 25:311–316.
34. McConathy WJ, Trieu VN, Koren E, et al. Triglyceride-rich lipoprotein interactions with Lp(a). *Chem Phys Lipids* 1994;6768:105–114.
35. Marcovina SM, Morrisett JD. Structure and metabolism of lipoprotein[a] *Curr Opin Lipid* 1995;6:136–145.
36. Jones PH, Pownall HJ, Patsch W, et al. Effect of Gemfibrozil on fasting and post-prandial levels of lipoprotein[a] in type II hyperlipoproteinemic subjects. *J Lipid Res* 1996;37:1298–1308.

Chapter 19

Do Progestins Attenuate Estrogen's Beneficial Effects on the Cardiovascular System?

Leon Speroff, MD

Postmenopausal hormone therapy deserves consideration as a legitimate component of preventive health care for older women. One can argue convincingly that protection against cardiovascular disease is the major benefit of postmenopausal estrogen treatment, and the magnitude of this benefit is considerable. There is a sound rationale for this protection in the link between cardiovascular disease and the sex hormones.

During the reproductive years, women are "protected" from coronary heart disease. For this reason, women lag behind men in the incidence of coronary heart disease by 10 years, and for myocardial infarction and sudden death, women have had a 20-year advantage. The reasons for this are complex, but a significant contribution to this protection can be assigned to the higher high-density lipoprotein (HDL) levels in younger women, an effect of estrogen. Throughout adulthood, the blood HDL cholesterol (HDL-C) level is ~10 mg/dL higher in women, and this difference continues through the postmenopausal years. Total and low-density lipoprotein cholesterol (LDL-C) levels are lower in premenopausal women than in men, although the levels gradually increase with aging, and after menopause they rise rapidly. In men. the LDL-C levels increase gradually until about age 50 when, in contrast to women, the levels stop rising. After menopause, the risk of coronary heart disease doubles for women as the atherogenic lipids about age 60 reach levels greater than those in men. At all ages, however, HDL-C values in women are 10 mg/dL higher than in men.

From: Forte TM, (ed). *Hormonal, Metabolic, and Cellular Influences on Cardiovascular Disease in Women.* Armonk, NY: Futura Publishing Company, Inc.; © 1997.

The higher HDL levels in women compared with men represent the net effect of estrogen (HDL elevating) in women and androgens (HDL lowering) in men. Athough the exact mechanism of protection provided by HDL is not totally understood, it is fair to say that HDL promotes the efflux of cholesterol from macrophages and the intimal wall of the arteries. At roughly the age of menopause (48–55), the average cholesterol level in women rises higher than the average level in men as HDL declines and LDL increases.[1] In women, data from two large prospective studies indicate that HDL-C is related more closely to cardiovascular disease than is LDL-C.[2,3]

The importance of HDL-C in women is a major reason that clinicians are concerned about the impact of a progestational agent. The addition of a progestational agent to postmenopausal estrogen therapy is now accepted as a standard part of the treatment program. The obvious objective for this combined estrogen-progestin approach is the need to prevent the increased risk of endometrial cancer associated with exposure to unopposed estrogen. But, in protecting the uterus, have we sacrificed (attenuated) some of estrogen's beneficial actions on the cardiovascular system? To address this question, we must consider the many activities of estrogen in the cardiovascular system, and place the effect on the lipid profile in perspective.

Mechanisms for Estrogen's Protection Against Cardiovascular Disease

A Favorable Impact on Lipids and Lipoproteins

The most important lipid effects of postmenopausal estrogen treatment are the reduction in LDL-C and the increase in HDL-C. Although it is recognized now that this is not the sole mechanism for estrogen's beneficial impact on cardiovascular disease, the lipid effects still play a substantial role.[4]

Estrogen increases triglyceride levels and increases LDL catabolism as well as lipoprotein receptor numbers and activity, resulting in decreasing LDL levels.[5–7] The increase in HDL levels, particularly due to the HDL_2 subfraction, is to an important degree the consequence of the inhibition of hepatic lipase activity, that converts HDL_2 to HDL_3. LDL particle size gets smaller (potentially a more atherogenic adverse effect) with estrogen treatment, a change that is associated with an increase in the triglyceride content of LDL;

however, it is not certain to what degree this change is related to dose nor is the clinical significance understood.[8,9] Furthermore, because small LDL is more atherogenic because it is oxidized more easily, this change in LDL particle size may be compensated by the antioxidant activity of estrogen that protects against atherosclerosis by inhibiting lipoprotein oxidation.[10] The changes in circulating apoprotein levels mirror those of the lipoproteins: apolipoprotein (apo) B (the principal surface protein of LDL) levels diminish in response to estrogen, and apo A-I (the principal apo of HDL) increases. The HDL and triglyceride increase induced by estrogen treatment is attenuated if progestins are added in sufficient doses.[11] Both estrogen and exercise favorably affect the lipid and lipoprotein profile; however, in a comparison of exercise and estrogen treatment, combining estrogen and exercise did not produce a synergistic outcome.[12]

Apo E is the ligand for the LDL receptor and exists in different isoforms. Individuals exhibit different apo E phenotypes according to which isoforms are expressed. Specific phenotypes are associated with specific LDL-C levels. This association is greater in women than in men and greater in postmenopausal women compared with premenopausal women.[13] Modulation of the interaction between the apo E phenotype and LDL-C levels by the sex hormones remains to be well studied. Nevertheless the presence of specific apo E phenotypes accelerates the postmenopausal increase in LDL-C. A linkage between the apo E phenotype and late onset Alzheimer's disease has also been reported.[14]

Direct Anti-Atherosclerotic Effects

An important study in monkeys supported the protective action of estrogen against atherosclerosis, but by a mechanism independent of the cholesterol profile. Oral administration of a combination of estrogen and a high dose of progestin to monkeys fed a high-cholesterol diet decreased the extent of coronary atherosclerosis despite a reduction in HDL-C levels.[15-17] In somewhat similar experiments, estrogen treatment markedly prevented arterial lesion development in rabbits, and this effect was not reduced by adding progestin to the treatment regimen.[18-21] This suggests that women with already favorable cholesterol profiles would benefit through this additional action. And, in considering the impact of progestational agents, lowering of HDL is not necessarily atherogenic if accompanied by an increased estrogen impact.

The monkey colony studies have been extended to a postmenopausal model (ovariectomized monkeys). Compared with no hormone treatment, treatment with either estrogen alone or estrogen with progesterone in a sequential manner, significantly reduced atherosclerosis, once again independently of the circulating lipid and lipoprotein profile.[22] A direct inhibition of LDL accumulation and an increase in LDL metabolism in arterial vessels could be demonstrated in these monkeys being fed a highly atherogenic diet.[23]

Thus, estrogen exerts a protective effect directly on the arterial wall independent of its effects on circulating lipoproteins. The presence of sex steroid receptors in arterial endothelium and smooth muscle lends support for the importance of this direct action; however, the mechanisms involved remain unknown.[24] One important mechanism may be coronary artery remodeling. Atherosclerosis is associated with a compensatory change in coronary artery size that increases the magnitude of the lumen (a process called remodeling). It is important to note that the addition of a progestin did not attenuate the beneficial effect of estrogen on coronary remodeling in monkeys.[25] Involvement of estrogen and estrogen receptors is supported by the observation that atherosclerotic coronary arteries in premenopausal women demonstrate diminished expression of estrogen receptors compared to normal premenopausal arteries.[26]

Endothelium-dependent Vasodilatation and Antiplatelet Aggregation

Endothelium modulates the degree of contraction and function of the surrounding smooth muscle, primarily by the release of endothelium-derived relaxing and contracting factors (EDRFs and EDCFs). In hypertension and other cardiovascular diseases, the release of EDRFs [which is probably one factor, nitric oxide (NO)] is blunted, and the release of EDCFs (the most important being endothelin-1) is augmented. The endothelins are a family of peptides that act in a paracrine fashion on smooth muscle cells. Endothelin-1 appears to be exclusively synthesized by endothelial cells. Endothelin-induced vasoconstriction is a consequence of a direct action on vascular smooth muscle cells, an action that is reversed by NO. Impaired release of NO, therefore, enhances endothelin action. Hypertension and atherosclerosis are believed to be influenced by the balance among these factors. In vitro, both estradiol and progesterone attenuate coronary artery contractions in response to the epithelial vasoconstrictor, endothelin.[27] Women have lower circulating levels of endothelin, and the levels are even lower during pregnancy and decrease in response to estrogen treatment.[28]

NO (and estrogen) also inhibits the adhesion and aggregation of platelets in a synergistic manner with prostacyclin (also a potent vasodilator derived from the endothelium).[29] These local actions are a likely site for sex steroid involvement; the vasodilating and antiplatelet action of estrogen, especially in the coronary arteries, is probably a consequence of endothelial response. In addition, postmenopausal women experience greater stress-induced neuroendocrine and blood pressure responses that are ameliorated by estrogen treatment.[30,31] However, the addition of medroxyprogesterone acetate (10 mg for 10 days) attenuates the beneficial effects of estrogen on measures of cardiovascular reactivity.[32]

Increased blood flow due to vasodilatation and decreased peripheral resistance can be observed to occur rapidly after the administration of estrogen. This response can be produced by both transdermal and oral administration.[33,34] The synthesis and secretion of NO (the potent epithelial vasodilating product) can be directly stimulated by estrogen in in vitro experimental preparations of coronary arteries.[35]

The synthesis of NO is involved in the regulation of vascular (and gastrointestinal) tone, and in neuronal activity. A family of isozymes (NO synthases) catalyze the oxidation of L-arginine to NO and citrulline. The action of NO synthase in the endothelium is calcium dependent, and its synthesis is mediated specifically by estrogen.[36] The NO synthase gene contains estrogen response elements, however conflicting expression (no response vs. stimulation) of this gene in response to estradiol has been reported.[37,38] In animal experiments, the endothelial basal release of NO is greater in females, a gender difference that is mediated by estrogen.[39,40]

Acetylcholine induces vasoconstriction in coronary arteries, however, the direct administration of estradiol in physiological doses into the coronary arteries of postmenopausal women with and without coronary heart disease converts acetylcholine-induced vasoconstriction into vasodilatation with increased flow.[41] This same estrogen-associated response is observed in women with coronary atherosclerosis comparing estrogen users to nonusers.[42] This is an endothelium-dependent response. The acute administration of estradiol to women delays the onset of signs of myocardial ischemia on electrocardiograms and increases exercise tolerance.[43] This is consistent with an effect that results in vasodilatation and increased blood flow. In both normal postmenopausal women and women with hypertension, hypercholesterolemia, diabetes mellitus, or coronary artery disease, the intra-arterial infusion of physiological amounts of estradiol into the forearm potentiates endothelium-dependent vasodilatation.[44]

Endothelium-Independent Vasodilatation

Estrogen causes relaxation in coronary arteries that are de-nuded of epithelium.[45] This response is not prevented by the presence of inhibitors of NO synthase or prostaglandin synthase. Thus this vasodilatation is achieved through a mechanism independent of the vascular endothelium, perhaps acting upon calcium-mediated events. The vasodilatation produced by sodium nitroprusside is endothelium-independent. In normal postmenopausal women and postmenopausal women with risk factors for atherosclerosis (hypertension, hypercholesterolemia, diabetes mellitus, coronary artery disease), the administration of physiological levels of estradiol increases forearm vasodilatation induced by sodium nitroprusside.[44]

Inotropic Actions on the Heart

Estrogen treatment increases left ventricular diastolic filling and stroke volume.[46–48] This effect is probably a direct inotropic action of estrogen which delays the age-related change in compliance that impairs cardiac relaxation.[49] In a 3-month study, medroxyprogesterone acetate (5 mg daily for 10 days each month) did not attenuate the increase in left ventricular output (systolic flow velocity) observed with estrogen treatment.[50]

Improvement of Glucose Metabolism

An age-related decline in the basal metabolic rate begins at menopause, associated with an increase in body fat, especially central (android) body fat.[51] Insulin resistance and circulating insulin levels increase in women after menopause, and impaired glucose tolerance predicts an increased risk of coronary heart disease.[52,53] Estrogen (with or without progestin) prevents the tendency to increase central body fat with aging.[54,55] This would inhibit the interaction among abdominal adiposity, hormones, insulin resistance, hyperinsulinemia, blood pressure, and an atherogenic lipid profile. Hyperinsulinemia also has a direct atherogenic effect on blood vessels, perhaps secondary to insulin propeptides. In addition to its vasoconstrictive properties, endothelin-1 exerts a mitogenic effect and therefore contributes to the atherosclerotic process. Insulin directly stimulates the secretion of endothelin-1 in endothelial cells, and the circulating levels of endothelin-1 are correlated with insulin levels.[56]

Postmenopausal women being treated with oral estrogen have lower fasting insulin levels and a lesser insulin response to glucose, indicating another mechanism for the protection against cardiovascular disease.[11,57,58] There is an important dose-response relation; 0.625 mg conjugated estrogens improve insulin sensitivity, 1.25 mg does not.[59] The addition of a progestational agent can attenuate this beneficial response to oral estrogen, but the clinical impact and variation with dose are unknown.[59,60] Nonoral administration of estrogen has little effect on insulin metabolism, unless a dose is administered that is equivalent to 1.25 mg conjugated estrogens.[60,61] Because a lower oral dose produces a beneficial impact, this suggests that the hepatic first-pass effect is important in this response.

Consistent with this salutary impact of estrogen, the Nurses' Health Study has documented a 20% decreased risk of noninsulin dependent diabetes mellitus in current users of estrogen.[62]

Inhibition of Lipoprotein Oxidation

The oxidation of LDL particles is a step (perhaps the initial step) in the formation of atherosclerosis, and smoking is associated with a high level of lipoprotein oxidation. In animal experiments, the administration of large amounts of antioxidants inhibits the formation of atherosclerosis and causes the regression of existing lesions. Vitamin E and beta carotene (the prohormone of Vitamin A) are antioxidants. Studies indicate that the risk of myocardial infarction in smokers is higher in men and women with the lowest carotene levels, and supplementary intake of vitamin E decreases the risk of coronary heart disease.[63–65] The Nurses' Health Study has reported a decreased risk of coronary heart disease in women with high-carotene levels.[65] Thus treatment with antioxidants may reduce the risk of cardiovascular disease and the risk of complications in those who already have cardiovascular disease.[66]

Estrogen is an antioxidant. Estradiol directly inhibits LDL oxidation in response to copper and decreases the overall formation of lipid oxides.[10,67] Importantly, this antioxidant action of estradiol is associated with physiological blood levels.[68] In addition, estrogen may regenerate circulating antioxidants (tocopherols and beta carotene) and preserve these antioxidants within LDL particles. This antioxidant action of estrogen preserves endothelial-dependent vasodilator function by preventing the deleterious effect that oxidized LDL has on endothelial production of vasoactive agents.[69]

A Favorable Impact on the Clotting Mechanism

The increased incidence of thromboembolic disease, hypertension, and altered carbohydrate metabolism during older, high-dose oral contraceptive use is well documented. Because of the lower dosage in a postmenopausal hormone program, these metabolic effects are not seen in postmenopausal therapy.

Clinical data on the association between postmenopausal estrogen therapy and the risk of venous thrombosis are limited. Older case-control studies failed to find a link between postmenopausal doses of estrogen and venous thrombosis.[70,71] However, these studies excluded cases with pre-existing risk factors for thrombosis. A well-designed case-control study of older women unselected for other thrombotic risk factors indicated that postmenopausal doses of estrogen did not increase the risk of venous thrombosis.[72] Others have also failed to find an increase in venous thromboembolism associated with postmenopausal hormone therapy.[73] Because venous thrombosis occurs later in life and is relatively infrequent in younger women, the cohort studies have had insufficient experience with this clinical problem to provide us with data.

Reduced levels of fibrinogen, factor VII, and plasminogen activator inhibitor have been observed in premenopausal women compared with postmenopausal women, and estrogen alone or combined with a progestin prevents the usual increase in these clotting factors associated with menopause.[74-76] This would be consistent with increased fibrinolytic activity, another possible cardioprotective mechanism probably mediated, at least partially, by NO and prostacyclin. Platelet aggregation is also reduced by postmenopausal estrogen treatment, and this response is slightly attenuated by medroxyprogesterone acetate.[29] However, in a randomized 1-year trial, the addition of medroxyprogesterone acetate, either sequentially or continuously, produced a more favorable change in coagulation factors compared to unopposed estrogen.[77] The transdermal and oral routes of administration of estrogen (combined with medroxyprogesterone acetate) do not have important differences in the effect on hemostatic risk factors, such as factor VII, fibrinogen, and antithrombin III; appropriate doses of hormone therapy do not have an adverse impact on the clotting system.[77-79]

It is important to recognize the importance of the dose-response relation between estrogen and the risk of thrombosis. High doses of estrogen cause thrombosis. Low doses of estrogen even may protect against thrombosis. The doses of estrogen that should be used for postmenopausal hormone therapy are possibly beneficial, and doses greater than those that protect against cardiovascular disease and osteoporosis (equivalent to 0.625 conjugated estrogens) should be avoided.

Inhibition of Vascular Smooth Muscle Growth and Migration–Intimal Thickening

Hypertension and atherosclerosis are associated with increased proliferation of vascular smooth muscle cells. This growth of smooth muscle cells is also characterized by migration into the intima. Arterial intimal thickening is an early indicator of atherosclerosis. The proliferation and migration of human aortic smooth muscle cells in response to growth factors are inhibited by estradiol, and importantly, this inhibition is not prevented by the presence of progesterone.[80] NO, which is regulated by estrogen, also inhibits smooth muscle proliferation.

Inhibition of Macrophage Foam Cell Formation

A feature of atherosclerotic plaque formation is monocytic infiltration into the arterial wall and the formation of macrophage foam cells. In nonantioxidant activity, estrogen inhibits macrophage foam cell formation.

Therefore, the possible beneficial actions of estrogens on cardiovascular disease include all of the following: (1) A favorable impact on the circulating lipid and lipoprotein profile, especially a decrease in total cholesterol and LDL-C and an increase in HDL-C. (2) A direct antiatherosclerotic effect in arteries. (3) Augmentation of vasodilating and antiplatelet aggregation factors, specifically NO and prostacyclin (endothelium-dependent mechanisms). (4) Vasodilatation by means of endothelium-independent mechanisms. (5) Direct inotropic actions on the heart. (6) Improvement of peripheral glucose metabolism with a subsequent decrease in circulating insulin levels. (7) Antioxidant activity. (8) Favorable impact on the clotting mechanism, at least partially mediated by endothelial NO and prostacyclin synthesis. (9) Inhibition of vascular smooth muscle growth and migration—intimal thickening. (10) Inhibition of macrophage foam cell formation.

Cardiovascular Disease and Progestins

Because the public health benefit of estrogen therapy on cardiovascular disease is of such enormous impact, it is vital that we know whether the addition of progestin has an adverse effect on the lipid profile and ultimately on cardiovascular disease. A review of the literature on this question suggests a dose-response relation.[81–89]

It is likely that the daily dose of the progestational agent is associated with a threshold level below which endometrial protection can be insufficient. Currently, the sequential program uses 5 or 10 mg medroxyprogesterone acetate and the combined daily method uses 2.5 mg. The dose of norethindrone that is comparable with 2.5 mg medroxyprogesterone acetate is 0.25 mg.[90] Although lower doses of progestational agents are effective in achieving target tissue responses (such as reducing the nuclear concentration of estrogen receptors), the long-term impact on endometrial histology has not yet been firmly established. The question of dose is an issue of major importance, especially in terms of the cardiovascular system and compliance because of progestin-induced side effects.

A decrease in HDL-C has been noted with 10-day monthly treatment with norethindrone (5 mg), megestrol acetate (5 mg), levonorgestrel (250 μg), and even medroxyprogesteron acetate (10 mg). No significant change was noted with micronized progesterone (200 mg). The lack of an effect noted with micronized progesterone was observed with a dose (200 mg daily), which yields a normal luteal phase blood level of progesterone. A similar "physiological" dose of synthetic progestins may be free of an adverse impact on HDL-C. Barrett-Connor and colleagues have been studying the adult residents of Rancho Bernardo, California. The women using both estrogen and progestin demonstrated the same favorable impact on cardiovascular risk factors as estrogen-only users when compared to the nonusers.[91] On the other hand, a well-designed study indicated that although the sequential estrogen plus progestin program had a favorable impact on lipids and the lipoprotein profile, the impact (as measured 1 year later) was less than that achieved by estrogen alone.[92]

Conclusions regarding the impact of progestational agents on cardiovascular disease are very much influenced by dose and duration of administration of the progestational agent involved. Although short-term studies suggest a negative impact of progestin (ie, subtracting from the beneficial effect of estrogen), long-term studies indicate that this short-term effect disappears.

Studies with the combination of an estrogen and a low dose of a progestational agent administered continuously (every day without a break) are emerging and documenting a favorable impact on lipids and lipoproteins. The various formulations include estradiol and levonorgestrel,[93] estradiol and 1 mg norethindrone acetate,[94] estradiol and dydrogesterone,[95] estradiol valerate and levonorgestrel or cyproterone acetate,[96] ethinyl estradiol and 0.5–1.0 mg norethindrone acetate,[97] and 0.625 conjugated estrogen and 2.5–5.0 mg medroxyprogesterone acetate.[98] Christiansen has documented the maintenance of a favorable lipid profile during a period of 5 years of treatment with continuous, combined estradiol and 1 mg norethindrone acetate.[94]

A large, prospective, 1-year randomized clinical trial compared sequential and combined regimens of conjugated estrogens and medroxyprogesterone acetate to unopposed estrogen.[58] Although the increase in HDL-C, HDL$_2$, and apo A-I levels was greater with unopposed estrogen, there was still a significant increase with combined estrogen-progestin treatment. Importantly, the decrease in total cholesterol, LDL-C, apo B, and lipoprotein(a) [Lp(a)] was equivalent, comparing unopposed estrogen with either sequential or daily, combined estrogen-progestin. Fasting glucose and insulin levels were improved in all treatment groups. Similar results have been observed in a 2-year randomized trial with 2 mg estradiol and 1 mg norethindrone acetate.[99] In a large cross-sectional study of 4,958 postmenopausal women, a favorable impact on the lipoprotein profile and fasting insulin levels was observed in users of unopposed estrogen and combined estrogen-progestin compared with nonusers.[11]

In Spain, 8 months of uninterrupted treatment with a daily dose of 2.5 mg medroxyprogesterone acetate in a combined estrogen-progestin program produced a favorable effect on the lipoprotein profile not substantially different from that achieved with estrogen alone.[100] A large multicenter trial in the United States produced a favorable lipoprotein profile during a 12-month period of time in women receiving daily 0.625 mg conjugated estrogen and 2.5 mg medroxyprogesterone acetate (and the positive effect was more pronounced in women with lower baseline HDL levels).[101]

Studies in women of arterial vascular resistance by Doppler ultrasound flow patterns have indicated no detrimental effects of exogenous progesterone or medroxyprogesterone acetate to the beneficial decrease in resistance (and increase in blood flow) produced by estrogen administration.[102,103]

Clinical Events–Epidemiological Data

How accurately do surrogate endpoints (such as the lipid profile) reflect and predict clinical events? Ultimately, only clinical event data (myocardial infarctions and strokes) will provide an accurate assessment. Such data are just beginning to emerge, and thus far, are reassuring, although limited by small numbers. In chronological order, they are as follows.

Two follow-up reports based upon a cohort of English women were focused primarily on cancer mortality.[104,105] Nevertheless, there was a statistically significant lower mortality rate due to ischemic heart disease and cerebrovascular disease associated with estrogen-progestin therapy; however, data were insufficient to compare estrogen alone with combined treatment.

In a case-control study of women with strokes or myocardial infarctions, the use of combined estrogen-progestin (specific drugs not indicated) was associated with a 14% reduced relative risk; however, this conclusion was based upon 12 cases and 28 controls, and the confidence interval (0.43–1.74) did not achieve significance, reflecting the lack of statistical power.[106]

A report from the cohort study from Uppsala, Sweden, provides information from the follow-up of ~23,000 women who were prescribed hormone therapy.[107] Overall there was a 30% reduction in myocardial infarction in women prescribed estradiol valerate or conjugated estrogens. What is especially noteworthy was a 50% reduced risk of myocardial infarction in women exposed to a sequential estrogen-progestin regimen consisting of 2 mg estradiol valerate and 10 days each month of levonorgestrel (250 mg). Treatment with this combined estrogen-progestin product was also associated with a 39% reduced risk of stroke, a statistically significant finding based on 27 cases compared to an expected incidence in the population (confidence interval: 0.40–0.88).[108]

In a case-control study from Massachusetts, no significant impact of estrogen-progestin treatment was noted; however, the authors indicated that the data were insufficient for evaluation (23 cases and 30 controls).[109]

A case-control study from the United Kingdom concluded that combined estrogen-progestin therapy was associated with a 32% statistically significant reduced risk of myocardial infarction (76 cases and 361 controls with a confidence interval of 0.47–0.97).[110]

In a population-based case-control study (502 cases and 1,193 controls) from Seattle, unopposed current use of estrogen was associated with a 31% reduction in the risk of myocardial infarction, and the current use of estrogen-progestin (largely a sequential regimen) with a 32% reduced risk.[111] Although this risk reduction was almost, but not quite statistically significant, there certainly was no evidence of attenuation secondary to the addition of a progestin. It is worth observing that the duration of treatment was relatively short, averaging <2 years.

In a comparison of postmenopausal women in Finland receiving unopposed estrogen or a sequential regimen of estradiol valerate and levonorgestrel (250 g for 10 days), both treatment groups had an equal reduction in ultrasonographically observed atherosclerotic plaques in the aorta and in the carotid and iliac arteries, despite a lesser increase in HDL-C with estrogen-progestin compared with unopposed estrogen (as in all of the studies reviewed above).[112]

These clinical event data (although still limited by small numbers) do not support the contention that exposure to a progestin (even the most androgenic of progestins) attenuates the cardiovascular benefit of estrogen.

The Postmenopausal Estrogen/Progestin Interventions (PEPI) Trial

PEPI was a randomized, double-blind, placebo-controlled 3-year trial of 875 postmenopausal women conducted in 7 clinical centers in the United States.[113] The participants were assigned randomly to the following treatment groups: placebo; estrogen alone, 0.625 mg conjugated estrogens daily; sequential estrogen and progestin, 0.625 mg conjugated estrogens daily and 10 mg medroxyprogesterone acetate days 1–12; sequential estrogen and progesterone, 0.625 mg conjugated estrogens daily and 200 mg micronized progesterone days 1–12; and continuous combination estrogen and progestin, 0.625 mg conjugated estrogens and 2.5 mg medroxyprogesterone acetate daily.

The statistical analysis indicated that an increase in HDL-C levels was greater with unopposed estrogen (mean increase 5.6 mg/dL) and with sequential estrogen and micronized progesterone (mean increase 4.1 mg/dL), compared with women receiving estrogen and medroxyprogesterone. However, as in the trials reviewed above,[58,99] the decrease in LDL-C was essentially the same in all treatment groups and significantly improved compared with the placebo group. There were no significant differences in systolic blood pressure, although all groups gradually increased systolic blood pressure with aging. There were no differences in diastolic blood pressure, and no changes with aging. The mean change in the 2-hour insulin levels did not differ significantly according to the treatment groups. The fasting insulin levels decreased slightly (compared with an increase in the placebo group) but did not achieve statistical significance in the treatment groups; however, all treatment groups demonstrated a significant decrease in fasting glucose levels. The placebo group demonstrated the well-recognized increase in fibrinogen (a risk factor for cardiovascular disease) that occurs after menopause. All treatments prevented this increase in fibrinogen.

The PEPI trial demonstrated a favorable impact on cardiovascular risk factors in women taking estrogen as well as combinations of estrogen and progestins. A major question is whether it is justified to interpret the results as indicating that a combination of estrogen plus micronized progesterone is clinically better because of the HDL-C responses. Observational studies have indicated that in women there is a 2–3% decrease in heart disease with a 1 mg increase in HDL-C. If this is accurate, then potentially the difference between estrogen and micronized progesterone compared with estrogen plus medroxyprogesterone acetate (a 3 mg HDL-C difference) would amount to a 9% difference in the risk of heart disease. However, the story is not that simple. Many of the beneficial actions of estrogen in terms of cardiovascular disease are dynamic effects on blood flow, atherosclerosis, the clotting system, and insulin levels. Given this complicated and multifactorial impact, the small difference in HDL-C is reduced in importance. It is worth emphasizing that the PEPI trial revealed the same beneficial effects in all treatment groups on LDL-C, fibrinogen, insulin levels, and glucose levels. In the Finnish ultrasonographic study, women receiving estradiol valerate and levonorgestrel had as great a reduction in large artery atherosclerotic plaques as those women on unopposed estrogen, despite a similar attenuation in HDL-C levels as observed in the PEPI trial.[112]

One of the important contributions of PEPI is to provide a good response to the criticism that the reason estrogen users have less cardiovascular disease is because clinicians give estrogen to healthier women. The results of this randomized trial demonstrate that estrogen has a greater impact compared to a placebo group, thus the design compensated for this criticism.

Conclusion

More than 30 published studies have addressed postmenopausal estrogen use and cardiovascular disease. Only a handful of studies have failed to find evidence for a protective effect of estrogens, most noteworthy the 1978 and 1985 reports from the Framingham study, the only prospective cohort study to report an increased risk among estrogen users.[114,115] However, the Framingham reports adjusted the data for total and HDL-C levels, an inappropriate adjustment since an impact on these variables is a major effect of estrogen. Reanalysis of the Framingham data (excluding angina as an endpoint) indicated a protective effect among women 50–59 years old, with too few estrogen users to estimate risk among older women.[116] Because this analysis still adjusted for HDL, it probably underestimated the benefit of postmenopausal use of estrogen.

Most impressive, therefore, are the uniformity and consistency of the literature on this subject. All the population-based case-control studies and (with the reanalysis of the Framingham Heart Study) all of the prospective studies conclude that postmenopausal use of estrogens protects against cardiovascular disease. Indeed, the studies probably all underestimate the protective effect because of the high percentage of postmenopausal women who discontinue their treatment. Sophisticated assessment and analysis (using the methods of information synthesis and meta-analysis) indicate that the effect of estrogen on heart disease is not controversial or ambiguous, but there clearly exists a protective benefit.[117,118] We have such uniformity and consistency among the epidemiological studies that the argument is very convincing. There remains, therefore, the important question of the nature and degree of impact due to the addition of progestational agents.

Evidence is accumulating to indicate that a progestational dose that protects the endometrium is available that avoids a significant impact on lipids and the lipoprotein profile. Furthermore, the growing appreciation for an impact of estrogen on mechanisms independent of lipids and the lipoprotein profile makes the presence of the progestin less concerning. With growing confidence we can offer and support combined estrogen-progestin therapy as an important contribution to good health for postmenopausal women.

References

1. Matthews KA, Meilahn E, Kuller LH, et al. Menopause and risk factors for coronary heart disease. *N Engl J Med* 1989;321:641.
2. Jacobs DR Jr, Mebane IL, Bangdiwala SI, et al. High density lipoprotein cholesterol as a predictor of cardiovascular disease mortality in men and women: The follow-up study of the Lipid Research Clinics Prevalence Study. *Am J Epidemiol* 1990;131:32.

3. Wilson PW, Garrison RJ, Castelli WP, et al. Prevalence of coronary heart disease in the Framingham offspring study: Role of lipoprotein cholesterols. *Am J Cardiol* 1980;46:649.
4. Manolio TA, Furberg CD, Shemanski L, et al. for the CHS Collaborative Research Group. Associations of postmenopausal estrogen use with cardiovascular disease and its risk factors in older women. *Circulation* 1993;88(part 1):2163.
5. Eriksson M, Berglund L, Rudling M, et al. Effects of estrogen on low density lipoprotein metabolism in males. Short-term and long-term studies during hormonal treatment of prostatic carcinoma. *J Clin Invest* 1989;84:802.
6. Walsh BW, Schiff I, Rosner B, et al. Effects of postmenopausal estrogen replacement on the concentrations and metabolism of plasma lipoproteins. *N Engl J Med* 1991;325:1196.
7. Muesing RA, Miller VT, LaRosa JC, et al. Effects of unopposed conjugated equine estrogen on lipoprotein composition and apolipoprotein-E distribution. *J Clin Endocrinol Metab* 1992;75:12150.
8. Granfone A, Campos H, McNamara JR, et al. Effects of estrogen replacement on plasma lipoproteins and apolipoproteins in postmenopausal dyslipidemic women. *Metabolism* 1992;41:1193.
9. Campos H, Sacks FM, Walsh BW, et al. Differential effects of estrogen on low-density lipoprotein subclasses in healthy postmenopausal women. *Metabolism* 1993;42:1153.
10. Rifici VA, Khachadurian AK. The inhibition of low-density lipoprotein oxidation by 17-beta estradiol. *Metabolism* 1992;41:1110.
11. Nabulsi AA, Folsom AR, White A, et al. Association of hormone-replacement therapy with various cardiovascular risk factors in postmenopausal women. *N Engl J Med* 1993;328:1069.
12. Lindheim SR, Notelovitz M, Feldman EB, et al. The independent effects of exercise and estrogen on lipids and lipoproteins in postmenopausal women. *Obstet Gynecol* 1994;83:167.
13. Schaefer EJ, Lamon-Fava S, Johnson S, et al. Effects of gender and menopausal status on the association of apolipoprotein E phenotype with plasma lipoprotein levels: Results from the Framingham Offspring Study. *Arterioscler Thromb* 1994;14:1105.
14. Corder EH, Saunders AM, Strittmatter WJ, et al. Gene dose of apolipoprotein E type 4 allele and the risk of Alzheimer's disease on late onset families. *Science* 1993;261:921.
15. Adams MR, Clarkson TB, Koritnik DR, et al. Contraceptive steroids and coronary artery atherosclerosis in cynomolgus macaques. *Fertil Steril* 1987;47:1010.
16. Clarkson TB, Adams MR, Kaplan JR, et al. From menarche to menopause: Coronary artery atherosclerosis and protection in cyanomolgus monkeys. *Am J Obstet Gynecol* 1989;160:1280.
17. Clarkson TB, Shively CA, Morgan TM, et al. Oral contraceptives and coronary artery atherosclerosis of cynomolgus monkeys. *Obstet Gynecol* 1990;75:217.
18. Kushwaha RS, Hazzard WR. Exogenous estrogens attenuate dietary hypercholesterolemia and atherosclerosis in the rabbit. *Metabolism* 1981;30:57.
19. Hough JL, Zilversmit DB. Effect of 17 beta estradiol on aortic cholesterol content and metabolism in cholesterol-fed rabbits. *Arteriosclerosis* 1986;6:57.

20. Henriksson P, Stamberger M, Eriksson M, et al. Oestrogen-induced changes in lipoprotein metabolism: Role in prevention of atherosclerosis in the cholesterol-fed rabbit. *Eur J Clin Invest* 1989;19:395.
21. Haarbo J, Leth-Espensen P, Stender S, et al. Estrogen monotherapy and combined estrogen-progestogen replacement therapy attenuate aortic accumulation of cholesterol in ovariectomized cholesterol-fed rabbits. *J Clin Invest* 1991;87:1274.
22. Adams MP, Kaplan JR, Manuck SB, et al. Inhibition of coronary artery atherosclerosis by 17-beta estradiol in ovariectomized monkeys. Lack of an effect of added progesterone. *Arterioscerosis* 1990;10:151.
23. Wagner JD, St Clair RW, Schwenke DC, et al. Regional differences in arterial low density lipoprotein metabolism in surgically postmenopausal Cynomolgus monkeys: Effects of estrogen and progesterone replacement therapy. *Arterioscler. Thromb* 1992;12:717.
24. Ingegno MD, Money SR, Thelmo W, et al. Progesterone receptors in the human heart and great vessels. *Lab Invest* 1988;59:353.
25. Williams JK, Anthony MS, Honoré EK, et al. Regression of atherosclerosis in female monkey. *Arterioscler Vasc Biol*. 1995;15:827.
26. Losordo DW, Kearney M, Kim EA, et al. Variable expression of the estrogen receptor in normal and atherosclerotic coronary arteries of premenopausal women. *Circulation* 1994;89:1501.
27. Lamping KG, Nuno DW. Estradiol and progesterone attenuate contractions to endothelin in coronary microvessels in vitro. Abstract. *Circulation* 1993;88(suppl):2535.
28. Polderman KH, Stehouwer CD, van Kamp GJ, et al. Influence of sex hormones on plasma endothelin levels. *Ann Intern Med* 1993;118:429.
29. Bar J, Tepper R, Fuchs J, et al. The effect of estrogen replacement therapy on platelet aggregation and adenosine triphosphate release in postmenopausal women. *Obstet Gynecol* 1993;81:261.
30. Lindheim SR, Legro RS, Bernstein L, et al. Behavioral stress responses in premenopausal and postmenopausal women and the effects of estrogen. *Am J Obstet Gynecol* 1992;167:1831.
31. Saab PG, Matthews KA, Stoney CM, et al. Premenopausal and postmenopausal women differ in their cardiovascular and neuroendocrine responses to behavioral stresses. *Psychophysiology* 1989;26:270.
32. Lindheim SR, Legro RS, Morris RS, et al. The effect of progestins on behavioral stress responses in postmenopausal women. *J Soc Gynecol Invest* 1994;1:79.
33. Hillard TC, Bourne TH, Whitehead MI, et al. Differential effects of transdermal estradiol and sequential progestogens on impedance to flow within the uterine arteries of postmenopausal women. *Fertil Steril* 1992;58:959.
34. Ganger KF, Vyas S, Whitehead MI, et al. Pulsatility index in the internal carotid artery is influenced by transdermal oestradiol and time since menopause. *Lancet* 1991;338:839.
35. Collins P, Jiang C, Shay J, et al. *In vitro* EDRF-dependent coronary artery relaxation to physiologic concentrations of 17β-estradiol: Modulation by *in vivo* sex hormone status. Abstract. *Circulation* 1993; 88(suppl):410.
36. Weiner CP, Lizasoain I, Baylis SA, et al. Induction of calcium-dependent nitric oxide synthases by sex hormones. *Proc Natl Acad Sci USA* 1994;91:5212.

37. Sayegh HS, Ohara Y, Navas JJP, et al. Endothelial nitric oxide synthase regulation by estrogens. Abstract. *Circulation* 1993;88(suppl):415.
38. Schray-Utz B, Zelher AM, Busse R. Expression of constitutive NO synthase in cultured endothelieal cells is enhanced by 17β-estradiol. Abstract. *Circulation* 1993;88(suppl):416.
39. Hayashi T, Fukuto JM, Ignarro LJ, et al. Basal release of nitric oxide from aortic rings is greater in female rabbits than in male rabbits: Implications for atherosclerosis. *Proc Natl Acad Sci USA* 1992;89:11259.
40. Collins P, Shay J, Jiang C, et al. Nitric oxide accounts for dose-dependent estrogen-mediated coronary relaxation after acute estrogen withdrawal. *Circulation* 1994;90:1964.
41. Gilligan DM, Quyyumi AA, Cannon RO III. Effects of physiological levels of estrogen on coronary vasomotor function in postmenopausal women. *Circulation* 1994;89:2545.
42. Herrington DM, Braden GA, Williams JK, et al. Endothelial-dependent coronary vasomotor responsiveness in postmenopausal women with and without estrogen replacement therapy. *Am J Cardiol* 1994;73:951.
43. Rosano GMC, Sarrel PM, Poole-Wilson PA, et al. Beneficial effect of oestrogen on exercise-induced myocardial ischaemia in women with coronary artery disease. *Lancet* 1993;342:133.
44. Gilligan DM, Badar DM, Panza JA, et al. Acute vascular effects of estrogen in postmenopausal women. *Circulation* 1994;90:786.
45. Chester A, Jiang C, Sarrel P, et al. 17β-Estradiol induces endothelium-independent relaxation in human coronary arteries *in vitro*. *Circulation* 1993;88(suppl):407.
46. Pines A, Fishman EZ, Levo Y, et al. The effects of hormone replacement therapy in normal postmenopausal women: Measurements of Doppler-derived parameters of aortic flow. *Am J Obstet Gynecol* 1991; 164:806.
47. Pines A, Fisman EZ, Ayalon D, et al. Long-term effects of hormone replacement therapy on Doppler-derived parameters of aortic flow in postmenopausal women. *Chest* 1992;102:1496.
48. Voutilainen S, Hippelainen M, Hulklo S, et al. Left ventricular diastolic function by Doppler echocardiography in relation to hormone replacement therapy in healthy postmenopausal women. *Am J Cardiol* 1993;71:614.
49. Giraud GD, Morton MJ, Wilson RA, et al. Effects of estrogen and progestin on aortic size and compliance in postmenopausal women. *Am J Obstet Gynecol* 1996;174:1708.
50. Prelevic GM, Beljic T. The effect of oestrogen and progestogen replacement therapy on systolic flow velocity in healthy postmenopausal women. *Maturitas* 1994;20:37.
51. Poehlman ET, Goran MI, Gardner AW, et al. Metabolic determinants of the decline in resting metabolic rate in aging females. *Am J Physiol* 1993;264:E450.
52. Walton C, Godsland IF, Proudler AJ, et al. The effects of the menopause on insulin sensitivity, secretion and elimination in non-obese, healthy women. *Eur J Clin Invest* 1993;23:466.
53. Proudler AJ, Godsland IF, Stevenson JC. Insulin propeptides in conditions asociated with insulin resistance in humans and their relevance to insulin measurements. *Metabolism* 1994;43:46.

54. Haarbo J, Marslew U, Gotfredsen A, et al. Postmenopausal hormone replacement therapy prevents central distribution of body fat after menopause. *Metabolism* 1991;40:1323.
55. Ley CJ, Lees B, Stevenson JC. Sex- and menopause-associated changes in body-fat distribution. *Am J Clin Nutr* 1992;55:950.
56. Ferri C, Pittoni V, Piccoli A, et al. Insulin stimulates endothelin-1 secretion from human endothelial cells and modulates its circulating levels *in vivo. J Clin Endocrinol Metab* 1995;80:829.
57. Cagnacci A, Soldani R, Carriero PL, et al.Effects of low doses of transdermal 17 beta-estradiol on carbohydrate metabolism in postmenopausal women. *J Clin Endocrinol Metab* 1992;74:1396.
58. Lobo R, Pickar JH, Wild RA, et al. for The Menopause Study Group, Metabolic impact of adding medroxyprogesterone acetate to conjugated estrogen therapy in postmenopausal women. *Obstet Gynecol* 1994;84:987.
59. Lindheim SR, Presser SC, Ditkoff EC, et al. A possible bimodal effect of estrogen on insulin sensitivity in postmenopausal women and the attenuating effect of added progestin. *Fertil Steril.* 1993;60:664.
60. Godsland IF, Ganger K, Walton C, et al. Insulin resistance, secretion, and elimination in postmenopausal women receiving oral or transdermal hormone replacement therapy. *Metabolism* 1993;42:846.
61. Lindheim SR, Duffy DM, Kojima T, et al. The route of administration influences the effect of estrogen on insulin sensitivity in postmenopausal women. *Fertil Steril* 1994;62:1176.
62. Manson JE, Rimm EB, Colditz GA, et al. A prospective study of postmenopausal estrogen therapy and subsequent incidence of non-insulin dependent diabetes mellitus. *Ann Epidemiol* 1992;2:665.
63. Kardinaal AFM, Kok FJ, Ringstad J, et al. Antioxidants in adipose tissue and risk of myocaridal infarction: The EURAMIC study. *Lancet* 1993;342:1379.
64. Gey KF, Stähelin HB, Eichholzer M. Poor plasma status of carotene and vitamin C is associated with higher mortality from ischemic heart disease and stroke: Basel Prospective Study. *Clin Invest* 1993;71:3.
65. Stampfer MJ, Hennekens CH, Manson JE, et al. Vitamin E consumption and the risk of coronary disease in women. *N Engl J Med* 1993;328:1450.
66. Gaziano JM, Manson JE, Ridker PM, et al. Beta carotene therapy for chronic stable angina. *Circulation* 1990;82:201.
67. Zhu, X-D, Knopp RH. Effect of sex hormones on oxidative modification of low density lipoproteins by placental macrophages and trophoblast and their susceptibility to cytotoxicity. Abstract. *Circulation* 1993;88(suppl):160.
68. Sack MN, Rader DJ, Cannon RO III. Oestrogen and inhibiton of oxidation of low-density lipoproteins in postmenopausal women. *Lancet* 1994;343:269.
69. Keaney JF, Shwaery GT, Xu A, et al. 17β-Estradiol preserves endothelial vasodilator function and limits low-density lipoprotein oxidation in hypercholesterolemic swine. *Circulation* 1994;89:2251.
70. Boston Collaborative Drug Surveillance Program. Surgically confirmed gallbladder disease, venous thromboembolism, and breast tumors in relation to postmenopausal estrogen therapy. *N Engl J Med* 1974;290:15.

71. Pettiti DB, Wingerd J, Pellegrin F, et al. Risk of vascular disease in women. *J Am Med Assoc* 1979;242:1150.
72. Devor M, Barrett-Connor E, Renvall M, et al. Estrogen replacement therapy and the risk of venous thrombosis. *Am J Med* 1992;92:275.
73. Lowe GDO, Greer IA, Cooke TG, et al. Risk and prophylaxis for venous thromboembolism in hospital patients. *Br Med J* 1992;305:567.
74. Gebara OCE, Mittleman MA, Sutherland P, et al. Association between increased estrogen status and increased fibrinolytic potential in the Framingham Offspring Study. *Circulation* 1995;91:1952.
75. Meilahn EN, Kuller LH, Matthews KA, et al. Hemostatic factors according to menopausal status and use of hormone replacement therapy. *Ann Epidemiol* 1992;2:445.
76. Scarabin PY, Flu-Bureau G, Bara L, et al. Haemostatic variables and menopausal status: Influence of hormone replacement therapy. *Thromb Haemost* 1994;70:584.
77. Nulsen JC, De Souza MJ, Walker FJ, et al. Progesterone influence on estrogen-induced changes in coagulation factors in postmenopausal women. Abstract. Annual Meeting, North American Menopause Society, 1994;P-60.
78. Boschetti C, Cortellaro M, Nencioni T, et al. Short- and long-term effects of hormone replacement therapy (transdermal estradiol vs oral conjugated equine estrogens, combined with medroxyprogesterone acetate) on blood coagulation factors in postmenopausal women. *Thromb Res* 1991;62:1.
79. Saleh AA, Dorey LG, Dombrowski MP, et al. Thrombosis and hormone replacement therapy in postmenopausal women. *Am J Obstet Gynecol* 1993;169:1554.
80. Brosselli M, Keller PJ, Kern F, et al. Estradiol inhibits mitogen-induced proliferation and migration of human aortic smooth muscle cells: Implications for cardiovascular disease in women. Abstract. *Circulation* 1994;90:I-87.
81. Hirvonen E, Malkonen M, Manninen V. Effects of different progestogens on lipoproteins during postmenopausal therapy. *N Engl J Med* 1981;304:560.
82. Mattsson L, Cullberg LG, Samsioe G. Influence of esterified estrogens and medroxyprogesterone on lipid metabolism and sex steroids. A study in oophorectomized women. *Horm Metab Res* 1982;14:602.
83. Silferstolpe G, Gustafsson A, Samsioe G, et al. Lipid metabolic studies in oophorectomized women: Effects on serum lipids and lipoproteins of three synthetic progestogens. *Maturitas* 1983;4:103.
84. Ylostalo P, Kauppila A, Kivinen S, et al. Endocrine and metabolic effects of low-dose estrogen-progestin treatment in climacteric women. *Obstet Gynecol* 1983;62:682.
85. Mattsson L, Cullberg G, Samsioe G. A continuous estrogen-progestogen regimen for climacteric complaints. *Acta Obstet Gynecol Scand* 1984;3:673.
86. Ottosson UB, Carlstrom K, Damber JE, et al. Serum levels of progesterone and some of its metabolites including deoxycorticosterone after oral and parenteral administration. *Br J. Obstet Gynaecol* 1984;91:1111.
87. Wren B, Garrett D. The effect of low-dose piperazine oestrogen sulphate and low-dose levonorgestrel on blood lipid levels in postmenopausal women. *Maturitas* 1985;7:141.

88. Ottosson UB, Johansson BG, von Schoultz B. Subfractions of high-density lipoprotein cholesterol during estrogen replacement therapy: A comparison between progestogens and natural progesterone. *Am J Obstet Gynecol* 1985;151:746.

89. Obel EB, Munk-Jensen N, Svenstrup B, et al. A two-year double-blind controlled study of the clinical effect of combined and sequential postmenopausal replacement therapy and steroid metabolism during treatment. *Maturitas* 1993;16:13.

90. King RJB, Whitehead MI. Assessment of the potency of orally administered progestins in women. *Fertil Steril* 1986;46:1062.

91. Barrett-Connor E, Wingard DL, Criqui MH. Postmenopausal estrogen use and heart disease risk factors in the 1980s. *JAMA* 1989;261:2095.

92. Sherwin BB, Gelfand MM. A prospective one-year study of estrogen and progestin in postmenopausal women: Effects on clinical symptoms and lipoprotein lipids. *Obstet Gynecol* 1989;73:759.

93. Wolfe BM, Huff MW. Effects of combined estrogen and progestin administration on plasma lipoprotein metabolism in postmenopausal women. *J Clin Invest* 1989;83:40.

94. Christiansen C, Riis BJ. Five years with continous combined oestrogen/progestogen therapy. Effects on calcium metabolism, lipoproteins, and bleeding pattern. *Br J Obstet Gynaecol* 1990;97:1087.

95. Voetberg GA, Netelenbos JC, Kenemans P, et al. Estrogen replacement therapy continuously combined with four different dosages of dydrogesterone: Effect on calcium and lipid metabolism. *J Clin Endocrinol Metab* 1994;79:1465.

96. Marslew U, Overgaard K, Riis BJ, et al. Two new combinations of estrogen and progestogen for prevention of postmenopausal bone loss: Long-term effects on bone, calcium and lipid metabolism, climacteric symptoms, and bleeding. *Obstet Gynecol* 1992;79:202.

97. Williams SR, Frenchek B, Speroff T, et al. A study of combined continuous ethinyl estradiol and norethindrone acetate for postmenopausal hormone replacement. *Am J Obstet Gynecol* 1990;162:438.

98. Weinstein L, Bewtra C, Gallagher JC. Evaluation of a continuous combined low-dose regimen of estrogen-progestin for treatment of the menopausal patient. *Am J Obstet Gynecol* 1990;162:1534.

99. Munk-Jensen N, Ulrich LG, Obel EB, et al. Continuous combined and sequential estradiol and norethindrone acetate treatment of postmenopausal women: Effect on plasma lipoproteins in a two-year placebo-controlled trial. *Am J Obstet Gynecol* 1994;171:132.

100. Cano A, Fernandes H, Serrano S, et al. Effect of continuous oestradiol-medroxyprogesterone administration on plasma lipids and lipoproteins. *Maturitas* 1991;13:35.

101. Gibbons WE, Judd HL, Luciano AA, et al. Comparison of sequential versus continuous estrogen/progestin replacement therapy on serum lipid patterns. Abstract 491. Society for Gynecological Investigation, Annual Meeting, 1991.

102. de Ziegler D, Bessis R, Frydman R. Vascular resistance of uterine arteries: Physiological effects of estradiol and progesterone. *Fertil Steril* 1991;55:775.

103. Penotti M, Nencioni T, Gabrielli L, et al. Blood flow variations in internal carotid and middle cerebral arteries induced by postmenopausal hormone replacement therapy. *Am J Obstet Gynecol* 1993;169:1226.

104. Hunt K, Vessey M, McPherson K, et al. Long-term surveillance of mortality and cancer incidence in women receiving hormone replacement therapy. *Br J Obstet Gynaecol* 1987;94:620.
105. Hunt K, Vessey M, McPherson K. Mortality in a cohort of long-term users of hormone replacement therapy: An updated analysis. *Br J Obstet Gynaecol* 1990;97:1080.
106. Thompson SG, Meade TW, Greenberg G. The use of hormonal replacement therapy and the risk of stroke and myocardial infarction in women. *J Epidem Community Health* 1989;43:173.
107. Falkeborn M, Persson I, Adami HO, et al. The risk of acute myocardial infarction after oestrogen and oestrogen-progestogen replacement. *Br J Obstet Gynecol* 1992;99:821.
108. Falkeborn M, Persson I, Terent A, et al. Hormone replacement therapy and the risk of stroke. *Arch Intern Med* 1993;153:1201.
109. Rosenberg L, Palmer JR, Shapiro S. A case-control study of myocardial infarction in relation to use of estrogen supplements. *Am J Epidemiol* 1993;137:54.
110. Mann RD, Lis Y, Chukwujindu J, et al. A study of the association between hormone replacement therapy, smoking and the occurrence of myocardial infarction in women. *J Clin Epidemiol* 1994;47:307.
111. Psaty BM, Heckbart SR, Atkins D, et al. The risk of myocardial infarction associated with the combined use of estrogens and progestins in postmenopausal women. *Arch Intern Med* 1994;154:1333.
112. Punnonen RH, Jokela HA, Dastidar PS, et al. Combined oestrogen-progestin replacement therapy prevents atherosclerosis in postmenopausal women. *Maturitas* 1995;21:179.
113. The Writing Group for the PEPI Trial. Effects of estrogen or estrogen/progestin regimens on heart disease risk factors in postmenopausal women: The Postmenopausal Estrogen/Progestin Interventions (PEPI) Trial. *JAMA* 1995;273:199.
114. Gordon T, Kannel WB, Hjortland MC, et al. Menopause and coronary heart disease: The Framingham Study. *Ann Intern Med* 1978;89:157.
115. Wilson PWF, Garrison RJ, Castelli WP. Postmenopausal estrogen use, cigarette smoking, and cardiovascular morbidity in women over 50. The Framingham Study. *N Engl J Med* 1985;313:1038.
116. Eaker ED, Castelli WP. Coronary heart disease and its risk factors among women in the Framingham Study. In: Eaker ED, Packard B, Wenger NG, eds. *Coronary Heart Disease in Women.* New York: Haymarket Doyma; 1987:122–130.
117. Speroff T, Dawson N, Speroff L. Is postmenopausal estrogen use risky? Results from a methodologic review and information synthesis. *Clin Res* 1987;35:362A.
118. Stampfer MJ, Colditz GA. Estrogen replacement therapy and coronary heart disease: A quantitative assessment of the epidemiological evidence. *Prev Med* 1991;20:47.

Chapter 20

Clinical Findings Related to Arterial Effects of Ovarian Steroids

Philip M. Sarrel, MD

Ovarian hormones play an integral role in the control of arterial blood flow in women.[1] Estrogens and progesterone produced in the body appear to act at all levels of arterial structure—the endothelial cell, the vascular smooth muscle cell and in nerve cells in the arterial adventitia.[2] Hormone receptors have been identified in the walls of arterial systems throughout the body, and there is considerable evidence for genomically mediated hormone effects on hemodynamic mechanisms.[3-5] Nongenomic hormone actions have also been described with estrogens and progestins having effects on ionic channels in vascular smooth muscle[6,7] and affecting neurotransmitter synthesis, release and uptake at presynaptic junctions.[8,9] Hemodynamic parameters supported by normal estradiol levels include arterial tone and stability, velocity of blood flow, and vasodilator reserve capacity.[1]

Arterial dysfunction and disease have been associated with acute and chronic estradiol-17β deficiency and with progestin antagonism of estrogenic effects. Most women, at some time in their lives, suffer from one or more vascular conditions that have been related to change in ovarian hormone production.

These conditions include vasomotor instability (hot flushes),[10] migraine headaches,[11,12] angina pectoris in the presence of normal coronary arteries (Syndrome X),[13,14] and myocardial infarction.[15] Myocardial infarction with onset of menstruation is an interesting and particularly relevant phenomenon that will be described in this chapter.

Estrogens have been used to treat vasomotor instability (VMI)in menopausal women and have proved efficacious.[16] Progestins have also been shown to restore vasomotor stability in women suffering

From: Forte TM, (ed). *Hormonal, Metabolic, and Cellular Influences on Cardiovascular Disease in Women.* Armonk, NY: Futura Publishing Company, Inc.; © 1997.

from hot flushes.[17] Estrogens have been used to treat migraine headaches associated with hormonal changes in the menstrual cycle[18] and in women diagnosed with Syndrome X.[14] Women with a history of myocardial infarction subsequently treated with estrogens have shown reduced mortality rates compared with untreated matched control women.[19]

This chapter will briefly review hemodynamic actions in arteries that are affected by estrogen deficiency and that have been associated with arterial dysfunctions and disease. Clinical experience evaluating ovarian hormones in women with vascular conditions will be summarized. Case presentations will be used to illustrate circulatory findings in women with these conditions and to show examples of circulatory responses to hormonal treatment.

Background: Hemodynamic Effects of Ovarian Steroids

Hemodynamic responses associated with estrogen deficiency include increased vascular resistance and decreased blood flow, loss of vasodilator reserve capacity, and increased vascular reactivity and vasomotor instability. There are numerous reports in the animal and human research literature describing the arterial blood flow effects of estrogens and progestins. Estrogens induce vasodilation and increased blood flow,[20] whereas progestins inhibit these responses.[21-23] Infusion of estrogens into an artery leads to a reduction in vascular resistance and an increase in flow. For example, Magness and Rosenfeld[20] showed, in sheep, that estradiol-17β introduced into a uterine artery induced increased flow and decreased vascular resistance starting within 30 minutes. Bourne et al.[24] used transdermal estradiol-17β and showed a decrease in pulsatility index in uterine arteries in women after 9 weeks of unopposed estrogen. Similar findings were reported by Gangar et al.[25] in measurements of carotid artery pulsatility index in women also treated with transdermal estradiol-17β. Reis et al.[26] assessed coronary blood flow and vascular resistance in postmenopausal women before and 15 minutes after intravenous administration of 35 μg of ethinyl estradiol. Eleven women were taking estrogens and six were not. An acute increase in coronary flow index and a decrease in coronary vascular resistance was seen in the women receiving estrogen for the first time and not seen in the women already receiving chronic estrogen treatment. Volterrani et al.[27] also showed an acute effect of estradiol-17β to increase peripheral blood flow. Collins et al.[28] showed that acute withdrawal of estradiol induces vasoconstriction reflecting a decrease in nitric oxide (NO) production.

There is evidence that estrogens stimulate endothelial cell NO production through genomic-mechanisms. For example, Caulin-Glaser et al.[29] found increased NO production from human endothelial cells grown in cell culture after exposure to estradiol-17β. The response was inhibited by a receptor antagonist. Estrogen potentiates endothelium-dependent vasodilator response to acetylcholine. Williams et al.[30] described this effect in coronary arteries of ovariectomized monkeys, and others have documented similar responses in women. For example, Gilligan et al.[31] studied coronary artery response to acetylcholine in 20 postmenopausal women including 7 with angiographic evidence of significant atherosclerotic disease. Coronary artery diameter measurements and blood flow velocity calculations showed physiological levels of estradiol-17β acutely and selectively potentiated endothelial-dependent vasodilation. Collins et al.[32] recently reported the effects of estradiol-17β infused into the coronary arteries in nine postmenopausal women and seven men with coronary artery disease. After 20-minutes infusion of estradiol-17β pretreatment vasoconstrictor responses to acetylcholine converted to vasodilator responses in the women with concomitant increase in blood flow velocity. The men did not show a response to the acute infusion of estradiol.

Estrogens affect catecholamine synthesis, release, and uptake in the arterial wall.[8,9] Acute and chronic estradiol deficiency are associated with vasomotor instability with rapid changes in serum catecholamine levels during events. For example, Kronenberg et al.[33] found increased levels of epinephrine and decreased levels of norepinephrine during hot flushes. Hot flushes are accompanied by peripheral vasodilatation, tachycardia, decreased skin resistance, and, often, sweating. Laser Doppler recordings of hand blood flow during hot flushes show marked vasodilation with two- to threefold increases in flow velocity during the episodes.[34] Rees and Barlow[35] studied hyperemic response in the forearm of women who were having hot flushes. Their findings support the concept of a dysautonomia induced by estradiol deficiency. Ginsburg and her associates[36] have also used forearm hyperemic response to assess peripheral vasoreactivity, concluding the menopausal hot flush "indicates an alteration in peripheral vascular control determined by adrenergic factors." Owens et al.[37] measured catecholamine levels and blood pressure changes in postmenopausal and premenopausal women and men during mental and physical stress. They concluded "menopause is associated with enhanced stress-induced cardiovascular responses. . .". For example, they found postmenopausal women had larger stress-induced systolic and diastolic blood pressure increases than either of the comparison groups.

One or more of these hemodynamic changes associated with estrogen deficiency, vasomotor instability, vasoconstriction, and loss of vasodilator reserve capacity, have been described in women experiencing hot flushes, migraine headaches, Syndrome X, and myocardial infarction.

Vasomotor Instability

Hot flushes are experienced by $\geq 75\%$ of women at menopause.[38] For 50%, the phenomena continue for up to 5 years. In a total-population study carried out in Sweden, among women who were 10 year postmenopause, 27% continued to have hot flushes.[10] The cardiovascular implications of a continuing state of vasomotor instability for ≥ 10 years remains to be determined. Preliminary findings, however, indicate that VMI for this length of time is a predisposing factor to myocardial infarction.[39]

During a hot flush, peripheral vessels alternately expand and contract with considerable shunting of blood volume from the central to the peripheral circulation. Catecholamine measures during hot flushes reported from different studies are contradictory. Whereas Kronenberg et al.[33] found an increase in epinephrine levels and a decrease in norepinephrine levels during flushing episodes, Caspar et al.[40] did not find such changes. Laser Doppler monitoring of skin blood flow and hyperemic response measures during flushing episodes are consistent with Kronenberg's findings of hot flushes being an event involving adrenergic surge with central arterial vasoconstriction and peripheral vasodilation and destabilized flow. A laser Doppler recording of skin blood flow during a hot flush shows an episode lasting 90 seconds with an increase of red cell velocity indicative of significant vasodilation and blood shunting.

Kronenberg[41] described other signs of vascular disturbance during hot flushes including chest pressure and pain, vascular type headaches, increased heart rate, and shortness of breath. VMI is associated with both chronic and acute estradiol deficiency. Most studies have been carried out in postmenopausal women who have been in a state of estradiol deficiency for ≥ 6

months, if not much longer. In addition, acute withdrawal of estradiol can induce severe VMI. As an example, a laser Doppler study of skin blood flow in a patient experiencing severe flushes is presented. The patient, a 56-year-old woman using daily estradiol-17β had not taken any tablets for 48 hours when she began to experience flushes and palpitations. During the next 24 hours, she developed anginal-type chest pain with radiation down her left arm. She also developed a severe left-sided throbbing headache and nausea. On admission for study, her blood pressure was 178/110 with a pulse of 96. She was in acute distress complaining of severe chest pain. Pupil dilation was significant and consistent with adrenergic surge activity. The laser Doppler recording indicates peripheral vasodilation with extremely unstable blood flow. Blood for serum estradiol was drawn (subsequently reported to be <25 pg/mL) and 1 mg of micronized estradiol-17β was administered sublingually. During the next 40 minutes, the VMI stabilized with an overall decrease in skin blood flow. Chest and head pain disappeared and hot flushes stopped. By 27 minutes after drug administration, the blood pressure was 124/78, consistent with levels recorded in her chart at previous visits. The usual oral dose of 1 mg estradiol-17β twice a day was restarted, and the patient remained well and asymptomatic during the next 72 hours. She has not suffered a recurrence of symptoms and has not missed any estrogen tablets since. Kronenberg's study indicates perimenopausal women with hot flushes experience the highest incidence of symptoms of concomitant vascular disturbance.[41] Among these women, 42.1% experienced chest pressure, 47.4% shortness of breath, and 36.4% head pain when they were having flushes. Rosano et al.[42] have recently reported these phenomena in menstruating women occur most often during the luteal phase of their menstrual cycle. Recognition of the occurrence of luteal phase angina, luteal phase vascular headaches, and luteal phase asthma suggests the phenomena reflect progesterone downregulation of the vasodilator effects of estradiol. The findings also indicate the importance of determining the phase of the menstrual cycle a woman is in when evaluating arterial function. For example, women whose exercise treadmill testing has shown ischemic changes during their luteal phase have shown nonischemic results when tested during a subsequent follicular phase.

Vasomotor instability should be regarded as a pathophysiological state secondary to acute and chronic estradiol deficiency and possibly to progesterone downregulation of estrogen arterial effects. The occurrence of other vascular phenomena such as migraine headaches and angina in women having hot flushes suggests the pathophysiology of the hot flush has more far-reaching and significant implications than previously recognized.

Migraine Headaches

Twenty-five million Americans suffer from migraine headache attacks each year.[12] Three out of four migraineurs are women with 25% of all women experiencing migraine headaches at some time during their reproductive years. Menstrually related or catamenial migraines occur just before or after the onset of menstruation or at ovulation-during times that coincide with acute decline in serum estradiol-17β levels. Somerville[43] correlated migraine attacks with acute depletion of estradiol-17β, response of the attack to estradiol treatment, and recurrence of an event as soon as the treatment estrogens wore off. Injections of long-acting estradiol valerate given 3–10 days before menses delayed the onset of migraine, but attacks set in when the estradiol levels fell to the usual menstrual levels. Welch et al.[44] hypothesized that menstrual migraine results from the effect of estradiol-17β withdrawal on the sympathetic nervous system resulting in altered cerebral vessel tone. Arteriolar tone is modified via adrenergic activity at α-2 receptors, ordinarily blocked by estradiol-17β. Estradiol acts to maintain low-norepinephrine levels and estradiol-17β withdrawal leads to norepinephrine-induced vasoconstriction in the preheadache "aura" stage. Vasodilation of the cerebral vessel is then thought to be a reaction to the resultant oligemia. The withdrawal of estradiol-17β and progesterone premenstrually leads to hyperreactive vessels susceptible to spasm.

Continuous treatment with exogenous estrogens has been demonstrated to prevent migraine attacks. Magos et al.[18] used subcutaneous estrogen implants, and several authors have used transdermal estrogens to demonstrate that migraine attacks could be prevented in susceptible women. Tamoxifen has also been shown to decrease migraine frequency and intensity in women suffering from cyclical attacks.[45] Brass et al.[46] and Sarrel[34] have reported success in treating migraine attacks with sublingual estradiol-17β. Transcranial Doppler measurement of cerebral blood flow during estradiol treatment showed a correlation between serum estradiol-17β levels and arterial blood flow.

Measurement of peripheral blood flow, using laser Doppler velocimetry, indicates migraine headaches and peripheral vasomotor instability coincide at times of estradiol-17β withdrawal. The migraine attacks, therefore, may be regarded as a sign of more widespread arterial disturbance and not an event isolated to a particular cerebral vessel.

Angina Pectoris

Women experience angina pectoris twice as often as men. First described by William Osler in 1896,[47] the frequency of diagnosed angina in women has been recently documented by La Croix et al.[48] in a national study of >12,000 men and women. The increased female-to-male ratio is seen in white women ages 25–54 compared with age-matched men. Black women showed even higher prevalence rates.

Estrogen deficiency has been associated with the development of atherosclerotic cardiovascular disease in women after menopause.[49,50]

Estrogen deficiency has also been associated in women with diagnosed angina pectoris who have subsequently been found to have normal coronary arteries as demonstrated by coronary angiography (Syndrome X). Rosano et al.[13] studied the gynecologic features of 107 women (aged 53 ± 9 years) with Syndrome X.

The women represented 80% of all patients diagnosed with Syndrome X at two major London teaching hospitals. All patients showed typical exertional angina pectoris, a positive exercise test, and normal coronary arteriograms in the absence of coronary artery spasm, systemic hypertension, left ventricular hypertrophy (LVH), or valvular heart disease. In 95/107 patients, chest pain began either during the perimenopausal period or after menopause; 43/63 menopausal patients had undergone hysterectomy at an average of 8 ± 6 years before the onset of the chest pain. The 40% incidence of hysterectomy was four times greater than that of an age-matched population. Estradiol-17β levels were all found to be ≤100 pmol/L with FSH >40 mIU/mL. The findings confirm an earlier study reported by Sarrel et al.[14] that also found a high-hysterectomy rate. Most of these women had retained ovaries and had not been given estrogen replacement therapy. The earlier study indicated all of the women had daily hot flushes with severe vasomotor instability documented by laser Doppler velocimetry. The study also reported diminished hyperemic response in the Syndrome X women that responded to estradiol-17β therapy. Symptomatic response subsequently was reported by Rosano et al.[42]

The following case is representative of the women evaluated in the two studies.

JG was first seen on 12/18/91 with a chief complaint of "I want to find out why I have this terrible feeling in my chest. Is it due to hormone imbalance?" At her initial visit, Mrs. G described a 4-year history of daily chest pain and/or pressure. The pain was precordial in location, radiated to the left shoulder, and occasionally extended down her left arm. Walking on any incline induced the chest symptoms as did climbing half a flight of stairs. The pressure was accompanied by severe shortness of breath. As many as 15–20 episodes occurred in a 24-hour period with a daily average of between 5 and 10 episodes. Accompanying the chest symptoms were hot flushes, severe headaches, awakening at night, numbness in hands and feet, occasional attacks of extreme anxiety, and, sometimes, psychological depression.

S-T depression of 1.2 mm was seen in leads 4–6 at the time of exercise testing. An acute episode in April, 1991, led to hospitalization for possible myocardial infarction. Coronary angiography at that time showed normal vessels and no enzyme changes occurred. She was treated with Xanax, 0.25 mg taken daily. A calcium channel blocking agent and a β-blocking agent were prescribed but proved ineffective in controlling symptoms. Cardiac medication at the time of her initial visit was GTN tablets. She was taking as many as six tablets per day with some relief of chest pain.

The past gynecologic history was significant for hysterectomy with left salpingo-oophorectomy in May, 1983. No hormone replacement was prescribed.

Physical examination showed a somewhat anxious woman, well developed, well nourished. Blood pressure was 98/62, pulse was 84 beats per minute; weight was 142 pounds. Initial laboratory studies included estradiol-17β (29 pg/mL), FSH (80.3 mIU/mL), and total cholesterol (157 mg/dL). Mrs. G was asked to maintain a daily diary of symptoms for the next 4 weeks. No estrogen replacement was prescribed at this visit.

At her second visit (1-29-92), Mrs G showed a diary with daily symptoms (those reported in the initial history) of moderate to severe intensity.

She discussed her anxiety about taking estrogens as she most feared the development of breast cancer. Information was provided, and the patient appeared to be somewhat reassurred. A hyperemic response study was carried out on 2-5-92. It indicated the high-peripheral flow levels seen in a chronically vasodilated state. Vasodilator response was shortened and diminished as compared with control studies in asymptomatic, age-matched women. The hyperemic response was measured using a laser Doppler velocimeter (Moor Instruments-MBF 3D) with finger blood flow measured before and after 5 minutes of brachial occlusion. Treatment with transdermal estradiol-17β was initiated. Within 4 months of continuous estradiol-17β treatment, anginal symtoms essentially disappeared. Thus, on 6/3/92 Mrs. G, reported she had not used any sublingual nitrates in more than 1 week's time and that she was able to move furniture without any exertional discomfort. Hyperemic response testing showed marked changes during the 4 months. For example, on 6/3/92 a low-baseline, pre-occlusion level is seen (1/4 the initial levels) and hyperemic response is increased markedly and sustained.

Follow-up has occurred at 6-month intervals for a total of 42 months through 9/95. Nitrate medication has not been used in >3 years. No medication has been used for cardiac symptoms other than the transdermal estradiol-17β. Previously reported symptoms of hot flushes, headaches, sleep disturbance, anxiety, and depression essentially have disappeared. At her last visit, she described her ability to walk uphill for 3–4 miles each day without chest pressure or pain. The occasional development of chest pressure is viewed as a signal to change her estrogen patch as the fresh patch invariably leads to subsidence of the symptoms. An echocardiogram in 1995 was normal as was an exercise tolerance test. Cholesterol levels have remained in the 150–160 mg/dL range. Hyperemic response testing has reconfirmed the lowered peripheral flow levels and enhanced hyperemic response.

The findings seen in the case presented are consistent with those previously reported.[13,14] A total of 20 women diagnosed with Syndrome X were studied before and after treatment with estradiol-17β. Cessation of hot flushes coincided with decrease or disappearance of chest pain. Hyperemic response was impaired in all the women at baseline. Postocclusion blood flow almost doubled after estradiol-17β treatment for 2 months, reaching levels approximating those of the untreated, asymptomatic control population.

The prognosis for patients with Syndrome X is thought to be good with many patients' symptoms subsiding within 2 or 3 years. Long-term follow-up studies do not show an increase in cardiovascular mortality compared with the general population. However, symptoms can be disabling and cause extreme mental stress and usually do not respond to usual anti-anginal medications. Response to estrogen treatment has been encouraging and may well turn out to be a treatment of choice for women with Syndrome X who also show other signs and symptoms of estrogen deficiency.

There is another issue worth mentioning, the problem of myocardial infarction in women with normal coronary arteries. We have seen a series of patients who have experienced a myocardial infarction with onset of menstruation and who subsequently have shown minimal or no atherosclerotic coronary artery disease. Findings in these women, of whom six have been studied in detail, include associated signs and symptoms of estradiol deficiency, eg, diminished and irregular menstruation, hot flushes, and severe migraine headaches. Estradiol levels measured within 24 hours of infarction have all been <30 pg/mL. Laser Doppler measures of peripheral flow show high-baseline levels and impaired hyperemic response. Subsequent treatment with estradiol has proved effective in controlling anginal symptoms and in restoring vasodilator capacity as measured with laser Doppler velocimetry.

Rosano et al.[51] have reported the effects of sublingual estradiol-17β on exercise-induced myocardial ischemia in women with coronary artery disease (CAD). Eleven women with CAD were studied 40 minutes after taking 1 mg of micronized estradiol-17β (Estrace 1 mg, Mead Johnson Laboratories, Princeton, New Jersey) or placebo. Each woman had two tests on different days at the same time of the day. The treatment sequence (estradiol or placebo) was assigned randomly. The women had been evaluated within 3 months of the study and met the following study criteria: a reproducible positive exercise test; proven CAD (>70%), diameter stenosis of one or more coronary arteries; and clinical signs and symptoms of estrogen deficiency.

All of the patients developed chest pain on exertion after placebo compared with 6 of 11 after estradiol-17β. All patients showed ≥1 mm ST segment depression during the placebo exercise test whereas seven had a positive exercise test after estradiol-17β. Time to 1-mm ST segment depression and total exercise time were increased by estradiol-17β. The authors concluded that acute administration of estradiol-17β had a beneficial effect on myocardial ischemia in women with CAD. That experience plus that of others which have shown that chronic administration reduces myocardial infarction in women who are at high risk[19] has led to our prescribing estrogen treatment for the women with normal arteries and myocardial infarction when in a state of estradiol-deficiency.

Actions of Progestins

The preceeding discussion has focused on the hemodynamic effects of estrogens that support normal arterial function and appear to contibute to the cardioprotective effects of estrogens that have been reported by others. Although it is clear that estrogens act through a variety of nongenomic as well as genomic mechanisms, actions through the estradiol receptors in the arterial wall appear to be of great significance. The observation that estrogen-enhanced NO production is primarily receptor-mediated raises the concern that progestin downregulation of the estradiol receptor could impair the vasodilator effects of the estrogen. There is evidence that progestins added to estrogen treatment regimes can induce arterial vasconstriction. This has been reported in primate studies[52] and human cerebral vessels.[53] A case is presented of coronary artery vasoconstriction in a postmenopausal woman 4 hours after taking combined estrogen and progestin treatment. The patient had experienced recurrent chest pain during each of two prior monthly treatment cycles during the days when she added progestin to her daily estrogen. On the estrogen-only days she was asymptomatic. She had no prior history of cardiac disease or of any significant coronary risk factors. Vasoconstriction seen with angiography was reversed in the catheterization laboratory with intracoronary nitrate. Subsequently, treatment with estrogen alone proved effective in controlling chest pain. The progestin treatment was not necessary as the patient was posthysterectomy. At present there is preliminary epidemiological evidence to indicate that postmenopausal women receiving progestins do not show a loss of the cardioprotective effects of estrogens. However, basic science findings of the importance of estrogen-receptor-mediated actions and clinical experiences serve to raise awareness that patients receiving combined estrogen/progestin treatment who experience signs or symptoms of ischemia should be evaluated carefully.

Conclusions

The vasoactive effects of estrogens demonstrated in laboratory research appear to bear clinical significance. The hormonal status of women experiencing a variety of vascular disturbances—vasomotor instability, migraine headaches, angina pectoris—should be determined, and if estradiol-17β deficiency is detected, consideration should be given to corrective ovarian hormonal therapy. The anti-estrogenic effects of progestins should be weighed in consideration of hormonal therapy for women at risk of vascular disorder.

References

1. Sarrel PM. Ovarian hormones and the circulation. *Maturitas* 1990; 12:287–298.

2. Sarrel PM, Lufkin EG, Oursler MJ, et al. Estrogen actions in arteries, bone and brain. *Sci Med* 1994;1:44–53.
3. Horwitz KB, Horwitz LD. Canine vascular tissues are targets for androgens, estrogens, progestins, and glucocorticoids. J Clin Invest 1982; 69:750–758.
4. Ingegno MD, Money SR, Thelmo W, et al. Progesterone receptors in the human heart and great vessels. *Lab Invest* 1988;59:353–356.
5. Padwick ML, Whitehead M, Coffer A, et al. Demonstration of oestrogen receptor related protein in female tissues. In: Studd JWW, Whitehead MI, eds. *The Menopause.* Oxford: Blackwell Scientific Press; 1988: 227–233.
6. Collins P, Rosano GMC, Jiang C, et al. Hypothesis: Cardiovascular protection by oestrogen: A calcium antagonist effect? *Lancet* 1993;341: 1264–1265.
7. Jiang C, Sarrel PM, Lindsay DC, et al. Endothelium-independent relaxation of rabbit coronary artery by 17B-oestradiol in vitro. *Br J Pharmacol* 1991;104:1033–1037.
8. Hamlet MA, Rorie DK, Tyce GM. Effects of estradiol on release and disposition of norepinephrine from nerve endings. *Am J Physiol* 1980; 239:H450–H456.
9. Altura BM. Sex as a factor influencing the responsiveness of arterioles to catecholamines. *Eur J Pharmacol* 1982;20:281.
10. Hammar M, Berg M, Fahreus L, et al. Climacteric symptoms in an unselected sample of Swedish women. *Maturitas* 1984;6:345–350.
11. Welch KM, Darnley D, Simins RTR. The role of estrogen in migraine: A review and hypothesis. *Cephalalgia* 1984;4(4):227–236.
12. Stewart WF, Lepton RB, Celentano DD, et al. Prevalence of migraine headache in the United States: Relation to age, income, race and other sociodemographic factors. *JAMA* 1992;267(1):64–69.
13. Rosano GMC, Collins P, Kaski JC, et al. Syndrome X in women is associated with oestrogen deficiency. *Eur Heart J* 1995;16:610–614.
14. Sarrel PM, Lindsay DC, Rosano GMC, et al. Angina and normal coronary arteries in women: Gynecologic findings. *Am J Obstet Gynecol* 1992;167:467–471.
15. Barrett-Connor E, Bush TL. Estrogen and coronary heart disease in women. *JAMA* 1991;265:1861–1867.
16. Lauritzen C. The female climacteric syndrome: Significance, problems, treatment. Acta Obstet Gynecol Scand 1976:51(suppl):47–61.
17. Albrecht BH, Schiff I, Tulchinsky D,, et al. Objective evidence that placebo and oral medroxyprogesterone acetate therapy diminish menopausal vasomotor flushes. *Am J Obstet Gynecol* 1981;139:631–635.
18. Magos AL, Zilkha KJ, Studd JW. Treatment of menstrual migraine by oestradiol implants. *J Neurol Neurosurg Psych* 1983;46(11):1044–1046.
19. Sullivan JM, VanderZwaag R, Lemp GF, et al. Postmenopausal estrogen use and coronary atherosclerosis. *Ann Intern Med* 1988;108:358–363.
20. Magness RR, Rosenfeld CR. Local and systemic estradiol-17beta: Effects on uterine and system vasodilation. *Am J Physiol* 1989;256:E536–E542.
21. Resnik R, Brink GW, Plumer MH. The effect of progesterone on estrogen-induced uterine blood flow. *Am J Obstet Gynecol* 1977;128:251–254.
22. Sarrel PM. Progestogens and blood flow. *Int Proc J* 1989;1:266–271.
23. Sullivan JM, Shala BA, Miller LA, et al. Progestin enhances vasoconstrictor responses in post-menopausal women receiving estrogen replacement therapy. *Menopause* In press.

24. Bourne T, Hillard TC, Whitehead MI, et al. Oestrogen, arterial status and postmenopausal women. *Lancet* 1990;1470–1471.
25. Gangar KF, Vyas S, Whitehead MI, et al. Pulsatility index in carotid artery in relation to transdermal oestradiol and time since menopause. *Lancet* 1991;338:839–842.
26. Reis SE, Gloth ST, Blumenthal RS, et al. Ethinyl estradiol acutely attenuates abnormal coronary vasomotor responses to acetylcholine in postmenopausal women. *Circulation* 1994;89:52–60.
27. Volterrani M, Rosano GMC, Coats A, et al. Estrogen acutely increases peripheral blood flow in postmenopausal women. *Am J Med* 1995;99:119–122.
28. Collins P, Shay J, Jiang C, et al. Nitric oxide accounts for dose-dependent estrogen-mediated coronary relaxation following acute estrogen withdrawal. *Circulation* 1994;90:1964–1968.
29. Caulin-Glaser TL, Sessa W, Sarrel PM, et al. Estradiol stimulates NO production via transcriptional and non-transcriptional pathways. *Circulation* 1994;90 I–30.
30. Williams JK, Adams MR, Klopfenstein HS, et al. Estrogen modulates responses of atherosclerotic coronary arteries. *Circulation* 1990;81:1680–1687.
31. Gilligan DM, Quyyumi AA, Cannon RO III. Effect of physiological levels of estrogen on coronary vasomotor function in postmenopausal women. *Circulation* 1994;89:2545–2551.
32. Collins P, Rosano GMC, Sarrel PM, et al. 17β-Estradiol attenuates acetylcholine-induced coronary arterial constriction in women but not in men with coronary heart disease. *Circulation* 1995;92:24–30.
33. Kronenberg F, Cote LJ, Linki DM, et al. Menopausal hot flashes: Thermoregulatory, cardiovascular and circulating catecholamine and LH changes. *Maturitas* 1984;6:31–43.
34. Sarrel PM: Blood flow and ovarian secretions. In: Naftolin F, DeCherney A, Guttman JN, Sarrel PM, eds. *Ovarian Secretions and Cardiovascular and Neurological Function.* New York: Raven Press; 1990:81–90.
35. Rees M, Barlow D. Absence of sustained reflex vasoconstriction in women with menopausal flushes. *Hum Reprod* 1988;3:823–825.
36. Ginsburg J, Swinhoe J, O'Reilly B. Cardiovascular responses during the menopausal hot flush. *Br J Obstet Gynecol* 1982;88:925–930.
37. Owens JF, Stoney CM, Matthews KA. Menopausal status influences ambulatory blood pressure levels and blood pressure changes during mental stress. *Circulation* 1993;88:2794–2802.
38. McKinlay SM, Jeffreys M. The menopausal syndrome. *Br J Prev Soc Med* 1974;28:108–115.
39. Gerhard M, Ganz P. How do we explain the clinical benefits of estrogen? *Circulation* 1995;92:5–8.
40. Caspar RF, Yen SSE, Welkes MM. Menopausal flushes: A neuroendocrine link with pulsatile luteinizing hormone secretion. *Science* 1979;205:823–825.
41. Kronenberg F. Hot flashes: Epidemiology and physiology. *NY Acad Sci* 1990;592:52–86.
42. Rosano GMC, Lefroy DC, Peters NS, et al. Symptomatic response to 17B-estradiol in women with Syndrome X. Abstract. *J Am Coll Cardiol* 1994;24:6A.
43. Somerville BW. The role of estradiol withdrawal in the etiology of menstrual migraine. *Neurology* 1972;22(4):355–365.

44. Welch KM, Darnley D, Simkins RTR. The role of estrogen in migraine: A review and hypothesis. *Cephalalgia* 1984;4(4):227–236.
45. O'Dea JPK, Davies EH. Tamoxifen in the treatment of menstrual migraine. *Neurology* 1990;40(9):1470–1471.
46. Brass LM, Kisiel D, Sarrel PM. A correlation between estrogen and middle cerebral artery blood velocity at different times in the menstrual cycle in women with catamenial migraines. *J Cardiovasc Technol* 1990;9:68.
47. Osler W. *Lectures on Angina Pectoris and Allied States.* New York: Appleton 1901.
48. LaCroix AZ, Haynes SG, Savage DD, et al. Rose questionnaire angina among United States black, white, and Mexican-American women and men. *Am J Epidemiol* 1989;129:669–686.
49. Colditz GA, Willett WC, Stampfer MJ, et al. Menopause and the risk of coronary heart disease in women. *N Engl J Med* 1987;316:1105–1110.
50. Bush TL, Barrett-Connor E, Cowan LD, et al. Cardiovascular mortality and noncontraceptive use of estrogen in women: Results from the Lipid Research Clinics Program Follow-up Study. *Circulation* 1987;75:1102–1109.
51. Rosano GMC, Sarrel PM, Collins P, et al. Beneficial effect of oestrogen on exercise-induced myocardial ischemia in women with coronary artery disease. *Lancet* 1993;342:133–136.
52. Williams JK, Honore EK, Washburn SA, et al. Effects of hormone replacement therapy on reactivity of atherosclerotic arteries in cynomolgous monkeys. *J Am Coll Cardiol* 1994;24:1757–1761.
53. Sarrel PM, Albakri E, Auld E, et al. Oral progesterone therapy impairs cerebrovascular reactivity. American Heart Association 20th International Joint Conference on Stroke and Cerebral Circulation, Feb. 1995, Charleston, South Carolina.

Chapter 21

Hormone Replacement Therapy
Outlook for the Future

John C. LaRosa, MD

The last few years have seen intense interest in the effects of estrogen replacement therapy (ERT) and estrogen-progestin or hormone replacement therapy (HRT) in postmenopausal women. As a result, much has been learned and many questions have been answered. Inevitably, a number of questions remain and a number of new issues have been raised. The future of these regimens is contained in the answers to those questions. Some of the important yet unanswered issues include the following.

Who Should Be Taking ERT or HRT?

Most clinical experience with ERT and HRT and, indeed, most clinical trials to date, have involved women in the peri- and immediate postmenopausal state. There is little experience with effects in women >65 years. And yet it is in that age group where the incidence of vascular disease is greatest and the potential for benefit highest. It has even been suggested that because the absolute risk of vascular disease is relatively low in women <65, the optimal age for beginning hormones is after ≥65 years.[1] In this way, the maximum benefit on vascular disease could be attained while minimizing the risk of long-term exposure thought by some to promote breast cancer. A corollary question is whether or not hormones should be used from the time of menopause until death (or at least until a very old age) and whether such long-term exposure carries any risk. Because most women have taken hor-

From: Forte TM, (ed). *Hormonal, Metabolic, and Cellular Influences on Cardiovascular Disease in Women.* Armonk, NY: Futura Publishing Company, Inc.; © 1997.

mones for only a few years after menopause, there are no studies that address this issue, although current use of estrogen appears to be associated with a higher risk of breast cancer in older women.[2] The Women's Health Initiative, which will enroll older as well as younger postmenopausal women, should provide some information to address these important issues.

In Whom is ERT/HRT Clearly Contraindicated?

Observational studies of women with family history of breast cancer in first-degree families indicate that there is a strong association between ERT and risk of breast cancer.[3] Although such associations do not prove cause and effect, it is probably prudent that women with such family histories be discouraged from taking estrogen.

Recently, associations between ERT and ovarian cancer[4] and systemic lupus erythematosus have been reported.[5] This literature is sparce, however, and the incidence of these diseases is much lower than that of breast cancer, so that it is not clear at this point what influence these findings should have on clinical practice. Again, prudence dictates that women at risk of these disorders be evaluated carefully before being put on hormones and that their clinical course while on such therapy be monitored carefully. On the other hand, ERT has been associated with a diminished risk of colon cancer.[6] It is possible that at-high-risk patients might benefit from its prescription.

What Is the Effect of Adding Progestin to Postmenopausal ERT Regimens?

Primarily because of the risk of uterine cancer with unopposed estrogen, it has become accepted practice to add a progestin to protect the endometrium from hyperplasia. The long-term effect of adding a progestin to ERT in postmenopausal women is only now, however, being examined. Observational epidemiological data indicate that the effect on reducing heart attacks in postmenopausal women using unopposed estrogen is unaffected by the addition of medroxyprogesterone,[7] the most commonly used postmenopausal progestin in the United States. This is in keeping with the results of the Postmenopausal Estrogen/Progestin Interventions (PEPI) Trial, which indicated that medroxyprogesterone and, even more strikingly, micronized progesterone had little effect on the generally favorable impact of estrogen on lipoproteins and other risk factors.[8] Medroxyprogesterone reversed most of the increase in high-density lipoprotein cholesterol (HDL-C) produced by estrogen in that study, although it had virtually no effect on estrogen lowering of low-density lipoprotein cholesterol (LDL-C). Micronized progestin appeared to be essentially neutral.

At the cellular and subcellular levels, the effects of progestin are less clear. In a study of atherogenesis in rabbits,[9] progestins appeared to enhance the anti-estrogenic effects of estrogen. In studies of cholesterol-induced cytotoxicity,[10] smooth muscle cell proliferation,[11] and cholesterol accumulation of macrophages,[12,13] however, progestins appeared to oppose the beneficial effects of estrogen.

Most progestins have effects that are weakly androgenic. In female primates, androgenic effects on atherosclerosis are generally adverse.[14] It is not known how much of the postmenopausal acceleration of atherogenesis in humans might be related to the effect of "unopposed" androgens. It is clear that hyperandrogenic states, such as occur in women with polycystic ovaries, result in lower HDLs and higher LDLs than found in control subjects.[15]

On the other hand, in a small study of the lipoprotein effects of a combination of estrogen and testosterone, LDL levels were lowered further with the combination than with estrogen alone.[16]

It is unclear to what extent the androgenicity of progestins affect the progress of atherogenesis, particularly in postmenopausal women. In the PEPI Trial, as well as older trials of oral contraceptives (OC) in premenopausal women,[17] androgenic progestins (such as levonorgestryl), caused adverse effects on lipoproteins. Newer, less androgenic, progestins (such as norgestimate, desogestrel, gestodene),[18] do not have such effects but have not been widely examined in postmenopausal women.[19]

Contrary to some expectations, progestins do not appear to ameliorate the effect of estrogen, however slight, on breast cancer risk[2,20] and may even exacerbate it.[21] On the other hand, progestins do not appear to compromise the beneficial effects of estrogen in preventing atherosclerosis.[22,23]

The primary indication for adding progestin to postmenopausal regimens is protection of the endometrium. An estrogen that did not produce endometrial hyperplasia but did protect the vasculature against atherogenesis would be of great interest in the search for satisfactory HRT regimens.

How is the Effect of Estrogen on Vascular Disease Influenced by its Administration?

Despite the fact that many women take replacement estrogen by a nonoral route, none of the long-term observational studies or clinical trials of estrogen in postmenopausal women is designed to study the effect of nonoral estrogen. Aggregate results from a number of small clinical trials demonstrate that nonoral estrogen does not have the same quantitatively beneficial effects on circulating lipoproteins and clotting factors as does oral estrogen, although there is some question as to whether the effects of nonoral estrogen may be enhanced by longer term administration.[24,25] This is not surprising, given the fact that the effects on lipoproteins are probably mediated largely through the liver. Oral administration provides estrogen, concentrated in the portal circulation, to the liver.

Critics of oral estrogen point out with some justification, however, that the administration of estrogen orally is not physiological, because the ovaries do not drain into the portal vein but into the peripheral circulation. It is unknown whether the more direct effects of estrogen on various aspects of atherogenesis, including antioxidation,[26] interference with platelet adherence,[27] vasodilation,[28] and interference of vessel wall LDL-C uptake,[29] are influenced by the route of administration. It is unfortunate that this issue has not been more carefully studied, because it is likely that nonoral administration of estrogen will continue to be a popular regimen. Better information about the effects of nonoral estrogen on atherogenesis is critical because these effects, rather than those on coronary risk factors, may be the predominant ones determining estrogen's anti-atherosclerotic benefits.

Can the Beneficial Vascular Effects of Estrogen be Isolated?

Concern about estrogen relates not to its vascular effects but to its adverse effects on endometrium endothelium and perhaps on breast tissue as well. The propensity for unopposed estrogen to cause uterine hyperplasia is clearly established. Approximately one-half of patients in the PEPI study on unopposed estrogen could not be continued on that regimen because of the development of uterine hyperplasia.[8] Hyperplasia, in turn, predisposes to uterine cancer, although the absolute (as opposed to relative) risk of that disease is low, even in women on estrogen.

The effect of estrogen on breast hyperplasia and neoplasia, as noted previously, is less clear, although the weight of evidence indicates that exposure to estrogen is, overall, a weak-to-moderate risk factor for the development of breast cancer.[2,3] An estrogen that does not have hyperplastic effects, either on the uterus or the breast, but retained beneficial effects on inhibiting atherogenesis, would be ideal.

Tamoxifen appears to be a compound that fulfills two of the three requirements. Like estrogen, it has favorable effects on lipoprotein patterns,[30] including lowering lipoprotein (a) [Lp(a)][31]. In preliminary studies, it appears to inhibit the development of clinical coronary disease in women being given it for the treatment of breast cancer.[32] Larger-scale studies of tamoxifen's effect on breast cancer as well as vascular disease are currently underway. Tamoxifen, however, does not protect the uterus against hyperplasia and cancer,[33] so that a progestin of some kind is still required.

Preliminary studies of phytoestrogens, such as genistein, imply that these may be compounds with all the desired properties. Asian populations ingesting soy-containing diets, potent sources of phytoestrogens, have a lower risk of coronary disease, as well as breast and uterine cancers, than in western societies.[34] In animal studies, genistein has been demonstrated to retard rather than promote, experimentally induced mammary cancer.[35] Soy-containing diets have been shown to lower LDL and triglyceride levels without adversely affecting HDL levels.[36] Soy diets appear to have little effect, however, on endocrinologic parameters such as FSH, LH, and sex hormone-binding globulin (SHBG),[37] indicating either that they are weak estrogens or that their metabolic effects are more selective than gonadal estrogens.

Finally, little is known about differences in gender-specific or end-organ responses to estrogens, progestins, and other gonadal hormones. Studies done in men have demonstrated that, despite favorable lipoprotein changes, estrogens (in doses much higher than those currently used in most postmenopausal replacement regimens) are associated with an excess mortality.[38] This may simply be due to the thrombotic effect of very high-estrogen doses. It may also be due to the fact that males do not respond to estrogen in the manner predicted by experience in females.

How Can Compliance to Hormone Replacement Regimens Be Improved?

As is true of most chronic drug regimens, compliance to estrogen replacement regimens is surprisingly poor.[39] Most information about the effects of estrogen in postmenopausal women comes from epidemiological studies in which women studied during a 10-year period of time are divided into those who have "never" or "ever" used estrogen. The latter category is composed of women who may, on average, use estrogen for no more than 2 or 3 years after menopause.[40] Thus we have, in fact, relatively poor information about the long-term effects of estrogen, in part, because compliance to this as well as to so many other long-term drug regimens is not good. Reasons for poor compliance vary from fear of cancer to cessation of postmenopausal symptoms.[39] It is, nevertheless, sobering to realize that we know less about long-term effects of estrogen than might be first thought. On the other hand, if HRT regimens are beneficial, as they currently appear to be,[41] then it is critical that we better understand how to maintain women more consistently on these regimens throughout the postmenopausal period.

Summary

We know a great deal about HRT already. It is clear, even without clinical trials, that such regimens have a highly favorable effect on clinical atherosclerosis and that those effects are due both to generally beneficial effects on risk factors, including circulating lipoproteins, and on the process of atherogenesis itself. We know much less about the effect of added progestins. Information thus far from population studies implies that they do not have an adverse effect on atherosclerotic disease, but may have neutral or even promoting effects on breast cancer, although data are scant. To the extent that progestins may be seen as weak androgens, their effect on atherosclerosis should remain suspect. Although evidence is not extensive, androgens appear to have adverse effects both on lipoprotein risk factors and on atherogenesis itself. The role that "unopposed" androgens may play in the development of atherosclerosis in postmenopausal women is not clear but is potentially substantial. It is also an area that requires further investigation.

The effect of route of administration of HRT regimens has been understudied. The major clinical trials now in the field do not include treatment arms using non-oral estrogen or progestin. It is likely that, despite the fact that a substantial minority of women will continue to take estrogen via these routes, we will have little or no information, even at the completion of the trials currently in progress, addressing the long-term effects of such regimens.

The search for the ideal estrogens and progestins used in post-menopausal women will and should go on. The ideal estrogen would be one that has beneficial effects on atherogenesis but neutral or protective effects on hyperplasia on the reproductive organs, including the uterus and breast. Tamoxifen appears to protect the breast but not the uterus, and in preliminary experiments, appears to have a beneficial effect on vascular disease. Phytoestrogens, such as those found in soy-containing foods, may be anti-atherogenic without promoting uterine or breast hyperplasia. They have not, however, been studied widely. Considerable additional data must be gathered before any public health recommendations can be considered.

Assuming that the replacement of progestins continues to be required (and except for the beneficial effects on uterine hyperplasia, there seems to be no other indication for them), it will be necessary to find progestins that have as little androgenic potency as possible. In that regard, the newer progestins, already used in OCs, such as norgestimate, desogestrel, and gestodene, should be examined for their effects in postmenopausal replacement regimens.

Finally, in HRT as well as in other chronic drug regimens, the issue of compliance is critical but often ignored. Hormone replacement regimens are probably poorly adhered to. Until we are able to find better methods of ensuring compliance and continuance in these regimens, their full benefit cannot be realized. While much has been learned about HRT, then, much remains to investigate. These issues, potentially affecting one-half of the population for one-third of their lifespan, are of critical public health importance.

References

1. Prince RL, Geelhoed EA. When should postmenopausal women start taking oestrogen replacement therapy? *Med J Aust* 1995;162:173–174.
2. Colditz GA, Hankinson SE, Hunter DJ, et al. The use of estrogens and progestins and the risk of breast cancer in postmenopausal women. *N Engl J Med* 1995;332:1589–1593.
3. Steinberg KK, Thacker SB, Smith SJ, et al. A meta-analysis of the effect of estrogen replacement therapy on the risk of breast cancer. *JAMA* 1991;265:1985–1990.
4. Rodriguez C, Calle EE, Coates RJ, et al. Estrogen replacement therapy and fatal ovarian cancer. *Am J Epidemiol* 1995;141:828–835.
5. Sanchez-Guerrero J, Liang MH, Karlson EW, et al. Postmenopausal estrogen therapy and the risk for developing systemic lupus erythematosus. *Ann Intern Med* 1995;122:430–433.
6. Calle EE, Miracle-McMahill HL, Thun MJ, et al. Estrogen replacement therapy and risk of fatal colon cancer in a prospective cohort of postmenopausal women. *J Natl Cancer Inst* 1995;87:517–523.

7. Psaty BM, Heckbert SR, Atkins D, et al. The risk of myocardial infarction associated with the combined use of estrogens and progestins in postmenopausal women. *Arch Intern Med* 1994;154:1333–1339.
8. The Writing Group for the PEPI Trial. Effects of estrogen or estrogen/progestin regimens on heart disease risk factors in postmenopausal women. The Postmenopausal Estrogen/Progestin Interventions (PEPI) Trial. *JAMA* 1995;273:199–208.
9. Haarbo J, Hansen BF, Christiansen C. Hormone replacement therapy prevents coronary artery disease in ovariectomized cholesterol-fed rabbits. *APMIS* 1991;99:721–727.
10. Zhu X-D, Knopp RH. Effect of sex hormones on oxidative modification of low density lipoproteins by placental macrophages and trophoblast and their susceptibility to cytotoxicity. Abstract. *Circulation* 1993;88:I-30.
11. Hanke H, Hanke S, Dauble C, et al. Effect of estrogen and progesterone on smooth muscle cell proliferation in experimental atherosclerosis. Abstract. *Circulation* 1994;90:I-291.
12. Huber LA, Scheffler E, Poll T, et al. 17 beta-estradiol inhibits LDL oxidation and cholesteryl ester formation in cultured macrophages. *Free Radic Res Commun* 1990;8:167–173.
13. Mazzone T, Krishna M, Lange Y. Progesterone blocks intracellular translocation of free cholesterol derived from cholesteryl ester in macrophages. *J Lipid Res* 1995;36:544–551.
14. Adams MR, Williams JK, Kaplan JR. Effects of androgens on coronary artery atherosclerosis and atherosclerosis-related impairment of vascular responsiveness. *Arterioscler Thromb Vasc Biol* 1995;15:562–570.
15. Talbott E, Guzick D, Clerici A, et al. Coronary heart disease risk factors in women with polycystic ovary syndrome. *Arterioscler Thromb Vasc Biol* 1995;15:821–826.
16. Hickok LR, Toomey C, Speroff L. A comparison of esterified estrogens with and without methyltestosterone: Effects on endometrial histology and serum lipoproteins in postmenopausal women. *Obstet Gynecol* 1993;82:919–924.
17. Lipson A, Stoy DB, LaRosa JC, et al. Progestins and oral contraceptive-induced lipoprotein changes: A prospective study. *Contraception* 1986;34:121–134.
18. Speroff L, DeCherney A, and the Advisory Board for the New Progestins. Evaluation of a new generation of oral contraceptives. *Obstet Gynecol* 1993;81:1034–1047.
19. Porcile A, Gallardo E, Onetto P, et al. Very low estrogen-desogestrel contraceptive in perimenopausal hormonal replacement. *Maturitas* 1994;18:93–103.
20. Stanford JL, Weiss NS, Voigt LF, et al. Combined estrogen and progestin hormone replacement therapy in relation to risk of breast cancer in middle-aged women. *JAMA* 1995;274:137–142.
21. Bergkvist L, Adami H-O, Persson I, et al. The risk of breast cancer after estrogen and estrogen-progestin replacement. *N Engl J Med* 1989;321:293–297.
22. Falkeborn M, Persson I, Adami H-O, et al. The risk of acute myocardial infarction after oestrogen and oestrogen-progestogen replacement. *Br J Obstet Gynaecol* 1992;99:821–828.
23. Psaty BM, Heckbert SR, Atkins D, et al. The risk of myocardial infarction associated with the combined use of estrogens and progestins in postmenopausal women. *Arch Intern Med* 1994;154:1333–1339.

24. LaRosa JC. Metabolic effects of estrogens and progestins. *Fertil Steril* 1994;62(suppl 2)140S-146S.
25. Whitcroft SI, Crook D, Marsh MS, et al. Long-term effects of oral and transdermal hormone replacement therapies on serum lipid and lipoprotein concentrations. *Obstet Gynecol.* 1994;84:222–226.
26. Rifici VA, Khachadurian AK. The inhibition of low-density lipoprotein oxidation by 17-β estradiol. *Metabolism* 1992;41:1110–1114.
27. Bar J, Tepper R, Fuchs J, et al. The effect of estrogen replacement therapy on platelet aggregation and adenosine triphosphate release in postmenopausal women. *Obstet Gynecol* 1993;81:261–264.
28. Lieberman EH, Gerhard M, Yeung AC, et al. Estrogen improves coronary vasomotor responses to acetylcholine in post menopausal women. Abstract. *Circulation* 1993;88:I-79.
29. Wagner JD, Clarkson TB, St Clair RW, et al. Estrogen replacement therapy (ERT) and coronary artery (CA) atherogenesis in surgically postmenopausal cynomolgus monkeys. *Circulation* 1989:80(suppl II)331.
30. Dnistrian AM, Schwartz MK, Greenberg EJ, et al. Effect of tamoxifen on serum cholesterol and lipoproteins during chemohormonal therapy. *Clin Chim Acta* 1993;223:43–52.
31. Shewmon DA, Stock JL, Rosen CJ, et al. Tamoxifen and estrogen lower circulating lipoprotein(a) concentrations in healthy postmenopausal women. *Arterioscler Thromb* 1994;14:1586–1593.
32. Rutqvist LE, Mattsson A. for the Stockholm Breast Cancer Study Group. Cardiac and thromboembolic morbidity among postmenopausal women with early-stage breast cancer in a randomized trial of adjuvant tamoxifen. *J Natl Cancer Inst* 1993;85:1398–1406.
33. van Leeuwen FE, Benraadt J, Coebergh JWW, et al. Risk of endometrial cancer after tamoxifen treatment of breast cancer. *Lancet* 1994;343:448–452.
34. Goldin BR, Adlercreutz H, Gorbach SL, et al. The relationship between estrogen levels and diets of Caucasian American and Oriental immigrant women. *Am J Clin Nutr* 1986;44:945–953.
35. Lamartiniere CA, Moore J, Holland M, et al. Neonatal genistein chemoprevents mammary cancer. *Proc Soc Exp Biol Med* 1995;208:120–123.
36. Anderson JW, Johnstone BM, Cook-Newell ME. Meta-analysis of the effects of soy protein intake on serum lipids. *N Engl J Med* 1995;333:276–282.
37. Baird DD, Umbach DM, Lansdell L, et al. Dietary intervention study to assess estrogenicity of dietary soy among postmenopausal women. *J Clin Endocrinol Metab* 1995;80:1685–1690.
38. Gould AL, Rossouw JE, Santanello NC, et al. Cholesterol reduction yields clinical benefit: A new look at old data. *Circulation* 1995;91:2274–2282.
39. Wren BG, Brown L. Compliance with hormonal replacement therapy. *Maturitas* 1991;13:17–21.
40. Lobo RA. Treatment of the postmenopausal woman: Where we are today. In: Lobo RA, ed. *Treatment of the Postmenopausal Woman: Basic and Clinical Aspects.* New York: Raven Press; 1994:427–432.
41. Grady D, Rubin SM, Petitti DB, et al. Hormone therapy to prevent disease and prolong life in postmenopausal women. *Ann Intern Med* 1992;117:1016–1037.

Index

Index

affecting arterial LDL metabolism, 158–160
affecting coagulation, 310
metabolic effects of, 313
and endometrial protection, 312
Megestrol acetate, and decrease in HDLC, 312
Men Born in 1913 Study, 250
Methyltestosterone with estrogen, affecting arterial LDL metabolism, 160–162
Migraine headaches, and estrogen deficiency, 325, 330–331
Monitored Atherosclerosis Progression Study, 255
Monkey studies
  anti-atherosclerotic effects of estrogen, 305–306
  arterial constriction in response to acetylcholine, 126
  cardiovascular characteristics in, 21, 22
  estrogen affecting diet-induced atherosclerosis, 41–45
  lipoprotein metabolism affected by estrogen, 46–47
  in arterial LDL, 154–165
  plaque area reduction after hormone replacement, 179–180
  postmenopausal studies, 31–35
  premenopausal studies, 22–31
  protective effects of estrogen on atherosclerosis, 2, 3
Monocyte adhesion to endothelial cells
  and atherogenesis, 125, 127
  estrogen affecting, 8–9, 128–129

nitric oxide affecting, 127, 129–130
Monocyte chemoattractant protein-1, 129
  expression affected by estrogen, 9, 48
Mouse studies, 4, 9, 59, 62, 63

National Health and Nutrition Examination Survey
  NHANES I, 262, 263
  NHANES II, 264, 269
Natriuretic peptide, C-type, vascular relaxation from, in female and male pigs, 104–106
Necrotic core formation, estrogen affecting, 11
Nitric oxide, 126
  and atherosclerosis, 126–127
  and endothelin action, 306
  and monocyte adhesion to endothelial cells, 127, 129–130
  and platelet aggregation, 307
  estrogen affecting, 186
  synthesis affected by estrogen, 11, 119, 307, 327
  vascular responses to, estrogen and progesterone affecting, 102–104
  and vasodilator response to endothelial stimuli, 176
Norepinephrine levels in hot flushes, 327, 328
Norethindrone
  combined with estradiol, 313
  and decrease in HDLC, 312
Norgestrel in oral contraceptives, affecting lipoproteins, 290–297
Normative Aging Study, 251
North Karelia Project, 250